ANNALS OF THE NEW YORK ACADEMY OF SCIENCES

Volume 457

EDITORIAL STAFF

Executive Editor
BILL BOLAND

Managing Editor
JOYCE HITCHCOCK

Associate Editor
JUSTINE CULLINAN

The New York Academy of Sciences
2 East 63rd Street
New York, New York 10021

HOPE FOR A NEW NEUROLOGY

ANNALS OF THE NEW YORK ACADEMY OF SCIENCES
Volume 457

HOPE FOR A NEW NEUROLOGY

Edited by Fernando Nottebohm

The New York Academy of Sciences
New York, New York
1985

Library of Congress Cataloging-in-Publication Data

Main entry under title:

Hope for a new neurology.

(Annals of the New York Academy of Sciences, ISSN 0077-8923 ; v. 457)
Based on a conference entitled Hope for a new neurology, held in New York, N.Y. on Apr. 16-18, 1984, and sponsored by the Institute for Child Development Research.
Includes bibliographies and indexes.
1. Brain—Diseases—Congresses. 2. Nervous system—Regeneration—Congresses. 3. Neurology—Congresses. I. Nottebohm, Fernando. II. New York Academy of Sciences. III. Institute for Child Development Research (New York, N.Y.) IV. Series.

[DNLM: 1. Brain Diseases—congresses.
W1 AN626YL v.457 / WL 348 H791]
Q11.N5 vol. 457 500 s 85-28347
[RC386.2] [616.8]
ISBN 0-89766-309-8
ISBN 0-89766-310-1 (pbk.)

S/PCP
Printed in the United States of America
ISBN 0-89766-309-8 (cloth)
ISBN 0-89766-310-1 (paper)
ISSN 0077-8923

ANNALS OF THE NEW YORK ACADEMY OF SCIENCES

Volume 457
December 31, 1985

HOPE FOR A NEW NEUROLOGY[a]

Editor

FERNANDO NOTTEBOHM

CONTENTS

[a] This volume is the result of a conference entitled Hope for a New Neurology, which was held in New York, New York on April 16–18, 1984 under the sponsorship of the Institute for Child Development Research.

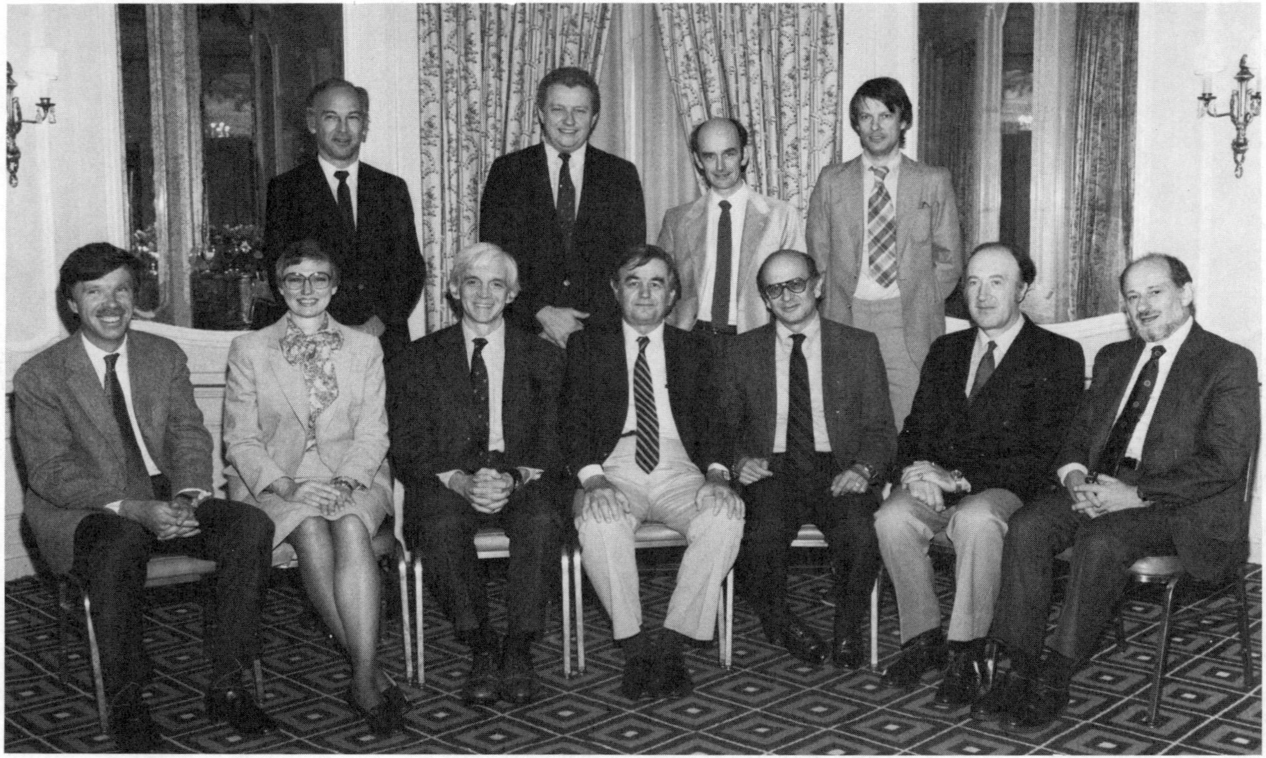

Conference Participants (left to right): *Seated*: F. Nottebohm, Shirley A. Bayer, Frank H. Duffy, Pasquale P. Graziadei, Pasko Rakic, Peter Behan, and Norman Geschwind. *Standing*: Carl W. Cotman, Donald L. Price, Anders Björklund, and Lars Olson.

Preface

FERNANDO NOTTEBOHM
Field Research Center for Ecology and Ethology
The Rockefeller University
Millbrook, New York 12545

This book comprises the proceedings of a conference organized to survey recent advances in the study of brain dysfunction and brain repair in humans and in animals.

A knowledge of the processes that lead to the formation of new synapses, growth of new axons, and formation of new brain cells is vital to an understanding of the repair of damaged circuits. These same processes could be related to the recovery from coma. A common prospect for a patient involved in an accident resulting in coma is that he or she may "wake up" after a period of some months, say four to six, with decreasing chances of this happening after then. Why do some patients regain consciousness and some do not? Why four to six months? There is plenty of time in those months for generating new neurons, for new axons to grow, and for millions of synapses to form. Are circuits rebuilt in this manner responsible for reinstating consciousness and voluntary control? We do not know if such rebuilding occurs, and if it occurred, what it might mean.

It is our vast lack of knowledge about all these questions that leads to the hopelessness associated with brain damage cases. Recent clinical and animal work points to new opportunities for the identification and correction of brain disorders.

Five of the participants in this conference directly address the study of brain damage in humans. These are Norman Geschwind, Peter Behan, Frank H. Duffy, Donald L. Price and Lars Olson.

The work on postpuberal neurogenesis has its roots in the pioneering observations of Dr. Joseph Altman, who was the first to suggest, in 1963, that neurons might continue to be generated in the adult mammalian brain. The impressive tradition and body of work from his laboratory are continued by Dr. Shirley Bayer, who presents her research in this volume. The other reports on neurogenesis in adulthood are those of P. P. Graziadei, M. S. Kaplan, F. Nottebohm, and P. Rakic.

There may be times when brains are incapable of self-repair. Neural grafts might offer the best alternative in this case. This extremely promising approach is evaluated by C. W. Cotman, A. Björklund, and L. Olson. Olson's presentation is noteworthy in that it describes the first attempts at correction of Parkinson's disease in humans by use of intracranial grafts of adrenal medullary tissue.

Another participant, Dr. Albert Aguayo, was unable to send his manuscript in time for publication. I deeply regret this loss, since his material on axonal regrowth is exceedingly novel and elegant. I have added a chapter on excellent *in vivo* and *in vitro* work on neurogenesis in adult fish spinal cord by Drs. Marilyn J. Anderson and Stephen G. Waxman.

Norman Geschwind contributed brilliantly to this conference. His store of neurologic information was endless, and his skill as a raconteur was highlighted by his wonderful sense of humor. He died on November 4, 1984. Norman made a very perceptive comment at this conference; he pointed out that brain dysfunction due to a known genetic disorder offered the greatest hope for prevention or cure because the product of a missing gene could be reintroduced and thus the handicap corrected. He was talking about that vast new frontier in the neurosciences, the molecular basis for understanding brain function and dysfunction, which he, in collaboration with Peter Behan, approached from the angle of immunodisorders. Our conference touched a little on this molecular theme (see the papers by Behan and Geschwind, and by Cotman and Nieto-Sampedro), and this is an approach that undoubtedly will grow enormously in the near future. However, even as we bow to the powers of reductionism and to the promise that molecular aproaches hold for brain repair, we should remember that brains are also more than vast arrays of molecules. Think of it: after six months of coma a person may regain conciousness. What is consiousness? How does one coax it back into existence? These questions are basic to our understanding of brain function, and yet were not discussed at this meeting. Other scientists, at another time, will have to take up where we left off.

This symposium—Hope for a New Neurology—would not have been possible without the help and enthusiasm of Jane and Peter Pattison. The conference was underwritten by the Institute for Child Development Research, which they founded and preside over.

This book will have succeeded if it conveys the idea that neurology is not an area of despair, but one of enormous opportunity. When I first considered the title "Hope for a New Neurology" for this conference, I asked Norm Geschwind whether he thought it was presumptuous. He mulled this over, and then said "No." Norm Geschwind was one of the great neurologists of this century and it is to his memory that this book is dedicated.

Mechanisms of Change after Brain Lesions[a]

NORMAN GESCHWIND[b]

Department of Neurology
Harvard Medical School, and
The Dana Research Institute
Beth Israel Hospital
Boston, Massachusetts 02215

Dramatic examples of recovery after the occurence of both clinical and experimental lesions of the nervous system have been recognized for at least a century. Even in the early literature on aphasia, references were made to unexpected recoveries. One of the most striking early experimental studies was carried out by W. T. Porter,[1] professor of physiology at the Harvard Medical School and the teacher of Walter Cannon. He hemisected the upper cervical cord in animals, which led to ipsilateral paralysis of the diaphragm, innervated by the phrenic nerve, which typically persisted in the absence of further interventions. After an interval, Porter transected the opposite phrenic nerve. Instead of finding total apnea, as he expected, he found that the diaphragm on the originally paralyzed side immediately began to function. The speed of this restoration of function was noteworthy. After electrotonic blockade of the phrenic nerve contralateral to the hemisection, the originally paralyzed diaphragm begins to contract within one respiratory cycle; with removal of the block contraction stops within the same interval.[2] If, however, the opposite phrenic nerve is transected within a short period after the hemisection, there is no recovery.

This important, although neglected, experiment illustrates several important principles. First, there must be many other cases in which the capacity for recovery is latent, and revealed only by some further manipulation, but experimenters have only rarely been zealous in their search for the right maneuver. Second, plasticity is not confined to more advanced structures, but occurs even at lower levels. This experiment also provides evidence against a common semi-philosophical argument advanced as an objection to therapy (e.g., thalamotomy for parkinsonism) by means of the placement of additional lesions, that is, that it makes no sense to try to treat a damaged nervous system by damaging it further. The crossed phrenic phenomenon also shows how difficult it can be to establish the mechanism of plasticity.

[a] This work was supported in part by grants from the National Institutes of Health and the National Science Foundation and from the Orton Dyslexia Society Research Fund and the Essel Foundation.

[b] Deceased November 4, 1984.

Porter believed that an alternative pathway crossing in the cord below the level of the transection became active after section of the opposite phrenic nerve. In later years Cannon and Rosenblueth[3] carried out several experiments, but could not clarify the mechanism. Finally, this phenomenon illustrates the risks of prematurely deciding that all the mechanisms of plasticity are known. Thus, a recent paper stated that there were only three such mechanisms, i.e., terminal and collateral sprouting and changes in receptors. Yet none of these could account for the instantaneous reappearance of activity in the originally paralyzed diaphragm after section of the opposite phrenic nerve.

This paper will review some factors involved in change in the nervous system after lesions. It is a salient principle that one can probably never speak of a *fixed* neurological lesion. Damage in every location is followed by a sequence of changes, both local and distant, some instantaneous and others proceeding over years. I will not confine myself to a discussion of *recovery*, which has received most emphasis because of its apparently great potential implications for therapy. It is likely that many changes, perhaps the majority, are unfavorable, serving to prevent the expression of latent restorative processes. Study of these unfavorable mechanisms may be even more important than investigation of spontaneous recovery in leading to improved methods of therapy. The stress on "recovery" rather than change was often the reflection of the Panglossian philosophical concept that the nervous system was designed to compensate for almost any injury. This view neglected the large number of permanently impaired patients. It also reflected unawareness that spontaneous recovery often provides little or no survival advantage. A cat may recover from hemiplegia after an interval, but in the wild it will not live long enough for the recovery to occur. Hence many forms of recovery have been sacrificed in evolution in return for other features that do provide survival advantage. The apparent increasing importance, as one moves up the evolutionary scale, of cerebral dominance, which obviously reduces recovery, reflects this principle. Unfortunately the excessive optimistic stress on recovery often led to failure to do research on neurologic mechanisms.

Let us consider two examples drawn from the clinic. The prototypical human neurologic impairment is the hemiplegia that occurs as a consequence of vascular occlusion. While the causative lesions are often large, it is surprising how frequently small lesions, difficult to find even at autopsy, lead to permanent paralysis. By contrast, in the cat, total hemispherectomy will lead to severe hemiplegia, which can lessen to the point that after a few months only an expert examiner can still find impairment. Even in the monkey, the permanent functional disability is far milder than that in the human. It is often said that lower animals always recover better than humans, but this is probably false. Some evidence suggests that the young human may tolerate cerebellectomy better than the kitten will. I suspect that the human often possesses restorative mechanisms similar to those of other species, and that lack of recovery reflects either failure to utilize latent mechanisms (such as those of the crossed phrenic phenomenon) or interfering processes which prevent possible recovery. There are, in fact, a few cases in which humans recover from hemiplegia as well as do other species, despite large lesions.

The higher functions, subserved to a great extent by the expansion of human association cortex, are often recovered better than in hemiplegia, but permanent severe aphasias are still common. In the child with aphasia from a unilateral lesion there is typically a degree of restoration of language that is uncommonly seen in the adult, although at the price of diminished cognitive capacities of other types. Why are comparable recoveries found so much less often in the adult? The explanations advanced have little support, and are vaguer than is apparent on casual consideration. It is often argued that the child recovers by "using the other side" for language. A brief reflection shows that this statement can have more than one meaning. It might mean that the homologous areas on the other side reacquire language. Against this possibility is, however, the fact that some children with a massive left hemisphere lesion recover significantly within a few months. It is unlikely that new language acquisition could take place with such remarkable speed.

Another possible meaning of "recovery with the other side" is that language is laid down to a very large extent bilaterally, and that left cerebral dominance may simply reflect use of the side with a larger memory store and more efficient processing. The right hemisphere language mechanisms could be made available after damage to the left side. If this accounts for good recovery from childhood aphasia, it becomes more difficult to understand the lack of adult recovery. The language store that exists at an early age may be erased later. Another possibility is that the store persists, but is available only to a limited extent. Several pieces of evidence are concordant with this possibility. Immediately after a large left hemisphere lesion, one typically finds severe aphasia, even in the child, and recovery takes a few months or years. It is possible that the time necessary to acquire access to the existing language store on the right is much longer in the adult and/or that there are factors preventing access. Most neurologists are gloomy about the prognosis of severe adult aphasia after a few weeks, and pessimism is reinforced by lack of prolonged follow-up in most cases. I have, however, seen patients severely aphasic for over a year who then made excellent recoveries, one patient even returning to work as a salesman, and another as a psychiatrist. Furthermore there are patients who continue to improve over many years, e.g., a patient whose aphasia, still quite evident 6 years after onset, cleared substantially by 18 years. Colleagues who have followed many cases over periods up to 40 years have reported several such examples. Recovery from aphasia illustrates another important principle, i.e., that the changes after damage may show great individual variations. Several investigators[4–6] have pointed out that left-handed persons are much more likely to make good recoveries from aphasia than are the right-handed; right-handers with first-degree left-handed relatives also tend to manifest better recovery than other dextrals. I also have the impression that childhood dyslexics, despite marked worsening of reading comprehension after an aphasia-producing stroke, recover more rapidly from disturbances of comprehension and production of spoken language. One cannot stress strongly enough the importance of individual differences in the nervous system, for these have received inadequate attention from both clinicians and animal experimentalists.

RAPIDITY OF CHANGES AFTER LESIONS

TABLE 1 lists the kinds of changes that occur after a lesion and the factors that seem to favor some of them. I found it impossible to classify the changes and the factors into exclusive categories. It is far better, however, to view this problem in its broadest aspect than to narrow it excessively. To argue, as some do, that the only mechanisms of change after lesions are sprouting and receptor changes is both to create a premature impression of a certainty that does not exist and to omit mechanisms that fit into none of these categories. In particular, those changes that occur instantaneously cannot be accounted for by these mechanisms.

Some changes occur immediately, while others are evident only after years. The immediate unfavorable effects and both the favorable and unfavorable changes that occur after a brief interval are likely to be noticed. Late changes, whether favorable or unfavorable, are likely to be overlooked in both the human and the animal because long follow-up study is uncommon. In addition, it may not occur to the clinician that the very late changes are connected with the original lesion. Those who experiment on animals are faced with a special problem since neither the experimental subject nor the family can point out impairments of function not included in the experimental protocol or which may even be unknown. In the human, unexpected changes may be brought to the attention of the physician by the patient or the family. Very early favorable changes are almost universally overlooked. If, after damage to structures involved in a given function, other structures take over either immediately or after a very short period, the observer may never be aware of the change. This explains why study of changes of this type has been so neglected, despite its obvious importance. Such instantaneous changes should be capable of detection by physiological methods. It is also likely that a more refined study of function will always reveal differences from the normal state. Some investigators have argued that there is, in the strict sense, no complete recovery after any destructive lesion in the central nervous system, and that the substituted mechanisms always lack some of the more refined capacities of the destroyed regions. It is easy to draw the conclusion that a monkey with destruction of one pyramidal system is not impaired, but more sensitive testing will reveal difficulties.

TYPES OF CHANGES AFTER BRAIN LESIONS

Brain lesions themselves can be characterized as being of two types, neither of which is necessarily mutually exclusive. In one form, there is actual

TABLE 1. Change after Lesions of the Nervous System

- I. Mechanisms (listings are not necessarily exclusive)
  - A. Biochemical
    - *Nonspecific*
      - Edema and disappearance of edema
      - Ischemia without destruction
      - Immune responses
      - Scarring
      - Pressure effects
    - *Specific*
      - Increase or decrease in numbers of receptors
      - Induction or inactivation of enzymes
      - Viral alterations of specific cell function
      - Immune responses to specific neural components
      - Alterations in transmitter release
      - Transmitter reuptake by inactive neurons (Zigmond effect)
      - Alterations in membrane properties
  - B. Structural
    - Disrupted organization
    - Sprouting—collateral and terminal
    - Anomalous connections
    - Demyelination
    - Transynaptic and transneuronal degeneration
    - Diminished cell death in other areas (in fetal and possibly early postnatal life).
  - C. Physiological
    - Changes in facilitation, inhibition, and occlusion
    - Loss of feedback effects
    - Pacemaker shifts
    - Slowed conduction
    - Changes of synchrony
    - Opening of ineffective synapses
    - Changes of spatial or temporal summation
    - Kindling and epilepsy
  - D. "Psychological"
    - Perception of change by intact regions
    - Alternate strategies
- II. Factors Influencing Late Change
  - Age
  - Species
  - Previous learning
  - Individual differences (type and size of structures, connections, biochemistry, individual talents, handedness)
  - Previous exposure to drugs, hormones, and so forth (pre- and postnatal)
  - Lesion size
  - Preceding lesions (pre- and postnatal)
  - Serial lesions
  - Epilepsy
  - Stimulation (such as skin lesions or deliberate stimulation)
  - Emotional effects—motivation, hormones, circulating transmitters, and so forth.
  - Susceptibility to immune attack of areas formed abnormally in prenatal life

destruction of cells or fibers. In the other, there is a purely biochemical disturbance, e.g., an alteration in synaptic transmission. One must remember that there are, however, instances in which both cell death and biochemical changes are normal. Cell death takes place prenatally and recent evidence suggests that it may continue for a long period after birth. Similarly, it is likely that blockage or potentiation of transmission at certain synapses is often a normal phenomenon, e.g., at puberty or during adaptation to change of climate.

While certain changes are the result of specific neurologic responses and adaptations, others are nonspecific or reflect the activity of other systems. In most cases, recovery from hemiplegia within three weeks after vascular occlusion depends on nonspecific factors, such as recovery of neurons temporarily inactivated by ischemia or the resolution of edema; but changes caused by vascular lesions persisting after this time probably reflect the disorder of specific mechanisms. Continuing or late deterioration after a lesion may be caused either by neurologic processes (such as transsynaptic degeneration) or by immune attack at the site of the lesion. Of course, even transsynaptic degeneration itself may be the result of immunologic mechanisms. Many diseases in adult life may be caused by immune attack at sites malformed *in utero*, a mechanism that I cannot discuss in adequate detail at this time.

Loss of function after a destructive lesion may depend on alterations in distant structures connected to the damaged region. Some investigators have attributed such distant functional changes to alterations in blood flow, often seen in the PET scan, although in many, if not most cases, blood flow changes are probably secondary to altered function rather than vice versa. Similarly, much of the recovery after the occurrence of a lesion may derive from the return of function in distant but intact structures that were transiently inactivated.

Structural alterations are induced by biochemical changes after lesions. The specificity of these changes may be striking; nerve fibers of one particular origin may sprout in preference to others in the vicinity of a denervated structure. The reasons for these hierarchical patterns are unknown, but they are of major importance for any study of late change. While sprouting may in some instances have favorable consequences, the selective character of sprouting may often lead to the exclusion of just those connections that would be most useful.

Some of the mechanisms listed in the table are not known at this time to occur in the central nervous system. Neurons that sprout can, of course, produce anomalous reinnervation, but they do not grow over long distances, in contrast to damaged peripheral nerves. Potential pacemakers in the heart become active immediately when there is destruction of the normal site of origin of the cardiac impulse or the cardiac conduction system.[7] It would not be surprising if a similar mechanism occurred in the central nervous system. The example of the crossed phrenic nerve phenomenon illustrates that the immediate physiological mechanisms of change have been too often overlooked.

Let us consider another rapid change which illustrates the power of the somewhat neglected physiological and anatomic approach. Denny-Brown and his coworkers[8,9] studied the strip of preserved sensation when several dorsal roots were cut above and below an intact root. The preserved strip widened when the lateral portion of Lissauer's tract was sectioned in the cord; it narrowed when the medial portion was lesioned, but widened again if L-dopa or strychnine was given systemically.

Let me comment on the category which, for want of a better term, has been labeled as "psychological." This term has a narrower and more definite referent than is usually ascribed to it. A trivial example of this "psychological" type is the successful use of the left hand for managing a spoon or hammer after the occurrence of a right hemiplegia. There are other more subtle forms of "psychological" deficit, which have sometimes misled observers. The apparent shift of the fovea postulated in some patients with hemianopia turned out to result from turning of the eyes toward the hemianopic side so that what lay directly in front of the patient was now in the spared field. In some patients, however, a grossly inappropriate strategy appears: the eyes are turned toward the intact field and the disability that results from the hemianopia is therefore magnified. This occurs when the lesion induces gross inattention to the opposite side.

Another form of this mechanism may be seen in patients with callosal lesions. As has been known since these syndromes were first described in the early 1900s by Hugo Liepmann,[10] patients with callosal disconnection typically fail to carry out verbal commands with the left limbs, but some patients appear at first to be striking exceptions to this rule. There are several different mechanisms that can account for this behavior. In some cases the movement is carried out by the left hemisphere itself by way of nonpyramidal motor systems, which are distributed bilaterally. In this case the movement is often crude since it lacks fine distal components, which are poorly represented in these motor systems. There is another possible mechanism, exemplified by the following case: On being given a verbal command, the patient first carried out the movement with the right limb and only then with the left. If the right limb was held by the examiner, the patient could not carry out the movement on the left. In this particular case, the left hemisphere understood the command and carried it out; the right hemisphere then observed the movement and imitated what it saw. Another example of a new strategy is that of patients with spinal transection who appear to have regained bladder function. In many cases, at least, the patient has simply learned to set off the bladder reflex by mechanical pressure.

A factor that may be extremely important in late change is the pattern of stimulation. It is known that in the infant animal covering one eye leads to loss of binocular units in the visual cortex. The possibility that stimulation or its withdrawal in adult life can modify late change has received less attention. The ordinary practice of rehabilitation is based on the implicit assumption that attempted stimulation is good. There is, however, remarkably little experimental evidence on the varying effects of application or withdrawal of external stimuli, or indeed of direct stimulation of structures in the nervous system. It is important to be aware of the diversity of mechanisms that may occur, since if one is to use the knowledge for the purposes of rehabilitation, different strategies may have to be employed.

RECRUITMENT OF OTHER SYSTEMS

In the vicinity of a damaged region one may find certain types of functional activity in cells in which it was not previously found, as shown by Glees and Cole.[11] They destroyed the sites in the precentral motor cortex of the monkey from which hand movements were evoked electrically. The subsequent severe hand weakness improved after a few weeks. At a second operation it was possible to elicit hand movements from previously unresponsive locations. Wall and Egger[12] described a similar phenomenon in sensory systems. It is likely (on the basis of data I will not discuss) that a similar phenomenon occurs in language areas. If a lesion destroyed all the sites in the frontal operculum in which electrical stimulation led to speech arrest, severe aphasia would result that would probably lessen to some extent after a few weeks. If cortical stimulation were then carried out, I suspect that there would be locations in which stimulation would now cause speech arrest, although this had not occurred before the lesion. It is probably this mechanism that accounts for the excellent recovery after small lesions in the anterior speech regions.

In addition to these local effects there are also cases in which alternative pathways open. Erickson[13] showed that if the normal path of spread of an epileptic seizure was blocked surgically, the seizure would eventually follow a new route.

Both of these mechanisms raise intriguing questions. Are the neurons that become available for a particular function after a lesion now unavailable for a different function, which therefore diminishes? If an alternate pathway is used for a function in which it was not previously involved, do other functions suffer? The answers are not clear. It is possible that in some cases no impairment of function would occur, since many neurons activated after a lesion may have been active during initial learning, but were withdrawn as the efficiency of function rose. (There is evidence supporting the existence of this type of mechanism.) Another possibility is that some of these neurons constitute a reserve which would have played a role in future learning. In the latter case, of course, there will be an impairment of future function, which would not be immediately obvious.

FACTORS INFLUENCING CHANGE AFTER LESIONS

TABLE 1 contains a list of factors that influence the events after a lesion. The number is very large, and the detailed mechanisms are often poorly known. I will make only a few comments.

One factor that may well play a major role in species differences is the extent to which cerebral dominance is present. The greater the difference between the functions of corresponding regions on the two sides, the more reasonable it seems that poor recovery would follow a unilateral lesion. This factor will show up not only in species differences, but also in individual differences. The higher rate of recovery from aphasia in left-handers probably depends on the fact that sinistrals have, on the average, more symmetrical brains than dextrals.[14]

The effects of previous lesions on the consequences of later lesions are interesting and still not adequately studied. These are of at least two types. The first is the serial lesion effect; that is, destruction of certain regions in separated stages produces much less impairment than similar destruction in one stage, an effect seen in certain systems, but which is not universal. Another type of effect, probably related, occurs when lesions occur at different times in different locations. This has been used therapeutically, as in the performance of ventrolateral thalamotomy for the treatment of parkinsonism, the causative lesions of which are thought to be in the substantia nigra. Many years ago Tracy Jackson Putnam[15] showed that sectioning the pyramidal tract in the spinal cord could abolish parkinsonism on the same side in the absence of significant paralysis. It is still not clear whether the fact that the patient was parkinsonian led to a lesser degree of paralysis after the pyramidal lesion. This possibility has generally been neglected. Thus, when Bucy *et al.*[16] showed that hemiballismus (usually the result of sudden destruction of the corpus Luysii) lessened after section of the pyramidal tract in the peduncle, they concluded that a pyramidal lesion did not cause paralysis. They did not entertain the other alternative, that is, that a pyramidal lesion did not lead to paralysis when there was a preceding lesion in the corpus Luysii.

PRENATAL AND POSTNATAL LESIONS

In the above discussion I have deliberately confined myself to lesions in the mature individual. The situation during fetal life and in the first few years after birth is, however, of special interest since at no other time is the nervous system so plastic. This reflects the endowment of the embryo with an excess of neurons, many of which die before birth (recent work suggests that even in the first decade of life cell death may continue to take place). The surplus of neurons provides options that are no longer available when the nervous system has its final complement of cells. If one group of neurons is destroyed during the period when cell death is going on, there may be no diminution in the total number of neurons in the mature nervous system, but there can be a profound effect on the numbers in different regions. The pattern of cell death is probably normally modified by a large number of external influences other than frankly destructive lesions.

It was the accepted opinion for a long time, and is probably still believed by a majority of neurologists, that early lesions constitute a single class, that is, the consequences of damage in childhood and in the fetus are thought to be similar, although possibly different in degree. It is more likely that there are qualitative differences in many cases between prenatal lesions and those occurring in childhood. Goldman and Galkin[17] have shown that an intrauterine unilateral cortical lesion may lead to an altered pattern of connections of the homologous region of the other side. Furthermore, with such lesions one may observe increased size in later life both of the corresponding region on the opposite side and of other regions in the same hemisphere. The lesion removes neurons that would have competed for targets with the neurons from these regions. More of the neurons from the spared regions form connections than they would have in the normal case and therefore survive. The larger size of the spared regions is thus the result of diminished cell death. This raises the very interesting possibility that while damage in the fetus, especially if delimited, may result in lowered function in one area, it may lead to superior function in others. Although I will not discuss this possibility in detail, I believe that it is a mechanism of this type that accounts for the superiority of right hemisphere functions that is common in childhood dyslexics and for the often remarkable musical and artistic talents of some patients with childhood autism.

Current evidence suggests that in the period after birth a different pattern emerges. Several investigators have pointed out that a child who suffers from a unilateral aphasia-producing lesion recovers well, but does so at the expense of other abilities. Postnatally the brain is apparently plastic enough to permit recruitment to participation in language of neurons originally destined for other functions, but the level of the other functions necessarily declines. Although an adequate study has not yet been carried out, it is generally believed that lesions in the adult diminish the functions of the lesioned areas without affecting those dependent on spared areas. It thus appears that the effects of lesions are quite different prenatally, in the early postnatal years, and in adult life.

An attempt has been made in this paper to present as broad as possible a picture of the events that may succeed a brain lesion. While much has been learned, we still know remarkably little about many of the important mechanisms of recovery, e.g., those involved in immediate changes. I have discussed elsewhere some of the other mechanisms not treated here in detail, and have also given several examples of late recovery of function observed in humans.[18]

REFERENCES

1. PORTER, W. T. 1894–1895. The path of the respiratory impulse from the bulb to the phrenic nuclei. J. Physiol. **17:** 455–459.
2. DOLIVO, M. 1953. "Crossed phrenic phenomenon" et phénomène phrénique bilatéral. Helvet. Physiol. Pharmacol. Acta **11:** 251–269.
3. CANNON, W. B. & A. ROSENBLUETH. 1949. Supersensitivity of Denervated Structures. Macmillan. New York, NY.
4. GLONING, I., K. GLONING, G. HAUB & R. QUATEMBER. 1969. Comparison of verbal behavior in right-handed and non right-handed patients with anatomically verified lesion of one hemisphere. Cortex **5:** 43–52.

5. Luria, A. R. 1970. Traumatic Aphasia.: 27–76. Mouton. The Hague.
6. Subirana, A. 1969. Handedness and cerebral dominance. *In* Handbook of Clinical Neurology, Vol. 4. P. J. Vinken & G. W. Bruyn, Eds.: 248–272. North Holland. Amsterdam.
7. Hoffman, B. F. & P. F. Cranefield. 1960. Electrophysiology of the Heart. Blakiston. New York, NY.
8. Denny-Brown, D., E. J. Kirk & N. Yanagisawa. 1973. The tract of Lissauer in relation to sensory transmission in the dorsal horn of spinal cord in the macaque monkey. J. Comp. Neurol. **151:** 175–200.
9. Kirk, E. J. & D. Denny-Brown. 1970. Functional variation of the dermatomes in the macaque monkey following dorsal root lesions. J. Comp. Neurol. **139:** 307–320.
10. Liepmann, H. 1908. Drei Aufsätze aus dem Apraxiegebiet. Karger. Berlin.
11. Glees, P. & J. Cole. 1950. Recovery of skilled motor functions after small repeated lesions in motor cortex in macaque. J. Neurophysiol. **13:** 137–148.
12. Wall, P. D. & M. D. Egger. 1971. Formation of new connexions in adult rat brains after partial deafferentation. Nature **232:** 542–545.
13. Erickson, T. C. 1940. Spread of the epileptic discharge. Arch. Neurol. Psychiat. **43:** 429–452.
14. Galaburda, A. M., M. LeMay, T. L. Kemper & N. Geschwind. 1978. Right-left asymmetries in brain. Science **199:** 852–856.
15. Putnam, T. J. 1940. Treatment of unilateral paralysis agitans by section of the lateral pyramidal tract. Arch. Neurol. Psychiat. **44:** 950–976.
16. Bucy, P. C., J. E. Keplinger & E. B. Siqueira, 1964. Destruction of the "pyramidal tract" in man. J. Neurosurg. **21:** 385–398.
17. Goldman, P. S. & T. W. Galkin. 1978. Prenatal removal of frontal association cortex in the fetal rhesus monkey: Anatomical and functional consequences in postnatal life. Brain Res. **152:** 451–485.
18. Geschwind. N. 1974. Late changes in the nervous system: An overview. *In* Plasticity and Recovery in the Nervous System. D. G. Stein, J. J. Rosen & N. Butters, Eds.: 467–508. Academic Press. New York, NY.

Dyslexia, Congenital Anomalies, and Immune Disorders: The Role of the Fetal Environment[a]

PETER BEHAN

Department of Neurology
Institute of Neurological Sciences
University of Glasgow
Glasgow G51 4TF, Scotland

NORMAN GESCHWIND[b]

Neurological Unit
Beth Israel Hospital
Boston, Massachusetts 02215

The papers in this volume are devoted to understanding the mechanisms of the modifiability of the nervous system and the possible implications of these mechanisms for prevention or treatment of disease. In this paper we consider another aspect of the capacity of the brain for reorganization. While certain forms of neural alteration in the adult are well documented, the period in which the possibilities for restructuring are at their highest level is in fetal life, and modifiability is indeed the hallmark of brain development *in utero*. We will present data on humans whose clinical picture, we believe, reflects the operation of important influences that act on multiple systems during development. The delineation of the processes involved may well lead to future interventions during this labile period, which in turn may prevent the occurrence of many unfavorable consequences for future function.

We have recently demonstrated in several studies on several thousand people the strong association of left-handedness with learning disabilites (which had already been suggested by many authors, although some others have disagreed) and have documented the surprising fact that in left-handers there is a much higher rate of immune disorders than in right-handers. Furthermore, the first-degree relatives of our sinistral subjects had a higher rate of both learning disabilities and immune disorders than that of the right-handers.[8–10,19]

The preliminary analysis of the data of another recent study carried out by us in collaboration with the Hyperactive Children's Support Group of Great Britain yields similar findings. The hyperactive or hyperkinetic syn-

[a] This work was supported in part by Grants 06209 and NS 17018 from the National Institute of Neurological and Communication Disorders and Stroke of the National Institutes of Health and by the Orton Research Fund and the Essel Foundation.

[b] Deceased November 4, 1984.

drome is a learning disorder. Eighty-three children with a severe hyperkinetic syndrome completed a questionnaire which included the Handedness Inventory of Oldfield.[14] As can be seen in TABLE 1 there was a preponderance of males, most of them fair-haired and blue-eyed. *All* of the affected children gave a history of atopic illnesses, and there was an elevated rate of left-handedness. Among the siblings of these children were eight cases of dyslexia and one of autism. Other studies have revealed similar data.[12,28] In our first paper[9] we offered a working hypothesis concerning these relationships: we raised the possibility that certain common factors in the course of fetal life act simultaneously to alter development of the brain and of the immune system.

TABLE 1. Findings in 83 Children with the Severe Hyperactive Syndrome

	Boys	Girls
Number	59	24
Age range	8–15 yr	8–15 yr
Hair color: fair to blonde	70%	67%
Eye color: blue	64%	58%
Atopy: Total	100%	100%
Mild	10%	8%
Moderate	71%	58%
Severe	19%	34%
[a] LQ: $-100 \leqslant 0$	19%	21%
Other disorders		
Dyslexia	7%	8%
Epilepsy	0%	8%

[a] Laterality quotient (LQ) of $-100 \leqslant 0$ = degrees of left-handedness up to complete sinistrality (LQ of -100).

From data obtained in a previous study, we received the clinical impression that siblings of dyslexic children showed an increased incidence of skeletal malformations. In an earlier study one of us (PB) had found midline skeletal abnormalities (that is, Arnold-Chiari malformations) in four patients with autoimmune diseases (eosinophilic fasciitis, polymyositis, systemic lupus erythematosus, and vasculitis, respectively). In a fifth patient the same skeletal abnormality was associated with a high titer of circulating antinuclear antibody. It is likely that some common factors adversely affect the developing thymus and skeleton simultaneously. A genetic component is suggested by the known association of certain antigens of the major histocompatibility complex (HLA) with skeletal malformations and neural tube defects.[5,15,17,24] Further study will be needed to see whether skeletal malformations and dyslexia are indeed related.

As a result of these observations, we decided to investigate further the occurrence of congenital anomalies in families of dyslexic persons. The members of 132 families, each with one or more dyslexic children, were interviewed and a Handedness Inventory and detailed medical history obtained. In nine families one child (not the dyslexic individual) had a congenital cardiac abnormality: three had transposition of the great vessels and six had other lesions including patent ductus arteriosus, and atrial and ventricular septal defects (one associated with a diphragmatic hernia). Two dyslexics, not in this series, had congenital vascular malformations (one was an adult with epilepsy resulting from an arteriovenous malformation of the left temporal region, and the other had a fatal hemorrhage from a similar malformation). We have also studied a pair of female twins, each dyslexic and left-handed, with congenital cardiac defects and midline skeletal abnormalities. The possible relationship between dyslexia and heart lesions is especially interesting because in one form of congenital heart damage (that is, endocardial fibroelastosis), the majority of patients who came to postmortem examination were found to have neuronal migration defects in the brain.[25]

We decided to investigate the mothers of dyslexic children in order to ascertain the presence of familial disorders which might suggest genetic effects and to determine whether maternal factors might alter the environment of the developing fetus. Because of the high prevalence of atopic illnesses in dyslexics, we decided to look first at immunologic factions and therefore studied maternal humoral autoantibodies. In the 132 mothers of the dyslexic children we found that antithyroglobulin antibodies were present at a frequency 2.5 times as high as that of age- and sex-matched controls.

Our next investigation was prompted by the knowledge that damage can be produced in the infant by auto antibodies that have crossed the placenta; these disorders include transient signs of immune disorder in infants of affected mothers, as in systemic lupus erythematosus (SLE),[16] neonatal myasthenia gravis, thrombocytopenic purpura, and thyrotoxicosis.[20] Another example is congenital complete heart block. In one series an antibody to a ribonucleoprotein (the Ro antigen) was found in 34 of 41 mothers (83%) who had given birth to infants with isolated complete heart block.[21]

The Ro antigen is a nonhistone nucleoprotein, pH-sensitive and heat-labile; its antigenicity is not destroyed by trypsin, DNase, or RNase.[22,26] Although originally thought to be principally cytoplasmic in origin, it is now known to be concentrated mainly in nuclei.[22] We and others have identified it in human tissues (spleen, thymus, liver, heart and brain), in calf thymus and brain, and in rat thymus and dog spleen. A recent study has shown that the antigen is found in highest concentration in the brain and heart.[27] The term Ro is derived from the name of the first patient, a Madame Robert, in whom the antibody was demonstrated. Antibodies to Ro are found in a number of conditions, including Sjögren's syndrome, SLE, and rheumatoid arthritis.[13] Although the antibody is often found in patients with autoimmune disorders, it should be stressed that, as shown in the study of mothers of infants with congenital heart block, in which it appears to have a pathogenetic role, it can occur in healthy women as well.[21]

We have examined the sera of 45 mothers of dyslexic children and compared the results with those from a variety of other disorders and a range of controls including normal pregnant women and healthy age-matched controls. The antigen was prepared from calf thymus[26] and the sera examined by double immunodiffusion. Positive results were confirmed by counterimmunoelectrophoresis.

The results are shown in TABLE 2. Four of the 45 mothers of dyslexics had anti-Ro antibody in their serum. One of them, the mother of two dyslexic children, had the highest titers we have recorded. We have in fact used this patient's anti-Ro antibody in our purification technique, separating the Ro antigen by affinity chromatography.[26]

We have also found a high frequency (46%) of anti-Ro antibody in patients with polymyositis, particularly those with cardiac symptoms. Two patients who died of cardiac arrhythmia had conducting system lesions similar to those found in infants with congenital heart block. The high frequency of cardiac arrhythmias in patients with polymyositis, the development in some cases of anti-Ro antibody at the time of onset of the arrhythmia, and the similarity between the histologic changes in the heart in polymyositis and congenital heart block all suggest that this antibody may affect cardiac tissue. Further supporting evidence is afforded by the finding of anti-Ro antibody in patients with myotonic dystrophy who have similar cardiac arrhythmias. In this condition there can be selective damage to the cardiac conducting system, with lesions similar to those of congenital heart block.[23]

These findings indicate that there is an association between damage to the cardiac conducting tissue and anti-Ro antibody. The data of Scott *et al.*[21] strongly suggest that this antibody is implicated in the pathogenesis of congenital heart block, and our findings indicate that it may play a similar role in the cardiac damage of myotonic dystrophy and polymyositis. In both these disorders, immunologic abnormalities are present, and, in myotonic dystrophy, neuronal migration abnormalities are often found in the brain.[1,2,11]

The finding of anti-Ro antibody in the mothers of our dyslexic patients is of significance for several reasons. The development of anti-Ro antibody suggests the presence of an immune disturbance. Furthermore it is reasonable to suggest that it may play a pathogenetic role in many of the disorders observed in the offspring. It is tempting to speculate that, since the highest concentration of Ro antigen is in brain and heart,[11] the antibody might cause cerebral lesions as well as cardiac lesions. These speculations will need to be tested experimentally because neuronal migration abnormalities occur very frequently in patients with congenital cardiac lesions.[25]

In this preliminary report, it is worth mentioning that we also found a high titer of anti-Ro antibody in an 18-year-old girl who had given birth to

TABLE 2. Frequency of Anti-Ro Antibody

Patient Group	No. of Cases	Percent Positive
Mothers of dyslexic children	45	9%
Polymyositis	45	46%
Myasthenia gravis	25	12%
Myotonic dystrophy	17	35%
Sjögren's syndrome	17	41%
Systemic lupus erythematosus	8	50%
Normal pregnant women	200	0%
Normal healthy controls	500	0%

a child with multiple congenital abnormalities. This girl was taking sodium valproate as an anticonvulsant, a substance that has been implicated as a cause of congenital abnormalities, including neural tube defects.[3,18] Its possible role, if any, in this case, is being investigated.

Finally, in preliminary animal experiments, we have shown that high titers of anti-Ro antibody can be produced in rabbits by immunizing them with semi-purified Ro antigen. Six pregnant rabbits with high antibody titers were sacrificed on the day prior to delivery. More than half of the fetuses were dead and one of these had a defective skull, low-set ears, an open abdominal wall, and no large intestine.

DISCUSSION

Galaburda and Kemper[7] demonstrated disturbances of neuronal migration in the brain of a dyslexic child and similar lesions have been found in four other cases[4,6] and no case studied has been free of such lesions. Our earlier work[9,10] has demonstrated a high rate of immunologic disorders in dyslexic persons. The studies reported here suggest that dyslexia can be associated with congenital lesions of the cardiovascular system especially and probably also of the skeletal system. In addition, we have found evidence that the mothers of dyslexic children frequently have immunologic abnormalities, as shown by an elevated frequency of anti-thyroid and anti-Ro antibodies.

The importance of genetic factors has long been recognized in dyslexia, as in many other neurologic disorders. We wish in no way to deny the importance of such factors, but it is important to point out that the intra-uterine environment plays a major role in many cases in determining the course of development of the nervous system and other bodily systems. The relative neglect of this possibility is surprising since at no period in life is the pattern of the brain and other systems so readily modified. Recent studies have made it clear that development is not rigidly determined, but rather that multiple scenarios are possible, depending on which genes are expressed or repressed. The implications of this for the new neurology are clearly hopeful. The more we learn the details of the mechanisms by which development can be modified, the more likely is the possibility that many diseases can be prevented and that methods will be devised for ensuring the development of maximum individual potential.

REFERENCES

1. Behan, W. M. H. & P. O. Behan. 1980. A comparison between human polymyositis and the putative animal model, experimental allergic myositis. *In* Animal Models of Neurological Disease. F. C. Rose & P. O. Behan, Eds.: 72–89. Pitman. London.
2. Behan, W. M. H. & P. O. Behan. 1984. Disturbance of regulatory lymphocyte subsets in polymyositis. Ann. Neurol. **15:** 112–114.

3. COMMITTEE ON SAFETY OF MEDICINES. January 1983. Sodium valproate (Epilim) and congenital abnormalities. Current Problems No. 9.: 1–2. HMSO. London.
4. DRAKE, W. E. 1968. Clinical and pathological findings in a child with development learning disability, J. Learn. Disabil. **1:** 9–25.
5. FEINGOLD, J., N. FEINGOLD & E. BOIS. 1980. Spina bifida and anencephaly. Geographic correlation with the HLA system. Tissue Antigens **15:** 318–324.
6. GALABURDA, A. M. 1983. Developmental dyslexia: Current anatomical research. Ann. Dyslexia **33:** 41–58.
7. GALABURDA, A. M. & T. L. KEMPER. 1979. Cytoarchitectonic abnormalities in developmental dyslexia: A case study. Ann. Neurol. **6:** 94–100.
8. GESCHWIND, N. 1984. Immunological associations of cerebral dominance. *In* Neuroimmunology. P. Behan & F. Spreafico, Eds.: 451–461. Raven Press. New York, NY.
9. GESCHWIND, N. & P. O. BEHAN. 1982. Left-handedness: Association with immune disease, migraine and developmental learning disorders. Proc. Natl. Acad. Sci. USA **79:** 5097–5100.
10. GESCHWIND, N. & P. O. BEHAN. 1984. Laterality, hormones and immunity. *In* Cerebral Dominance: the Biological Foundations. N. Geschwind & A. Galaburda, Eds.: 211–224. Harvard University Press. Cambridge, MA.
11. GROVE, D. I., S. J. O'CALLAGHAN, T. O. BURSTON, & I. J. FORBES. 1973. Immunological function in dystrophia myotonica. Br. Med. J. **3:** 81–83.
12. KOLATA, G. 1983. Math genius may have hormonal basis. Science **222:** 1312.
13. MADDISON, P., H. MOGAVERO, T. T. PROVOST & M. REICHLIN. 1979. The clinical significance of autoantibodies to a soluble cytoplasmic antigen in systemic lupus erythematosus and other connective tissue disorders. J. Rheumatol. **6:** 189–195.
14. OLDFIELD, R. C. 1971. The assessment and analysis of handedness: The Edinburgh inventory. Neuropsychologia **9:** 97–113.
15. PEITRZYK, J. J. & G. TUROWSKI. 1979. Immunogenetic basis of congenital malformations: Association of HLA-B27 with spina bifida. Pediat. Res. **13:** 879–883.
16. PROVOST, T. T. 1983. Commentary: Neonatal lupus erythematosus. Arch. Dermatol. **119:** 619–622.
17. RAPAPORT, F. T., F. H. BACH, R. J. BACHVAROFF, J. G. MCCARTHY, A. P. RAISBECK, B. EGELANDSDAL & J. M. CONVERSE. 1979. The major histocompatibility complex (HLA) as a genetic marker in human craniofacial anomalies. Tissue Antigens **14:** 407–421.
18. ROBERT, E. & P. GUIBAUD. 1982. Maternal valproic acid and congenital neural tube defects. Lancet **2:** 937.
19. SCHACTER, S. C., B. J. RANSIL & N. GESCHWIND. Neuropsychologica. In press.
20. SCOTT, J. S. 1977. Immunological diseases in pregnancy. *In* Progress in Allergy. P. Kallas *et al.* Eds. **23:** 321–366.
21. SCOTT, J. S., P. J. MADDISON, P. V. RAYLOR, E. ESSCHER, O. SCOTT & R. P. SKINNER. 1983. Connective-tissue disease, antibodies to ribonucleoprotein, and congenital heart block. New Engl. J. Med. **309:** 209–212.
22. TAN, E. M. 1982. Autoantibodies to nuclear antigens (ANA): Their immunobiology and medicine. Adv. Immunol. **33:** 167–240.
23. THOMPSON, A. M. P. 1968. Dystrophia cordis myotonica studied by serial histology of the pacemaker and conducting tissue. J. Pathol. Bacteriol. **96:** 285–295.
24. VANNIER, J. P., B. CAVELIER, J. P. MARTIN, J. LEFORT, L. RIVAT & J. FEINGOLD. 1980. HLA, Pi, G, and Km phenotypes in a spina bifida population with myelomeningocele. Tissue Antigens **15:** 501–504.
25. VEITH, G. & H-K. ZIEGLER. 1965. Fehlbildungen des Gehirnes bei Endokardofibroelastose. Beitr. Pathol. Anat. **132:** 160–187.
26. VENABLES, P. J. W., P. R SMITH & R. N. MAINI. 1983. Purification and characterization of the Sjögren's syndrome A and B antigens. Clin. Exp. Immunol. **54:** 731–738.
27. WOLIN, S. L. & J. A. STEITZ. 1984. The Ro small cytoplasmic ribonucleoproteins: Indentification of the antigenic protein and its binding site on the Ro RNAs. Proc. Natl. Acad. Sci. USA. **81:** 1996–2000.
28. WOOD, L. O. 1983. Presentation at the American Thyroid Association, New Orleans, 1983.

The BEAM Method for Neurophysiological Diagnosis

FRANK H. DUFFY

Department of Neurology
Harvard Medical School, and
Department of Developmental Neurophysiology
The Children's Hospital
Boston, Massachusetts 02115

The late 1930s and early 1940s were a period of great excitement in clinical neurophysiology. Hans Berger[1] had documented the presence of a cortical rhythm that occurred upon eye closure and vanished upon eye opening. Furthermore, Gibbs and others had demonstrated that unique electrical paroxysms lay beneath the mystery of epilepsy.[2] These early findings and the research that rapidly followed encouraged the belief that electroencephalography would form a major investigative tool and thereby enhance our understanding of both normal and abnormal brain function. It was commonly conceived that to decipher the workings of the brain in cerebral palsy, schizophrenia, and antisocial behavior, it would simply be a matter of gazing more intently at the erratic tracings from the brain on EEG recordings and eventually the "signature" of the pathologic process would become apparent.

As the years have passed, however, it has become clear that electroencephalography has failed to live up to the lofty expectations of the 1930s and 1940s. While EEG remains the primary diagnostic procedure for elucidation and categorization of the epilepsies, for other disease processes its contribution has proven less reliable. The mysteries of cerebral palsy, schizophrenia, and antisocial behavior, for example, have not been unraveled by studies of brain wave activity. Curiously, many electroencephalographers still strongly support the notion that EEG has much to tell; yet they and others are unable to use this potentially powerful tool in a more productive manner. Why should this be?

TRADITIONAL EEG INTERPRETATION

The extraction of information from a clinical electroencephalogram is a nontrivial matter. Some years ago it occurred to us that perhaps the limitation on the clinical and research value of electroencephalography lay not in the EEG itself, but in the means by which information was gleaned from it.

The EEG consists of a series of "squiggly" lines on paper reminiscent of the seismograph used in geologic exploration and research. Ordinarily, 16 such channels are displayed on a single page and the total record consists of fan-folded paper forming a "book" of approximately 1 to 3 cm in thickness.

The principal means of analysis has been and remains visual inspection, and the skilled electroencephalographer analyzes the 100–200 pages of a book in roughly a 10-minute period.

Electroencephalographers are usually physicians who have completed a residency in neurology and have had an additional year or two of training in the field of EEG. Electroencephalographic interpretation depends to no small degree upon the skill of the electroencephalographer. We have long believed that EEGs contain much more in the way of useful information than can be extracted even by skilled readers dependent on otherwise unaided visual inspection.

The process by which an electroencephalographer evaluates an EEG is worth reviewing. First, the record is screened for obvious diagnostic paroxysmal activity. An example of this is the spike or spike-and-wave signature of epilepsy, which, when found, raises the probability that the subject has an underlying seizure disorder. Such clinically important paroxysms must be carefully distinguished from such artifacts as eyeblink or electrode malfunction. In general, those diseases best diagnosed by EEG are those that produce clear-cut, often recurring, and unambiguous discontinuities of brain electrical activity. Unfortunately, there are not many diseases that do so.

In the normal subject or in the diseased subject who does not produce paroxysmal activity, the flow of information from the brain is reasonably continuous and will not be interrupted if his level of consciousness and alertness remain stable. Such ongoing, ambient brain activity is referred to as EEG "background"; this must also be interpreted by unaided visual inspection. Occasionally alterations of the frequency content of background are sufficient to be clinically meaningful. Nonetheless, it is painfully obvious to anyone who has attempted to read EEGs that it is much easier to deal with paroxysmal diagnostic discontinuities than it is to attempt to make a diagnosis on the basis of clinical evaluation of EEG background.

This background evaluation consists of three complex steps: First, the electroencephalographer mentally performs a decomposition of the activity within one channel into different frequency components. In doing so, the electroencephalographer attempts to assess the extent of delta (0–3 Hz), theta (4–8 Hz), alpha (8–12 Hz), and beta (over 12 Hz) wave activity that exists in a particular brain location. Next, the electroencephalographer determines how consistent that pattern of activity is over time. Finally, he or she mentally creates a map of the spatial distribution of the findings. In other words, interpretation of EEG background consists of spectral analysis, temporal summation, and spatial topographic mapping. Needless to say, this complex and skill-dependent process probably represents the major factor in the failure of EEG to achieve its full potential.

A related area of neurophysiology, evoked potentials (EPs), has also suffered from this deficiency. In 1950, Dawson[3] first recorded the brains's electrical response to external stimulation. This he termed the evoked potential. Great excitement was sparked by this finding and it was widely hoped that the use of evoked potentials would allow more accurate "interrogation" of areas of the brain so that normal functions and disease-related pathophysiologies could be elucidated. Whereas EEG represents an indication of ongoing brain electrical activity, evoked potentials represent the brain's transient electrical response to external stimulation. Evoked responses are not visible in most instances from a single external stimulation. Rather, they are approximately 1/10th to 1/100th of the amplitude of the background EEG. By the analytic process of signal averaging, however, it is possible to demonstrate their presence. Once obtained from a single channel, evoked response is heuristically considered to be the product of a single stimulus, although many EPs (20–2000) may have gone into the generation of the average response.

Unfortunately, evoked potentials suffer from problems quite similar to those of the EEG, that is, they vary widely from location to location around the head and there is no general agreement as to where they are generated. Evoked potentials may last up to 750 msec or longer from the time of stimulation. The mid- and late-latency ranges beyond 50 to 100 msec are believed to represent activity arising in cortex from sensory-specific and from more diffuse, cortex-activating pathways. Ironically, the high degree of sensitivity of EPs to stimulus parameters, level of consciousness, and selective attention have made them poorly reproducible and difficult to clinically evaluate. Accordingly, evoked potentials have not achieved the level of clinical acceptance now afforded the EEG.

An exception to this has been the observation that very early evoked response components, especially from auditory or somatosensory stimulation, may arise from discrete brainstem or thalamic structures. These short-latency or far-field evoked potentials, measured below 50-msec latency, have, in contrast, proven of great clinical value in the assessment of brain function at the subcortical level.[4] Longer-latency EPs (that is, those going beyond 50 msec) probably represent specific and nonspecific cortical activation, but the variable nature of these responses has severely limited their utility (see, for example, Refs. 5 and 6). Further complicating the issue of long-latency evoked responses is their highly topographically specific wave shapes. In other words, spatial distribution is difficult to assess by visual inspection of these brief transient responses on EEG recordings.

THE INITIAL USES OF TOPOGRAPHIC MAPPING AS AN APPROACH TO EEG INTERPRETATION

Within the past decade advanced computer techniques have been used in an attempt to improve the visibility of information within the EEG and evoked potential data. For the EEG, the most important of these techniques have incorporated computerized spectral analysis. Here, EEG background is decomposed into spectral (i.e., wavelength) components using Fourier analysis and the fast Fourier transform (FFT) algorithm.[7] This procedure is analogous to analyzing the music in an orchestral score into its components, determining what portion of the sound is contributed by the bass instruments, what portion by brass, the reeds, and so forth. Spectral analysis can be performed on as much, or as little, of the EEG as desired. Hence, this single operation automatically condenses time and extracts frequency-specific information. Early attempts at topographically displaying this information were found to be clinically useful, [8–13] but these early techniques failed to displace electroencephalography and have not been widely accepted.

BRAIN ELECTRICAL ACTIVITY MAPPING

Our approach to the extraction of further information from both EEG and evoked potential data has been termed *brain electrical activity mapping* (BEAM). As shown in FIGURE 1, data are gathered from each of twenty active electrodes. For EEG data, spectral analysis is performed and the amount of delta, theta, alpha, and beta activity is numerically quantified for each electrode. By means of the topographic method shown in FIGURE 1, displays are made of the spatial distribution of these different frequency ranges. Ordinarily more than 3 minutes of EEG are summarized in each topographic map. This is true for the evoked potential data specifically shown in FIGURE 1. Topographic images are made of the voltage distribution of evoked potentials for every 4 msec over a range of 512 msec. Thus, a set of 128 serial topographic maps are created. Initially in our research, these images were viewed in endless-loop cinematography, utilizing photographic techniques commonly employed in the formation of cartoons. Today, this process is done automatically, with the resulting image displayed at the computer terminal. For maps of both EEG and evoked potentials, the value of the variable being measured is displayed in "pseudo-color grey scale." The result is a picture that is easily and rapidly interpretable by the clinician. These images have proven of great value in the assessment of EEG and evoked potential background. Essentially, the spectral, temporal, and spatial analyses are performed by the computer, thereby relieving the clinician of the burden of having to perform these complicated processes in his own mind.

Our first attempts to employ this method for elucidation of clinical pathology dealt with assessment of electrophysiological differences in patients with supratentorial brain tumors. Essentially, these tumors constituted a benchmark pathology, since their size and location were clearly established by the new computerized skull x-ray, the now well-known CT scan.[14] We found that the topographic maps of EEG slow activity delineated tumors in a manner that one might anticipate from experience in classic EEG. Surprisingly, tumors were also evident on evoked potential studies. Early components of the evoked response were diminished, while late activity was augmented overlying these space-occupying lesions. Furthermore, nonspecific late central vertex activity was often diminished.

Recently we have extended our studies of supratentorial lesions to follow patients treated for brain tumor longitudinally over time. In conjunction with Dr. Fred Hochberg at the Massachusetts General Hospital in Boston, we have followed a series of patients who have received initial therapy with intracarotid injections of an antimetabolic agent for treatment of highly malignant brain tumors (glioblastoma multiforme). Characteristically, such patients are initially very responsive to treatment. However, their tumor eventually recurs. Often these patients respond well to second and third treatments, with good function between recurrence. Unfortunately, the CT scan, an important device in establishing the initial diagnosis, is not as useful in detecting tumor recurrence because of the localized anatomical debris left in place after the initial tumor chemotherapy. This debris obscures detection of tumor regrowth months or years later. We attempted to demonstrate whether longitudinal BEAM studies might be of value in better pinpointing the time of recurrence. We were pleased to discover that serial trend plots of brain activity based, for example, upon delta brainwave activity overlying the tumor site made evident the nature of clinical progression such that tumor regrowth could often be predicted 3 to 6 weeks in advance of obvious clinical recurrence. Progression could be shown equally well by BEAM analysis of EEG or evoked potential data and we are now regularly employing this technique for the longitudinal tracking of brain tumors, as well as other neurologic abnormalities.

SIGNIFICANCE PROBABILITY MAPPING

Early on it became clear that normal subjects often demonstrated a degree of asymmetry or focality of topographic brain wave distributions. The question often became whether or not an obvious focality or asymmetry constituted a clinical abnormality or whether the degree of asymmetry could be explained by normal variation. In 1981, in conjunction with Dr. Peter Bartels from the University of Arizona, we developed a technique known as significance probability mapping (SPM).[15,16] In this process a single subject's topographic image can be compared to that of a control or reference data set. This results in a new image in which the original data are replaced by the delineation of individual deviation from the collected data on normal subjects. Essentially, the subject's data are replaced by their Z transform, thus displaying an image of standard deviation from the norm. This fulfills the final and complicated step in the clinical evaluation of EEG and evoked potential data, namely, the delineation of regional abnormality. Clinically, the technique of SPM has proven singularly valuable in the diagnostic delineation of abnormalities in clinical subjects.

However, we saw at that time that the greatest value of our technique would clearly be in its ability to distinguish meaningful cortical abnormalities that were not simultaneously defined by discrete lesions visible by CT scan. Accordingly, our first approach was to investigate a series of adolescents known to have sociopathic behavior. Classical neurology and neuropsychology[17] would predict frontal lobe abnormalities in the subjects. Nonetheless, most such patients have normal neurologic exams and fail to show absolutely clear-cut abnormality by psychological testing. In an early study of four such subjects, large asymmetries were found overlying the frontal lobes

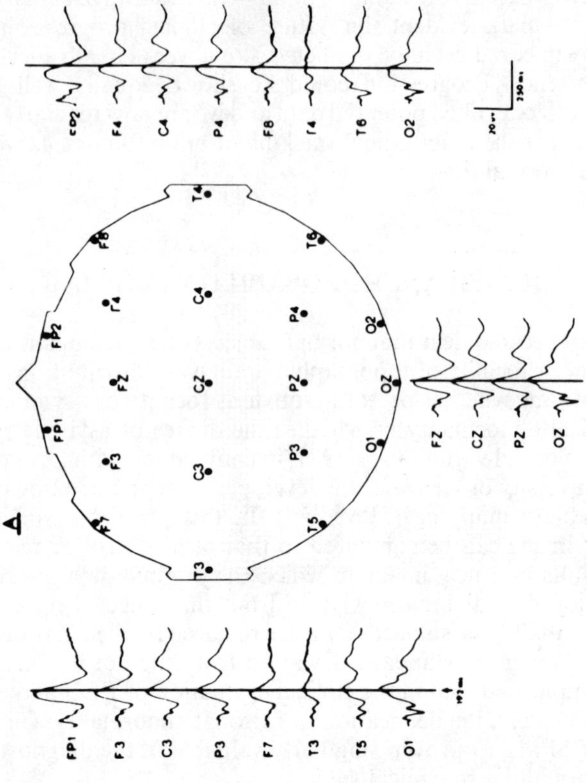
FP1
F3
C3
P3
F7
T3
T5
O1
F4
C4
P4
F8
T6
O2
FP2
FZ
CZ
PZ
OZ
T4
Q1
Q2

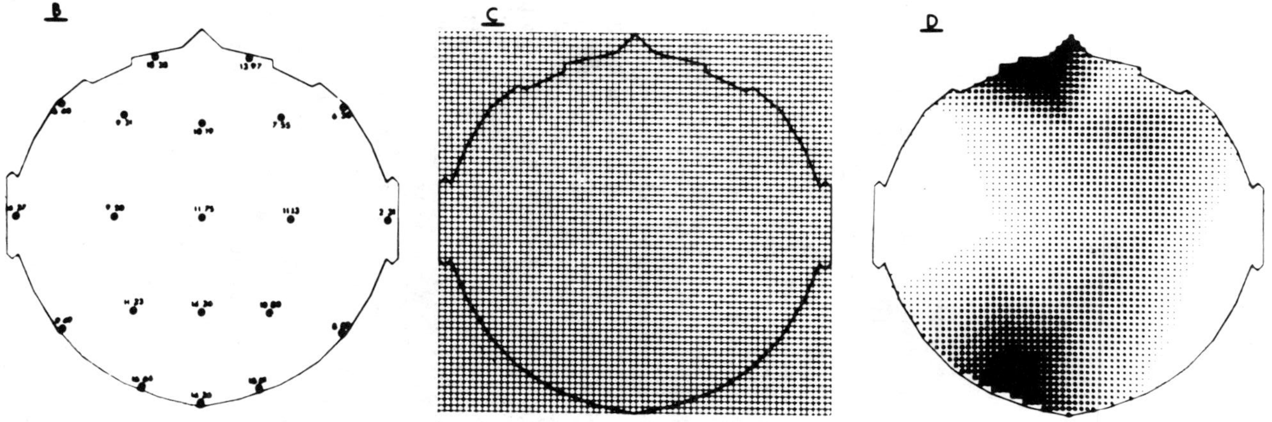

FIGURE 1. Construction of a topographic BEAM image for EP data. (A similar procedure is employed for the spatial map which ordinarily plots activity over a range of frequency bands.) Mean EPs are formed from each of 20 recording sites. Each EP is divided into 128 4-msec intervals, and the mean voltage value for each interval is calculated. **(A)** Individual EPs for the electrode locations are indicated on the head diagram. **(B)** Mean voltage values at these locations are shown for the interval beginning 192 msec after the stimulus (the vertical line in **[A]** indicates this time on the EPs). Next the head region is treated as a 64 × 64 matrix; the resulting 4096 spatial domains are illustrated in **(C)**. Each domain is assigned a voltage value by linear interpolation from the three known points. Finally, for display, the raw voltage values are fitted to a discrete-level equal-interval intensity scale as shown in **(D)**. The images are displayed on a color television screen using the gray scale in "pseudo color format." Sequential EP images can be viewed by computer-controlled cartooning of these images.

in the distribution of topographic activity produced by visual and auditory stimulation. Unfortunately, interest in these matters by the legal community prompted us to move into a less controversial area.

CHARACTERISTICS OF BRAIN DYSFUNCTION ASSOCIATED WITH DYSLEXIA

In concert with my colleague, Dr. Martha Denckla, we undertook an evaluation of children with specific reading disability, or dyslexia, an entity not known to have fixed lesions demonstrable by CT scan. To assess the potential of our technique, we attempted to look at a very restricted question: Would it be possible for us to determine meaningful regional topographic differences in brain electrical activity between control subjects and a very restricted group of dyslexic persons? To eliminate extraneous variables, we limited our study to boys aged 10–12 years, most of whom were right-handed, and all of whom suffered *only* from dyslexia. All selected children were more than $1\frac{1}{2}$ years retarded in age-expected reading ability, but were free of attentional deficit disorder or other forms of learning disability, "hard" neurologic findings, psychiatric disturbance, or epilepsy. We analyzed these children by means of both EEG and evoked potential paradigms ranging, in each condition, from the simple passive state to the highly activated state where cognitive or language tasks were demanded of the subject while under observation. To accomplish data analysis, we again relied upon the SPM technique. Instead of comparing a single subject to a group, as we had previously done, the task was now to compare two groups—normal boys and dyslexic boys. The appropriate statistical measure of between-group difference we chose to be the Student's *t* test; thus, controls and dyslexics were compared for a given condition by means of a topographic display of the *t* statistic, known as the *t*-SPM. The function of the *t*-SPM was to graphically delineate regions of between-group difference.[18,19]

We were pleased to find that regional differences were found in response to auditory stimulation. The differences occurred predominantly overlying the left posterior lateral hemisphere, regions most often associated with language function. Between-group difference was also found in the central parietal mid- and posterior temporal areas, extending back almost to the occipital region on the left, regions known to produce aphasia when lesioned. However, during some of the testing, through EEG spectral analysis, a large region of between-group difference was delineated in the medial frontal region, an area corresponding to the supplementary motor area. This was surprising since heretofore this region was not believed to have a major role in language function. Shortly after we completed our study, however, we became aware of the blood-flow mapping studies of Larsen and Lassen.[20,21] These researchers, using xenon-labeled regional cerebral blood-flow studies, demonstrated that the medial frontal supplementary motor area played an active role in normal subjects during language-related tasks. Whether the subjects were reading silently or verbally, the region shown to be activated by such language tasks coincided almost exactly with the regional differences indicated in our topographic maps of alpha activity. In other words, virtually the same regions involved in normal language production were found to be abnormal when dyslexic boys were compared with normal boys. We concluded from these results that dyslexia appears to represent dysfunction in the entire area normally involved in language function and that this system was more widely distributed than commonly appreciated. Furthermore, it appeared that the medial frontal supplementary motor area was unexpectedly involved and perhaps important in the generation of normal speech and thus in the pathophysiology of dyslexia. The alpha activity, which was augmented in this area in the dyslexic subjects, suggests a hypofunctionality. Patients who have cerebral infarctions in this area[22] are known to have specific difficulty in initiating reading and writing, although they can ultimately perform these tasks with difficulty.

Thus, topographic mapping of brain electrical activity seems to have proven useful in the delineation of functional abnormalities and specific reading disability. More recently, we have undertaken a partially completed study to investigate whether dyslexic patients constitute a homogeneous entity or whether there are electrophysiologically identifiable subcategories. Martha Denckla recognizes some five to seven clinically identifiable categories of "dyslexia-pure" patients, that is, those solely disabled by reading problems. Three of these categories occur with exceptional frequency and the remaining are rather rare. The three most common are "anomic disorder," "dysphonemic sequencing disorder," and a "global impaired category." These definitions are shown in TABLE 1. Anomic subjects have word-finding difficulty, but have excellent reading comprehension. Dysphonemic sequencers have complicated language dysfunction with comprehension difficulty. "Globals" are more universally impaired. In our study, these three groups were compared with each other. It became evident that the anomic group

TABLE 1. Definitions of Dyslexia Subtypes

Global-Mixed Language Disorder:
- (a) Below average performance on all or most language tests
- (b) Performance IQ of at least 95; verbal IQ of less than 90

Dysphonemic-Sequencing Disorder:
- (a) Decreased ability to perceive phonetic/phonemic detail resulting in misunderstandings of complex syntactical structures
- (b) Sequential order errors on sentence repetition and digit span
- (c) Naming errors of a phonemic nature

Anomic-Repetition Disorder:
- (a) Circumlocutory and paraphasic errors on confrontation naming
- (b) Reduced digit span and sentence repetition
- (c) Normal comprehension and articulation

was the most likely to demonstrate frontal dysfunction, whereas the dysphonemic group demonstrated bilateral central parietal dysfunction. Globals seemed to show a combination of both. Thus, the technique appears useful in marking off not only the pathophysiology of dyslexia in contrast to control subjects, but also *where* the subcategories of dyslexia differ from one another.

Dyslexia has been evaluated from an alternative standpoint in another study that we did. Instead of contrasting dyslexic and control subjects by means of *t*-SPM, the control subjects were contrasted with themselves as their state changed; dyslexic subjects were similarly studied. For example, we found that when normal controls move from passively sitting with eyes open to passively listening to a fairy tale, alpha activity is significantly reduced over the left temporal lobe. Conversely, when normal subjects listen to music, alpha activity is diminished over the right temporal lobe. Dyslexics, when they move from resting to listening to a fairy tale, also show a large reduction of alpha activity, but the activity, instead of being localized over the left temporal lobe, is seen to occur in the left posterior frontal area. Although listening to music reduces alpha waves over the right temporal lobe, it also reduces alpha activity in the midoccipital region. This curious pattern has been taken as evidence to suggest that these electrophysiological differences are suggestive of a different neural organization of the brain of the reading-disabled.

THE USE OF BEAM IN THE IDENTIFICATION OF COVERT EPILEPSY

Although epilepsy is primarily diagnosed by a unique paroxysmal pattern on the routine EEG, patients are occasionally seen who seem to have clinical seizures, but in whom spikes are not seen on the resting EEG nor can spikes be produced by various activating procedures. Topographic analyses of EEG background activity of these patients[24,25] have indicated a unique pattern. For example, background fast activity is often augmented directly over the region of epileptogenicity. This presumably derives from the fact that "sharp background," when spectrally analyzed, demonstrates an increased high-frequency component as a natural fallout of the fast Fourier transform algorithm. Occasionally in these same loci slow activity is also augmented. This constellation of increased background fast activity in a localized region has proven useful in the identification of potentially epileptogenic, "irritable" cortex. Often in these same regions evoked potential activity is markedly augmented. It appears that cortex may be ordinarily quiescent, but when invaded by specific or nonspecific sensory stimulation, there is an excessive response which is regionally specific to the irritable cortex. Thus the constellation of augmented evoked response activity and increased fast activity may signal irritative cortex. This discovery has proven useful in the identification of covert epilepsy.

SCHIZOPHRENIA STUDIES UTILIZING BEAM

In collaboration with Dr. John Morihisa at St. Elizabeth's Hospital in Washington, D.C., an investigation was undertaken of patients with schizophrenia.[26] These patients were evaluated both on and off medication. As has been previously demonstrated by many investigators,[27] we found a marked increase in frontal lobe slow activity. In this same area we also demonstrated augmentation of the late components of the visual evoked response. These findings come as no surprise, given the well-known theory of Dr. David Ingvar[28] that schizophrenia represents a "hypofrontality" with evidence of decreased metabolic function. In addition to these frontal lobe abnormalities, however, we showed a striking augmentation of beta activity in the left parietal and posterior temporal regions, and in this same locus an increase of the visual evoked response. These findings were highly reminiscent of those noticed in epilepsy. In another group of schizophrenics, studied with Dr. Robert McCarley and Dr. Ron Morstyn at the Massachusetts Mental Health Center, the P300 procedure was performed.[29] In this procedure the subject must indicate when, in a train of otherwise homogeneous stimuli, an "oddball" stimulus occurs. The evoked response to the oddball stimulus demonstrates a positive component between 300 and 500 msec that is lacking in the response to the frequently occurring stimulus evoked potential.[30] As opposed to extrapolations from scalp-recorded data, depth-recording studies have indicated that some or all of the P300 waveform may be generated from subcortical sources. In research using depth probes compared to scalp recordings, it was found that P300 activity increased with increasing distance from the scalp. Compatible with this finding was the fact that bilaterally implanted electrodes in the medial temporal lobe, particularly in the hippocampus, hippocampal gyrus, and amygdala, showed P300 activity of far greater amplitude than at the scalp. Okada *et al.*[31] have recently reported that, on the basis of neuromagnetic studies, the magnetic field associated with the P300 complex appears to arise in the hippocampal formation. Our finding was that schizophrenics demonstrate diminished P300 activity, again in the left posterior temporal region. Thus, there seems to be an unusual response in the left posterior hemisphere of schizophrenics, with a tendency for irritable activity to be evident, while at the same time, some of the normally occurring cognitive functions seem deficient. There are data to suggest that the P300 response originates deep within the brain rather than cortically; this is compatible with our findings of temporal abnormality. Both neurochemical evidence concerning limbic system disturbances in schizophrenia and cognitive psychological studies point to these regions. It is possible not only that the left temporal abnormality in our subjects might reflect an intrinsic limbic system disturbance, but also that this abnormality is secondary to abnormalities of activation and modulation from ascending aminergic systems.

It is interesting that Dr. Ira Sherwin[32] has shown that left temporal epileptics have a much higher instance of psychosis than do right temporal lobe epileptics. We are not suggesting here that schizophrenia is a form of epilepsy; rather, we speculate that left posterior hemisphere irritative processes may predispose patients to psychotic behavior and that further research is in order.

NORMATIVE AGING AND PRESENILE AND SENILE DEMENTIA

In conjunction with Dr. Marilyn Albert at the Massachusetts General Hospital in Boston, we have recently been evaluating patients with presenile dementia and senile dementia of the Alzheimer type.[33] We have attempted to contrast these pathologic processes with the effects of the normal aging process upon brainwave electrical activity. We were fortunate that this population of patients was well studied clinically and from all respects optimally healthy, except for disease of the central nervous system. Control subjects in these analyses had normal CT scans and normal neurologic exams, while the demented subjects demonstrated only the expected atrophic findings by CT scan.

One of our most surprising findings involved spectral analysis of the electroencephalogram in healthy normal subjects ranging in age from 30 to 80. In contrast to previous reports, we found no significant difference of peak alpha frequency or alpha frequency amplitude moving from the age of 30 to 80. The 30-year-old subjects demonstrated an alpha peak frequency at 9.7 Hz and the peak in the 70- to 80-year-old group was 9.1 Hz. Moreover, topographic distribution of delta and theta activity did vary with time and seemed, with age, to change predominantly and more rapidly over the temporal lobes, changing slightly more on the right side. Surprisingly, however, delta and theta slow activity diminished with age, a result that stands in marked contrast to previous reports.[34,35] Katz and Horowitz have suggested[36] that augmented slowing with age, reported by many observers, reflected not the normative aging process, but rather the fact that patients were included who had unsuspected medical diseases that had deleterious effects upon brain electrical activity. Fortunately our group was exceptionally healthy from a medical standpoint. Thus it appears that if one maintains good health, alpha frequency does not change over age and background slow activity not only fails to increase, but actually diminishes with age.

In contrast, patients with presenile dementia of the Alzheimer type demonstrated a marked augmentation of slowing over the temporal lobes. This finding alone suggests that the notion of Alzheimer's disease as a manifestation of accelerated aging is not accurate. Although changes in the temporal lobe were observed in both groups, the direction of change in background activity was quite different. The patients with presenile dementia as a group demonstrated increased theta slow activity, and decreased fast activity relative to controls, whereas the opposite was seen in the normative aging sample.

Patients whose dementia began well after the age of 65 (Alzheimer's of the senile type) likewise demonstrated marked augmentation of delta and theta slow activity attributable to their disease. The topographic distribution differed, however, from that of presenile dementia. In the senile group, changes were most prominent over the frontal and anterior temporal regions, whereas in the presenile group, changes were most common in the mid- and posterior temporal regions. The frontal area was unaffected. This suggested either that presenile dementia and senile dementia are different disease entities or that there is a marked disease–age interaction. Indeed, it is clinically known that presenile dementia seems predominantly to manifest itself by memory dysfunction, whereas with senile dementia classic frontal lobe findings are much more prominent.

ASSESSMENT OF BRAIN FUNCTION IN PREMATURE INFANTS

Here at Children's Hospital, in concert with Dr. Heidelise Als, we have been involved in the evaluation of electrophysiological function in the newborn infant. Dr. Als and her associates have developed a "synactive" model of development,[38] which outlines, as main dimensions of the human organism's uniqueness, the degree of differentiation and modulation of its behavioral organization. As the organism develops from the blastocyst all the way through birth and early childhood, it is in a state of continuous interaction with, and adjustment to, its environment. This process is dependent upon a consistent means of organismic change within the being. At birth, there are five *a priori* subsystems of functioning that must mutually coexist and support each other internally in order that the newborn infant maintain his primary developmental agendum at this point, i.e., alertness. These dimensions are: the autonomic system, the motor system, the state system, the attentional/interactive system, and the self-regulatory system. This model hypothesizes a developmental process of the infant that consists of a continuous balance between reaching out and moving towards, incorporating more and defending against, shutting off, avoiding, and withdrawing as necessary. It is clear that the premature infant is thrust into a situation wherein he is unprepared to integrate much of the extrauterine stimuli with which he is bombarded into his current developmental agenda. Much energy is expended in defensive, organism-protective activities.

Advances in medical technology have brought about a remarkable decrease in the mortality rate of premature and otherwise medically ill infants. It is suspected, moreover, that the survival of these infants may account to some degree for the apparent increase in the number of children with learning disabilities in the school-age years. Drillien, for example, suggests that more than 50% of the "small for gestational age" premature infants become learning-disabled, and that this cannot be explained on the basis of medical complications alone.[37] To help answer this question, Dr. Als developed a method known as the Assessment for Premature Infant Behavior (APIB).[39]

On the basis of her examination using this technique, she has found that it is possible for normal and premature infants to be clustered into identifiable categories that seem to have stability over time.[40] Taking advantage of this superior behavioral assessment method, we undertook some years ago a study of apparently normal infants living at home with their mother and without medical complications. Only half of the group scored very well on the APIB, while the other half did not score as well. These two "extreme" groups of normal infants were then contrasted by means of brain electrical activity mapping. The most prominent finding was that of a marked difference in the way in which delta activity changed when the infants moved from a drowsy to an alert state. In the higher functioning group, delta activity diminished as the degree of attentional demand increased. In contrast, the opposite change was observed in the less highly functioning group. Of interest is that this change of delta activity by SPM was largely limited to the frontal and central regions, especially on the left.[40] These data, on a small population, have led us to speculate that premature birth exerts a definite effect upon brain electrical activity, with the greatest impact being in the frontal lobes. Could this explain the higher incidence of attentional deficit disorder and reading disability in these poorer-functioning children? A study is presently in progress to evaluate this possibility.

BRAIN ELECTRICAL ACTIVITY MAPPING: ITS PROGRESS AND PROSPECTS

As can be seen, topographic mapping of brain electrical activity appears to be a clinically useful and powerful tool for the evaluation of a number of neurologic disorders. The dual characteristics of noninvasiveness and sensitivity to data that cannot be readily extracted by CT scan or conventional EEG analysis make topographic mapping a particularly powerful tool in clinical situations requiring repeated testing for longitudinal observations of degenerative or otherwise evolving disorders. We wish to stress, however, that the BEAM technique is not an exclusive diagnostic method capable of displacing the several other approaches to neurologic measurement. In our research on supratentorial brain tumors discussed earlier in this paper, diagnostic situations arose wherein the most powerful means of locating the offending lesions were different for different cases under differing clinical conditions. Depending upon the patient, the BEAM technique with SPM analysis, the CT scan, or the neuropsychological battery might be the preferred diagnostic strategy over the other two. It is our belief that in a number of instances topographic mapping of brain electrical activity has demonstrated a unique capability among this array of techniques, affording the clinician an improved diagnostic capability.

What then is the promise embodied in this new method of analyzing brain electrical activity? In addition to the extensions of the BEAM applications described here, we are beginning to look beyond the simple topographic map and have begun to trace the trajectories of electrical impulse through the brain. This approach, while simplifying the processes needed to collect and analyze data, has begun to expand our capabilities for the exploration of normal and pathologic brain function. By the simple expedient of relieving the electroencephalographer of the burdens of visual spectral analysis, temporal summation, and spatial topographic mapping, we are now in a position to rekindle the spark of enthusiasm that characterized those first developers of electroencephalography in the 1930s and perhaps to fulfill some of the promise then envisioned in understanding the intricate workings of the human brain.

REFERENCES

1. Berger, H. 1929. Uber das Elektrenkephalogram des Menshen. Arch. Psychiat. Nervenkr. **87:** 527–570.
2. Gibbs, F. A., E. L. Gibbs & W. G. Lennox. 1937. Epilepsy: A paroxysmal cerebral dysrhthmia. Brain **60:** 377.
3. Dawson, G. D. 1947. Cerebral responses to electrical stimulation of peripheral nerve in man. J. Neurol. Neurosurg. Psychiat. **10:** 134–140.
4. Yamada, T., J. Kimura, S. Young & M. Powers. 1978. Somatosensory evoked potentials elicited by bilateral stimulation of the median nerve and its clinical application. Neurology **28:** 218–223.
5. Stockard, J. E., J. J. Stockard, B. Westmoreland & J. Corfits. 1979. Brainstem auditory-evoked responses: Normal variation as a function of stimulus and subject characteristics. Arch. Neurol. **36:** 823–831.
6. Stockard, J. J., J. E. Stockard & F. W. Sharborough. 1978. Nonpathologic factors influencing brainstem auditory evoked potentials. Am. J. EEG. Technol. **18:** 177–209.
7. Tukey, J. W. 1977. Exploratory Data Analysis. Addison-Wesley.
8. Bechtereva, N. P., I. V. Vvedenskaia, Y. V. Dubikaitis, T. S. Stepanova, B. S. Ovnatov & V. V. Osov. 1963. Localization of focal brain lesions by electroencephalography. Electroencephalogr. Clin. Neurophysiol. **15:** 177–196.
9. Bickford, R. G. 1976. New trends in clinical electroencephalography. Practitioner **217:** 100–104.
10. Gotman, J., P. Gloor & W. F. Ray. 1975. A quantitative comparison of traditional reading of the EEG and interpretation of computer-extracted features in patients with supratentorial brain lesions. Electroencephalogr. Clin. Neurophysiol. **38:** 623–639.
11. Petsche, H. 1976. Topography of the EEG: survey and prospects. Clin. Neurol. Neurosurg. **79:** 15–28.
12. Vaughn, H. G., Jr. & W. Ritter. 1970. The sources of auditory evoked responses recorded from the human scalp. Electroencephalogr. Clin. Neurophysiol. **28:** 360–378.
13. Walter, W. G. & H. W. Shipton. 1951. A new toposcopic display system. Electroencephalogr. Clin. Neurophysiol. **3:** 281–292.
14. Giannitrapini, D. & L. Kayton. 1974. Schizophrenics and EEG spectral analysis. Electroencephalogr. Clin. Neurophysiol. **36:** 377–386.
15. Bartels, P. H. & J. Subach. Significance probability mapping and automated interpretation of complex pictorial scenes. *In* Proceedings of the U.S.–Japan Joint Technology Council Meeting on Image Processing, Pasadena, California, 1975.
16. Duffy, F. H., P. H. Bartels & J. L. Burchfiel. 1981. Significance probability mapping: An aid in the topographic analysis of brain electrical activity. Electroenceph. Clin. Neurophysiol. **51:** 455–462.
17. Portius, A. A. 1972. Neurological aspects in some types of delinquency, especially among juveniles. Adolescence **7:** 289–308.
18. Duffy, F. H., Denckla, M. B., Bartels, P. H. & G. Sandini. 1980. Dyslexia: Regional differences in brain electrical activity by topographic mapping. Ann. Neurol. **7:** 412–420.

19. DUFFY, F. H., M. B. DENCKLA, P. H. BARTELS, G. SANDINI & L. S. KIESSLING. 1980. Dyslexia: Automated diagnosis by computerized classification of brain electrical activity. Ann. Neurol. **7:** 421–428.

20. LARSEN, B., E. SKINHOJ, N. A. LASSEN. 1978. Variations in regional cortical blood flow in the right and left hemispheres during automatic speech. Brain **101:** 193–210.

21. LASSEN, N. A., D. H. INGVAR & E. SKINHOJ. 1978. Brain function and blood flow. Scientific American **239:** 62–71.

22. MASDEU, J. C., W. C. SCHOENE & H. FUNKENSTEIN. 1978. Aphasia following infarction of the left supplementary motor area: A clinicopathologic study. Neurology **28:** 1220–1223.

23. DUFFY, F. H., P. H. BARTELS & J. L. BURCHFIEL. 1981. Significance probability mapping: An aid in the topographic analysis of brain electrical activity. Electroencephalogr. Clin. Neurophysiol. **51:** 455–462.

24. LOMBROSO, C. T. & F. H. DUFFY. 1980. Brain electrical activity mapping as an adjunct to CT scanning. *In* Advances in Epileptology: XIth Epilepsy International Symposium. R. Canger, F. Angeleri & J. K. Perry, Eds.: 83–88. Raven Press. New York, NY.

25. LOMBROSO, C. T. & F. H. DUFFY, 1982. Brain electrical activity mapping in the epilepsies. *In* Advances in Epileptology: XIIIth Epilepsy International Symposium. H. Akimoto, H. Kazamatsuri, M. Seino & A. Ward, Eds.: 173–179. Raven Press. New York, NY.

26. MORIHISA, J. M., F. H. DUFFY & R. J. WYATT. 1983. Brain electrical activity mapping (BEAM) in schizophrenic patients. Arch. Gen. Psychiat. **40:** 719–728.

27. GRANNTRAPINI, D. & L. KAYTON. 1974. Schizophrenic and EEG spectral analysis. Electroencephalogr. Clin. Neurophysiol. **36:** 377–386.

28. INGVAR, D. H. 1980. Abnormal distribution of cerebral activity in chronic schizophrenia: A neurophysiological interpretation. *In* Perspectives In Schizophrenia Research. C. Baxter & T. Melnechuk, Eds. Raven Press. New York, NY.

29. MORSTYN, R., F. H. DUFFY & R. W. MCCARLEY. 1983. Altered P300 topography in schizophrenia. Arch. Gen. Psychiat. **40:** 729–734.

30. GOODIN, D. S., K. S. SQUIRES, B. H. HENDERSON, *et al.* 1978. Age-related variations in evoked potentials to auditory stimuli in normal human subjects. Electroencephalogr. Clin. Neurophysiol. **44:** 447–458.

31. KAUFMAN, L. & S. J. WILLIAMSON. 1982. Magnetic location of cortical activity. Ann. N.Y. Acad. Sci. **388:** 197–213.

32. SHERWIN, I., P. PERNON-MAGNAN, J. BANCAUD, *et al.* 1982. Prevalence of psychoses in epilepsy as a function of the laterality of the epileptogenic lesion. Arch. Neurol. **39:** 621–625.

33. DUFFY, F. H., M. S. ALBERT, G. B. MCANULTY & A. J. GARVEY. Age-related differences in brain electrical activity of healthy subjects. Ann. Neurol. In press.

34. CONSTANTINIDIS, J., M. KRASSOIEVITCH & R. TISSOT. 1969. Correlations entre les perturbations electroencephalographiques et les lesions anatomo-histologiques dans les demence. Encephale **58:** 19–52.

35. GORDON, E. G. & M. SIM. 1967. The EEG in presenile dementia. J. Neurol. Neurosurg. Psychiat. **30:** 285.

36. KATZ, R. & G. R. HOROWITZ. 1982. Electroencephalogram in the septuagenerian: Studies in a normal geriatric population. J. Am. Geriat. Soc. **3:** 273–275.

37. DRILLIEN, C. M., A. J. M. THOMPSON & K. BARGOYNE. 1980. Low birthweight children at early schoolage: A longitudinal study. Dev. Med. Child Neurol. **22:** 26–47.

38. ALS, H. 1982. Towards a synactive theory of development: Promise for the assessment of infant individuality. Infant Mental Health J. **3:** 229–243.

39. ALS, H. 1985. Patterns of infant behavior: Analogs of later organizational difficulties? *In* Dyslexia: A Neuroscientific Approach to Clinical Evaluation. F. H. Duffy & N. Geschwind, Eds. Little, Brown. Boston, MA.

40. DUFFY, F. H. & H. ALS. 1983. Neurophysiological assessment of the neonate; an approach combining brain electrical activity mapping (BEAM) with behavioral assessment (APIB). *In* New Approaches to Development Screening of Infants. T. B. Brazelton & B. M. Lester, Eds. Elsevier-North Holland. New York, NY.

Neurobiological Studies of Transmitter Systems in Aging and in Alzheimer-Type Dementia[a]

DONALD L. PRICE,[b,c,d,e] CHERYL A. KITT,[c]
ROBERT G. STRUBLE,[c] PETER J. WHITEHOUSE,[d,e]
LINDA C. CORK,[c] AND LARY C. WALKER[c]

Departments of [c]Pathology, [d]Neurology, and [e]Neuroscience
Neuropathology Laboratory
The Johns Hopkins University School of Medicine
Baltimore, Maryland 21205

INTRODUCTION

The adult-onset degenerative disorders of the nervous system, particularly those involving cognition, memory, and behavior, cause great human suffering and impose enormous financial burdens on society.[61] Among the most common of these disorders are Alzheimer's disease (AD) and Parkinson's disease (PD). For many years, these disorders were considered hopeless: the cellular pathology was not well understood; animal models were not available; and treatments were ineffective. In recent years, this situation has changed significantly, and this area is now one of the most active fields of research in clinical neuroscience. New information is available about the involvement of neurons in specific regions of brain, the character of the pathology (particularly as regards neurofibrillary tangles and senile plaques), and relationships of these pathologic processes to alterations in transmitter-specific markers. After a very brief discussion of the clinical syndrome of Alzheimer-type dementia and of the value and future prospects of diagnostic studies, the present review describes some of the recent advances in this area, focusing on: the nature and distribution of structural and chemical pathologies (especially those involving specific neuronal systems); the development of nonhuman primate models of aging and disease; and prospects for using these models to design and test new therapeutic approaches.

[a] This work was supported by grants from the U.S. Public Health Service (NIH NS 10580, AG 03359, NS 15721, NS 20471, and NS 07179) and The Johns Hopkins University School of Medicine, as well as fellowships from the Commonwealth Fund, the McKnight Foundation, and the Alfred P. Sloan Foundation, and a gift from Point of View, Inc. Dr. Cork is the recipient of a Research Career Development Award (NIH NS 00488).

[b] Address for correspondence: Donald L. Price, M.D., Neuropathology Laboratory, 509 Pathology Building, The Johns Hopkins University School of Medicine, 600 North Wolfe Street, Baltimore, Maryland 21205.

CLINICAL MANIFESTATIONS AND LABORATORY EVALUATIONS

Patients with Alzheimer's disease usually present with loss of memory, although many also show disorders of language, praxis, and visual perception. This progressive dementia can begin in midlife, but is most common after the age of 65. Cognitive disorders also occur in 30–50% of patients with Parkinson's disease, especially in older individuals with more rapidly evolving motor symptoms which are unresponsive to L-dopa.[13,69,72] At present, there are no premortem laboratory tests specific for Alzheimer's disease. However, in some patients, computerized tomographic scans demonstrate progressive reductions in brain volume (atrophy) in excess of that occurring in normal aging.[45] Imaging methods, like positron emission tomography (PET), can determine cerebral blood flow and cerebral metabolism: patients with AD have reduced metabolic rates, particularly in parietal/temporal regions, and secondary changes in regional cerebral blood flow.[41,42,57] Activities of neurotransmitter systems can be demonstrated by PET in living humans, e.g., dopamine and its receptors can be visualized using [^{18}F] 6-fluoro-L-dopa[47] and [^{3}N]-[^{11}C] methyl spiperone,[130] respectively. Using labeled markers, these approaches should be helpful in investigating a variety of degenerative disorders, including Alzheimer's and Parkinson's disease.

STRUCTURAL AND CHEMICAL CHANGES IN AGING AND IN ALZHEIMER-TYPE DEMENTIA

Neurofibrillary Tangles

Demonstrated by silver impregnation methods, neurofibrillary tangles are filamentous inclusions in neurons, particularly in the hippocampus,[9] neocortex,[124] substantia innominata,[55] amygdala,[59] and several brainstem nuclei, including the raphe nuclei and locus coeruleus.[55,124] Tangles occur in small numbers in aged humans and may be conspicuous in a variety of disorders not directly related to Alzheimer's disease.[139] Neurofibrillary tangles are made up of highly insoluble crosslinked peptides[113] arranged as 10-nm-diameter paired helical filaments with crossover points every 80 nm.[64,138] The presence of dementia in AD appears to correlate with the number of tangles in cortex,[135,136] suggesting that this cytoskeletal pathology may be associated with changes in the dynamic properties of neurons whose dysfunction and death are important in the clinical expression of disease.

Senile Plaques

Senile plaques are composed of abnormal axons/nerve terminals (neurites),[64,137] abnormal dendritic processes,[101] and extracellular deposits of polypeptide fibrils in a β-pleated sheet configuration (amyloid). Abnormal axons are enlarged, filled with filaments and membranous material, and frequently show secondary changes in the myelin sheath. Although senile plaques occur in small numbers in aged monkeys and humans, in AD they are usually abundant, particularly in the amygdala, hippocampus, and neocortex.[59,126] Correlative studies, although recently challenged,[135] suggest that cortical plaque densities are the most useful postmortem predictors of the presence of dementia.[94,125,126] Some, although not all, demented patients with PD also show cortical plaques.[12,13,50]

Changes in Neurotransmitter Markers

Despite some inconsistencies, evidence to date indicates that, in the normal aged human brain, mild alterations may occur in several neurotransmitter systems, including catecholaminergic, cholinergic, and gamma-aminobutyric acid (GABA)ergic systems.[10,15,63,73] In AD, abnormalities occur in somatostatinergic, catecholaminergic, and cholinergic systems[1,11,15,23,24,27,28,85,94,95,103,104,114] with less-certain evidence for degeneration of serotonergic, GABAergic, and aspartate/glutamate systems.[7,16,105] Demented individuals with PD also show chemical changes, including abnormalities of cholinergic, noradrenergic, dopaminergic, and somatostatinergic markers.[22,36,107]

RELATIONSHIPS OF STRUCTURAL AND CHEMICAL CHANGES IN TRANSMITTER-SPECIFIC SYSTEMS

Recent studies of aging, AD, and PD have focused on morphologic and neurochemical changes in specific neuronal populations, particularly those in cholinergic, catecholaminergic, and somatostatinergic systems. In this review, we first outline the normal anatomy of these systems, particularly in primates, and then discuss changes occurring in aging, Alzheimer's disease, and Parkinson's diseases.

Basal Forebrain and Brainstem Cholinergic Systems

Normal Brain

The basal forebrain cholinergic system in primates, recently termed the Ch1–4 system,[76] includes cholinergic neurons in the medial septum (Ch1), nucleus of the diagonal band of Broca (Ch2–3), and nucleus basalis of Meynert (nbM) (Ch4). These regions have high levels of ChAT activity[74] and contain moderately large bipolar and multipolar neurons[53] which synthesize acetylcholinesterase (AChE) and choline acetyltransferase (ChAT).[52,76] Ch1 and Ch2 neurons project via the fimbria/fornix predominantly to the hippocampus; Ch4 neurons project via a ventral pathway to the amygdala, by a medial pathway (septum and cingulum) to medial neocortex, and via a lateral pathway (beneath and lateral to the putamen) to dorsolateral neocortex.[65] Projections of different cell groups in Ch4 show a topographic organization.[76,90] AChE histochemistry and ChAT immunocytochemistry reveal regional heterogeneities of axons and terminals in the amygdala, hippocampus, and neocortex. For example, in the amygdala, the density of AChE- and ChAT-containing axons and terminals and muscarinic cholinergic receptors is greatest in the basolateral amygdala, a region known (on the basis of anterograde transport studies) to receive projections from Ch4 cells.[62,65] Regional variations occur in ChAT activity: precentral and temporal regions have high activities; prefrontal and parietal regions have intermediate values; and occipital cortex has the lowest activity.[68] In rodents, some neocortical cholinergic activity is due to intrinsic neurons,[56] but it is not yet clear whether such cells exist in primates. That Ch4 makes a major contribution to cholinergic innervation of primate neocortex is shown by unilateral ibotenic acid lesions in the nbM, which result in almost 70% reductions in ChAT activity ipsilateral to the lesion.[118] Although functions of the Ch1–4 system are not yet well understood, physiological investigations suggest that these nerve cells have distinct firing properties[31] and may be important in cortical activation.

In the brainstem, two groups of nonmotor cholinergic neurons have been identified: some are located in the pedunculopontine tegmental nucleus, while others are present in the lateral dorsal tegmental nucleus.[77] These cell groups project to the substantia nigra, subthalamic nucleus, thalamus, globus pallidus, neostriatum,[109] and, to a minor degree, to neocortex.[83]

Aging, Alzheimer's Disease, and Parkinson's Disease

Although there is evidence in nonhuman primates that the cholinergic system participates in plaque formation, to date there is no convincing evidence for major reductions in the number of Ch1–4 neurons in cognitively intact aged individuals. In AD and in some cases of PD, neurons in this system degenerate; changes are less severe in older individuals.[8,22,84,121,131–134] In older individuals with AD, ChAT activity appears to be more extensively reduced than might be predicted on the basis of reductions in numbers of nbM neurons[97]; in at least one AD case (with a relatively short clinical course), the size, but not the number, of neurons in the nbM was reduced.[92] We have suggested that dysfunction of Ch1–4 neurons may underlie the reductions in cholinergic markers that occur in AD and in demented patients with PD.[99,100] Consistent with the concept that dysfunction and eventual death of these cholinergic neurons are significant factors in the production of cholinergic deficits in the brains of individuals with AD is the observation that some neurites in senile plaques contain AChE activity,[44,96,116] a marker of axons from the Ch1–4 complex. Experimental tests of this hypothesis are described below.

Brainstem cholinergic neurons have not been critically examined in aging or disease. In some cases of AD, ChAT activity may be decreased in the basal ganglia, thalamus, and brainstem.[26,104] Perhaps reductions in ChAT activity in these regions are secondary to loss of afferents from brainstem cholinergic systems.

Catecholaminergic Systems

Normal Brain

Catecholaminergic projections to primate neocortex are primarily derived from noradrenergic neurons in the locus coeruleus and dopaminergic neurons in the ventral tegmental area.[38,70,78–81] Neurons of the locus coeruleus, located in the dorsolateral pontine tegmentum, show monoamine fluorescence and contain AChE, tyrosine hydroxylase (TH), and dopamine β-hydroxylase.[5,70,91] Within cortex, noradrenergic innervation varies from region to region and from lamina to lamina.[17,78,80,81] Dopaminergic neurons of the ventral tegmental area and substantia nigra, which synthesize TH and AChE but not dopamine β-hydroxylase,[67,91,110] innervate striatum and neocortex.[17,70,79]

Aging, Alzheimer's Disease, and Parkinson's Disease

In aged nonhuman primates, dopamine and norepinephrine are decreased in neocortex,[49] and structural changes occur in TH-immunoreactive cortical axons (see below). Disagreements exist regarding changes in catecholaminergic markers in various regions of brains of aged humans.[63,73] In several species, numbers of neurons within the locus coeruleus and substantia nigra appear to decline with age[73,129]

Some patients with AD show changes in noradrenergic, but not in dopaminergic, systems. Reductions occur in the number of neurons in the locus coeruleus, in concentrations of norepinephrine, and in the activity of dopamine β-hydroxylase.[2,14,22,24,39,58,95,127] Individuals with PD have dopaminergic deficiencies due to changes in neurons in the substantia nigra[6,40]; these patients also show abnormalities in nonnigral catecholaminergic pathways,[60] including reductions in neurons in the ventral tegmental area[128] and locus coeruleus.[40] Some of these PD patients are demented,[69,72] and some show neocortical plaques[13,50]; it is not known how these clinical and pathologic changes relate to catecholaminergic systems.

Somatostatinergic Systems

Normal Brain

Somatostatin, a tetradecapeptide neurotransmitter, is synthesized by neurons in many parts of the forebrain, including striatum, amygdala, hippocampus, and neocortex.[35,37,81,89] In cortex, some multipolar and modified pyramidal cells synthesize this peptide. Receptors for somatostatin-14 and somatostatin-28 have been identified by [^{125}I] radioligand binding; highest binding is present in hypothalamus, striatum, amygdala, and neocortex.[102,122] Microiontophoretically applied somatostatin causes a dose-dependent direct increase in firing rates in a large percentage of pyramidal neurons in neocortex.[87] Little is known about functional roles of somatostatin in the forebrain.

Aging and Disease

Somatostatinergic neurons may be altered in aged individuals, and these nerve cells certainly are severely affected in some cases of Alzheimer's and Parkinson's disease.[27,85,103,106,111] Counts of immunostained neurons have not been reported, but somatostatin concentrations show significant negative associations with plaque counts[106] and with estimates of neurofibrillary tangles in temporal cortex.[106] Since somatostatin is reduced in regions that contain intrinsic somatostatinergic neurons and also show plaques,[59] we have suggested that somatostatinergic axons and terminals could be potential sources for some of the neurites in senile plaques (see below for test of this hypothesis).

Other Neuronal Systems Affected in Aging, Alzheimer's Disease, and Parkinson's Disease

In elderly humans, the number of neurons is reduced in neocortex,[63,82,123] hippocampus,[9] putamen,[19] substantia nigra,[73] and locus coeruleus.[129] In AD, neurons (whose transmitter specificity is uncertain) are decreased in the amygdala, hippocampus, and neocortex.[99,54,82,123] Some affected neurons may be somatostatinergic (see above), while others may use glutamate or aspartate as neurotransmitters.[7,16]

NONHUMAN PRIMATE MODELS OF AGING, CORTICAL CHOLINERGIC DEFICIENCY, AND NIGROSTRIATAL DOPAMINERGIC DEFICIENCY

Primate models can be extraordinarily useful for studies designed to clarify the effects of aging on the brain and for investigations of behavioral, structural, and chemical pathologies occurring secondary to transmitter system abnormalities, particularly involving Ch1–4/cortical cholinergic and nigrostriatal dopaminergic systems.

Aged Nonhuman Primates

Aged macaques develop a variety of mild cognitive deficits, including reductions in short-term memory, which resemble features seen in elderly humans.[10,29,98] Although there is variation between individuals, macaques commonly develop senile plaques between 16 and 22 years of age.[115,119,120] Senile plaques are not randomly distributed but have predilections for certain areas, particularly prefrontal and temporal cortices. Plaques can be classified according to their relative proportions of neurites and amyloid. Initially, we used the plaque classifications of "immature, mature, and end-stage"[115,137]; however, more recently, we have adopted terms which do not imply a vector of evolution: "neurite" plaques have many neurites and little amyloid; "mixed" plaques contain neurites and amyloid; and "amyloid" plaques have abundant amyloid and relatively few neurites. At the end of the second decade of life, macaques show a predominance of neurite and mixed plaques. During the third decade, plaque numbers and regional densities increase, achieving values similar to those reported in nondemented aged humans[125]; in these old animals, the percentage of amyloid plaques is increased.[117]

Our histochemical and immunocytochemical studies have begun to clarify the evolution and transmitter specificities of these processes. In normal macaques, AChE-stained intracortical axons appear as slender linear profiles which show occasional branches.[51] In aged animals, several abnormalities in AChE-rich axons have been detected,[119] including increased tortuosity, multifocal enlargements, and clusters of neurites (neurite plaques). Some of these clusters are associated with amyloid deposits (mixed plaques). In the oldest animals, some amyloid cores are associated with weak AChE staining (amyloid plaques). With ChAT immunocytochemistry, we have demonstrated irregular swellings of intracortical axons and clusters of ChAT-immunoreactive neurites in proximity to amyloid. The presence of amyloid-associated, ChAT-immunoreactive processes which are the size and shape of silver-stained neurites in plaques indicates that cholinergic processes are present in some neocortical plaques. Many of these cholinergic neurites are presumably derived from neurons in Ch4.

However, since AChE is also synthesized by dopaminergic neurons of the ventral tegmental area, noradrenergic neurons of the locus coeruleus, and somatostatinergic and GABAergic neocortical neurons,[5,21,30,75] some AChE-stained neurites may be derived from noncholinergic systems.[100] Methods to visualize TH and somatostatin immunoreactivities disclosed both normal and abnormal axons in the amygdala and neocortex of old monkeys. Some axons had multiple enlarged varicosities, while others appeared to end in enlarged single swellings or clusters of distended neurites, some of which were in proximity to amyloid.

These studies demonstrate the usefulness of the aged nonhuman primate model for assessing abnormalities occurring in brain as a consequence of aging; similar processes may occur in the brains of individuals with AD and related forms of dementia.

Primates with Neocortical Cholinergic Deficiencies

In humans, changes in Ch1–4 neurons are associated with memory inpairment and with reduced cholinergic markers in amygdala, hippocampus, and neocortex. To test the hypothesis that cholinergic deficiencies may be related to impaired memory, monkeys with bilateral partial Ch4 lesions were examined in a visual recognition memory task.[3] The experimental group showed no significant impairment unless challenged by administration of scopolamine, a muscarinic receptor blocker, which lowered test scores in the experimental group. Reconstruction of lesions disclosed topographic relationships between reductions in the number of nerve cells in the nbM and reductions in neocortical ChAT activity. With more extensive lesions, animals show overt impairment on these tasks.[4] These results tentatively suggest that cholinergic systems projecting to amygdala, hippocampus, and neocortex play a role in memory processing. Similar studies could be done in animals in whom catecholaminergic or somatostatinergic systems are damaged by 6-hydroxydopamine or cystamine, respectively.[18,88,108]

Primates with Nigrostriatal Dopamine Deficiency

Individuals who are exposed to the meperidine analogue, 1-methyl-4-phenyl-1,2,3,6-tetrahydropyridine (MPTP), develop rigidity, akinesia, flexed posture, and tremor, which are responsive to dopamine agonists.[66] Although the neurochemical correlates of this syndrome are now fairly well established,[20] structural changes occurring in the brain are not well understood. To clarify these processes, we have begun (with Drs. Eduardo Eidelberg and Tong Joh) to examine MPTP-treated monkeys using immunocytochemical methods. Our studies in MPTP-treated macaques show decreased numbers of TH-immunoreactive neurons in substantia nigra and TH-immunoreactive axons in the striatum.[140]

Since MPTP rapidly and selectively damages neurons in the substantia nigra pars compacta with a concomitant loss of TH immunoreactivity in the striatum, the model should be useful for studies of dopaminergic deficiency. PET scans of the distribution of L-dopa or spiperone binding or of glucose metabolism could be used to study the evolution of changes in specific regions or systems, allowing correlations of metabolic activity, transmitter levels, and receptors with behavior and with analysis of structural/functional changes seen at autopsy. Moreover, the model can be exploited to delineate the consequences of different therapeutic strategies, including the usefulness of new pharmacotherapies and of transplanting embryonic nigral neurons into dopamine-denervated primate striatum.

NEW THERAPEUTIC APPROACHES

Although L-dopa is an effective therapy for some of the motor abnormalities occurring in PD, there are, to date, no methods of treatment for the cognitive memory deficits of Parkinson's or Alzheimer's disease. Using animal models, we can begin to test pharmacologic agents and to examine the efficacy of experimental biological strategies, including the use of neural grafts and trophic factors. Because biological therapies have already shown some promise in rodent models and because of their relevance to some of the issues described above, the potential applicability of treatments with neural grafts and trophic factors is briefly described below.

Neural Grafts

Aged Animals

Aged rats show motor deficits and impairments in memory and learning which have, in part, been attributed to changes in dopaminergic and cholinergic systems.[10,46] In aged rats, nigral or Ch1–2 neuronal grafts can be successfully implanted to innervate targets in the neostriatum or hippocampus, respectively. Nigral grafts appear to improve balance and coordination in some rats.[46]

Animals with Dopaminergic Deficiency

Lesions of the rodent nigrostriatal dopaminergic pathway (produced by unilateral injection of 6-hydroxydopamine) cause asymmetric motor abnormalities (turning away from the lesion after apomorphine administration).[93] When embryonic nigral neurons are grafted into denervated striatum, spiroperidol binding is normalized[43] and motor asymmetries are reversed.[32,93] Monkeys with MPTP-induced nigrostriatal lesions could prove a useful model for testing the efficacy of embryonic nigral cell implants in primates with dopaminergic denervation of striatum. Treatment could be monitored clinically and, in large primates, by PET imaging of dopamine and its receptors.

Animals with Forebrain Cholinergic Deficiencies

Cholinergic denervation syndromes may also respond to neural grafts. Rats with lesions of the fornix or of the Ch1–4 system show impairment in some behavioral tasks. In "lesioned" animals, embryonic septal grafts successfully reinnervate the hippocampus, and animals with grafts show some improvement in behavioral performance.[33,71]

Trophic Factors

These factors may be necessary to maintain normal function in a variety of neuronal systems in the brain.[25,34,48,86] Most of these trophic factors have not been well characterized, with the exception of nerve growth factor. After injection of [^{125}I]-labeled nerve growth factor into the hippocampus, label appears in neurons of the medial septum and diagonal band of Broca[112]; after nerve growth factor is injected into the ventricles of neonatal rats, ChAT activity is increased in the septum, hippocampus, and neocortex.[48] Similar studies in nonhuman primates would be of interest and might have implications for understanding pathogenetic mechanisms in human degenerative disorders.

SUMMARY

Dysfunction and death of specific neuronal systems are important processes occurring in aging and in Alzheimer's and in Parkinson's disease. The neuropathology and neurochemistry of some of the neuronal systems at risk in these settings are subjects of active research; the nature and consequences of these cellular pathologies have begun to be clarified. The availability of animal models (including aged monkeys, macaques with cholinergic deficiencies, and monkeys with MPTP-induced nigrostriatal pathology, all of which recapitulate certain features of human aging or disease) allow the opportunity to assess the efficacies of new pharmacotherapies, neural grafts, and trophic factors. These approaches can be monitored by behavioral testing and, in some instances, by *in vivo* imaging methods, which can in turn be correlated with morphologic and chemical analyses of brain. Demonstration of the efficacy of these procedures in nonhuman primates would have profound implications on the development of new therapies designed to alleviate the effects of aging and disease on the human brain.

ACKNOWLEDGMENTS

We acknowledge helpful discussions with Drs. Mahlon R. DeLong, Susan J. Mitchell, William C. Mobley, J. Lynn Rutkowski, George R. Uhl, Richard M. Zweig, Manuel F. Casanova, Joseph T. Coyle, John Lehmann, Piero G. Antuono, Gary L. Wenk, Thomas Aigner, Mortimer Mishkin, Eduardo Eidelberg, and Michael V. Johnston. Drs. Bruce H. Wainer, Allan I. Levey, Paul M. Salvaterra, and Garrett D. Crawford provided antiChAT antibodies and Dr. Tong H. Joh provided antiTH antibody for some of the cited studies. Mrs. Carla Jordon and Ms. Nancy Cook provided skilled assistance in the preparation of the manuscript. Mr. Mark Becher and Mr. Richard Altschuler provided excellent technical assistance.

REFERENCES

1. ADOLFSSON, R., C. G. GOTTFRIES, L. ORELAND, B. E. ROOS & B. WINBLAD. 1978. Reduced levels of catecholamines in the brain and increased activity of monoamine oxidase in platelets in Alzheimer's disease: Therapeutic implications. *In* Alzheimer's Disease: Senile Dementia and Related Disorders (Aging). R. Katzman, R. D. Terry & K. L. Bick, Eds., Vol. **7:** 441–451. Raven Press. New York, NY.
2. ADOLFSSON, R., C. G. GOTTFRIES, B. E. ROOS & B. WINBLAD. 1979. Changes in the brain catecholamines in patients with dementia of Alzheimer type. Br. J. Psychiatry **135:** 216–223.
3. AIGNER, T., J. AGGLETON, S. J. MITCHELL, D. PRICE, M. DELONG & M. MISHKIN. 1983. Effects of scopolamine on recognition memory in monkeys after ibotenic acid injections into the nucleus basalis of Meynert. Soc. Neurosci. Abstr. **9:** 826.
4. AIGNER, T., S. MITCHELL, J. AGGLETON, M. DELONG, R. STRUBLE, G. WENK, D. PRICE & M. MISHKIN. 1984. Recognition deficit in monkeys following neurotoxic lesions of the basal forebrain. Soc. Neurosci. Abstr. **10:** 386.
5. ALBANESE, A. & L. L. BUTCHER. 1979. Locus ceruleus somata contain both acetylcholinesterase and norepinephrine: Direct histochemical demonstration on the same tissue section. Neurosci. Lett. **14:** 101–104.
6. ALVORD, E. C., JR., L. S. FORNO, J. A. KUSSKE, R. J. KAUFFMAN, J. S. RHODES & C. R. GOETOWSKI. 1974. The pathology of parkinsonism: A comparison of degenerations in cerebral cortex and brainstem. *In* Second Canadian-American Conference on

Parkinson's Disease: Advances in Neurology. F. H. McDowell & A. Barbeau, Eds. Vol. **5:** 175–193, Raven Press. New York, NY.

7. Antuono, P. G., J. Lehmann, K. J. Koller, P. J. Whitehouse, A. W. Clark, R. G. Struble, D. L. Price & J. T. Coyle. 1984. Endogenous neurotransmitter amino acids (ENAA) in Alzheimer's disease (AD). Neurology (Suppl. 1) **34:** 119.
8. Arendt, T., V. Bigl, A. Arendt & A. Tennstedt. 1983. Loss of neurons in the nucleus basalis of Meynert in Alzheimer's disease, paralysis agitans, and Korsakoff's disease. Acta Neuropathol. (Berlin) **61:** 101–108.
9. Ball, M. J. 1977. Neuronal loss, neurofibrillary tangles and granulovacuolar degeneration in the hippocampus with ageing and dementia. A qualitative study. Acta Neuropathol. (Berlin) **37:** 111–118.
10. Bartus, R. T., R. L. Dean, III, B. Beer & A. S. Lippa. 1982. The cholinergic hypothesis of geriatric memory dysfunction. Science **217:** 408–417.
11. Bird, T. D., S. Stranahan, S. M. Sumi & M. Raskind. 1983. Alzheimer's disease: Choline acetyltransferase activity in brain tissue from clinical and pathological subgroups. Ann. Neurol. **14:** 284–293.
12. Bloxham, C. A., E. K. Perry, R. H. Perry & J. M. Candy. 1984. Neuropathological and neurochemical correlates of Alzheimer-type and parkinsonian dementia. *In* Alzheimer's Disease: Advances in Basic Research and Therapies. Proceedings of the Third Meeting of the International Study Group on the Treatment of Memory Disorders Associated with Aging. R. J. Wurtman, S. H. Corkin & J. H. Growdon, Eds.: 39–52. Zurich.
13. Boller, F., T. Mizutani, U. Roessmann, & P. Gambetti. 1980. Parkinson disease, dementia, and Alzheimer disease: Clinicopathological correlations. Ann. Neurol. **7:** 329–335.
14. Bondareff, W., C. Q. Mountjoy & M. Roth. 1982. Loss of neurons or origin of the adrenergic projection to cerebral cortex (nucleus locus ceruleus) in senile dementia. Neurology **32:** 164–168.
15. Bowen, D. M., C. B. Smith, P. White & A. N. Davison. 1976. Neurotransmitter-related enzymes and indices of hypoxia in senile dementia and other abiotrophies. Brain **99:** 459–496.
16. Bowen, D. M. 1983. Biochemical assessment of neurotransmitter and metabolic dysfunction and cerebral atrophy in Alzheimer's disease. Biological aspects of Alzheimer's disease. Banbury Rep. **15:** 219–231.
17. Brown, R. M., A. M. Crane & P. S. Goldman. 1979. Regional distribution of monoamines in the cerebral cortex and subcortical structures of the rhesus monkey: Concentrations and in vivo synthesis rates. Brain Res. **168:** 133–150.
18. Brozoski, T. J., R. M. Brown, H. E. Rosvold & P. S. Goldman. 1979. Cognitive deficit caused by regional depletion of dopamine in prefrontal cortex of rhesus monkey. Science **205:** 929–932.
19. Bugiani, O., S. Salvarani, F. Perdelli, G. L. Mancardi & A. Leonardi. 1978. Nerve cell loss with aging in the putamen. Eur. Neurol. **17:** 286–291.
20. Burns, R. S., C. C. Chiueh, S. P. Markey, M. H. Ebert, D. M. Jacobowitz & I. J. Kopin. 1983. A primate model of parkinsonism: Selective destruction of dopaminergic neurons in the pars compacta of the substantia nigra by *N*-methyl-4-phenyl-1,2,3,6-tetrahydropyridine. Proc. Natl. Acad. Sci. USA **80:** 4546–4550.
21. Butcher, L. L. & R. Marchand. 1978. Dopamine neurons in pars compacta of the substantia nigra contain acetylcholinesterase: Histochemical correlations of the same brain section. Eur. J. Pharmacol. **52:** 415–417.
22. Candy, J. M., R. H. Perry, E. K. Perry, D. Irving, G. Blessed, A. F. Fairbairn & B. E. Tomlinson. 1983. Pathological changes in the nucleus of Meynert in Alzheimer's and Parkinson's diseases. J. Neurol. Sci. **59:** 277–289.
23. Coyle, J. T., D. L. Price & M. R. DeLong. 1983. Alzheimer's disease: A disorder of cortical cholinergic innervation. Science **219:** 1184–1190.
24. Cross, A. J., T. J. Crow, E. K. Perry, R. H. Perry, G. Blessed & B. E. Tomlinson. 1981. Reduced dopamine-β-hydroxylase activity in Alzheimer's disease. Br. Med. J. **282:** 93–94.

25. CRUTCHER, K. A. & J. N. DAVIS. 1981. Sympathohippocampal sprouting is directed by a target tropic factor. Brain Res. **204:** 410–414.
26. DAVIES, P. 1979. Neurotransmitter-related enzymes in senile dementia of the Alzheimer type. Brain Res. **171:** 319–327.
27. DAVIES, P. & A. J. F. MALONEY. 1976. Selective loss of central cholinergic neurons in Alzheimer's disease. Lancet **2:** 1403.
28. DAVIES, P., R. KATZMAN & R. D. TERRY. 1980. Reduced somatostatin-like immunoreactivity in cerebral cortex from cases of Alzheimer disease and Alzheimer senile dementia. Nature **288:** 279–280.
29. DAVIS, R. T. 1978. Old monkey behavior. Exp. Gerontol. **13:** 237–250.
30. DELFS, J. R., C-H. ZHU & M. A. DICHTER. 1983. Coexistence of acetylcholinesterase and somatostatin-immunoreactivity in neurons cultured from rat cerebrum. Science **223:** 61–63.
31. DELONG, M. R. 1971. Activity of pallidal neurons during movement. J. Neurophysiol. **34:** 414–427.
32. DUNNETT, S. B., A. BJORKLUND, R. H. SCHMIDT, U. STENEVI & S. D. IVERSEN. 1983. Intracerebral grafting of neuronal cell suspensions. IV. Behavioural recovery in rats with unilateral 6-OHDA lesions following implantation of nigral cell suspensions in different forebrain sites. Acta Physiol. Scand. Suppl. **522:** 29–37.
33. DUNNETT, S. B., W. C. LOW, S. D. IVERSEN, U. STENEVI & A. BJORKLUND. 1982. Septal transplants restore maze learning in rats with fornix-fimbria lesions. Brain Res. **251:** 335–348.
34. EDGAR, D. & Y-A. BARDE. 1983. Neuronal growth factors. Trends Neurosci. **6:** 260–262.
35. EMSON, P. C., M. ROSSOR & C. M. LEE 1981. The regional distribution of chromatographic behavior of somatostatin in human brain. Neurosci. Lett. **22:** 319–324.
36. EPELBAUM, J., M. RUBERG, E. MOYSE, F. JAVOY-AGID, B. DUBOIS & Y. AGID. 1983. Somatostatin and dementia in Parkinson's disease. Brain Res. **278:** 376–379.
37. FINLEY, J. C. W., G. H. GROSSMAN, P. DIMEO & P. PETRUSZ. 1978. Somatostatin-containing neurons in the rat brain: Widespread distribution revealed by immunocytochemistry after pretreatment with pronase. Am. J. Anat. **153:** 483–488.
38. FOOTE, S. L., F. E. BLOOM & G. ASTON-JONES. 1983. Nucleus locus ceruleus: New evidence of anatomical and physiological specificity. Physiol. Rev. **63:** 844–914.
39. FORNO, L. S. 1978. The locus coeruleus in Alzheimer's disease. J. Neuropathol. Exp. Neurol. **37:** 614.
40. FORNO, L. S. & E. C. ALVORD, JR. 1971. The pathology of parkinsonism. Part I. Some new observations and correlations. *In* Recent Advances in Parkinson's Disease. F. H. McDowell & C. H. Markham, Eds.: 120–130. F. A. Davis. Philadelphia, PA.
41. FOSTER, N. L., T. N. CHASE, P. FEDIO, N. J. PATRONAS, R. A. BROOKS & G. DICHIRO. 1983. Alzheimer's disease: Focal cortical changes shown by positron emission tomography. Neurology **33:** 961–965.
42. FRACKOWIAK, R. S. J. & J. M. GIBBS. 1983. The pathophysiology of Alzheimer's disease studied with positron emission tomography. Biological aspects of Alzheimer's disease. Banbury Rep. **15:** 317–327.
43. FREED, W. J., G. N. KO, D. L. NIEHOFF, M. J. KUHAR, B. J. HOFFER, L. OLSON, H. E. CANNON-SPOOR, J. M. MORIHISA & R. J. WYATT. 1983. Normalization of spiroperidol binding in the denervated rat striatum by homologous grafts of substantia nigra. Science **222:** 937–939.
44. FRIEDE, R. L. 1965. Enzyme histochemical studies of senile plaques. J. Neuropathol. Exp. Neurol. **24:** 477–491.
45. GADO, M., C. P. HUGHES, W. DANZIGER & D. CHI. 1983. Aging, dementia, and brain atrophy: A longitudinal computed tomographic study. Am. J. Neuroradiol. **4:** 699–702.
46. GAGE, F. H., S. B. DUNNETT, U. STENEVI & A. BJORKLUND. 1983. Aged rats: Recovery of motor impairments by intrastriatal nigral grafts. Science **221:** 966–969.
47. GARNETT, E. S., G. FIRNAU & C. NAHMIAS. 1983. Dopamine visualized in the basal ganglia of living man. Nature **305:** 137–138.
48. GNAHN, H., F. HEFTI, R. HEUMANN, M. E. SCHWAB & H. THOENEN. 1983. NGF-mediated

increase of choline acetyltransferase (ChAT) in the neonatal rat forebrain: Evidence for a physiological role of NGF in the brain? Dev. Brain Res. **9:** 45–52.
49. GOLDMAN-RAKIC, P. S. & R. M. BROWN. 1981. Regional changes of monoamines in cerebral cortex and subcortical structures of aging rhesus monkeys. Neuroscience **6:** 177–187.
50. HAKIM, A. M. & G. MATHIESON. 1979. Dementia in Parkinson disease: A neuropathologic study. Neurology **29:** 1209–1214.
51. HEDREEN, J. C., S. J. BACON, & D. L. PRICE. 1985. A modified histochemical technique to visualize acetylcholinesterase-containing axons. J. Histochem. Cytochem. **33:** 134–140.
52. HEDREEN, J. C., S. J. BACON, L. C. CORK, C. A. KITT, G. D. CRAWFORD, P. M. SALVATERRA & D. L. PRICE. 1983. Immunocytochemical identification of cholinergic neurons in the monkey central nervous system using monoclonal antibodies against choline acetyltransferase. Neurosci. Lett. **43:** 173–177.
53. HEDREEN, J. C., R. G. STRUBLE, P. J. WHITEHOUSE & D. L. PRICE. 1984. Topography of the magnocellular basal forebrain system in human brain. J. Neuropathol. Exp. Neurol. **43:** 1–21.
54. HERZOG, A. G. & T. L. KEMPER. 1980. Amygdaloid changes in aging and dementia. Arch. Neurol. **37:** 625–629.
55. HIRANO, A. & H. M. ZIMMERMAN. 1962. Alzheimer's neurofibrillary changes. A topographic study. Arch. Neurol. **7:** 227–242.
56. HOUSER, C. R., G. D. CRAWFORD, R. P. BARBER, P. M. SALVATERRA & J. E. VAUGHN. 1983. Organization and morphological characteristics of cholinergic neurons: An immunocytochemical study with a monoclonal antibody to choline acetyltransferase. Brain Res. **266:** 97–119.
57. INGVAR, D. H. & N. A. LASSEN. 1979. Activity distribution in the cerebral cortex in organic dementia as revealed by measurements of regional cerebral blood flow. *In* Bayer-Symposium VII: Brain Function in Old Age, Evaluation of Changes and Disorders. F. Hoffmeister & C. Muller, Eds.: 268–277. Springer-Verlag. Berlin.
58. IVERSEN, L. L., M. N. ROSSOR, G. P. REYNOLDS, R. HILLS, M. ROTH, C. Q. MOUNTJOY, S. L. FOOTE, J. H. MORRISON & F. E. BLOOM. 1983. Loss of pigmented dopamine-β-hydroxylase positive cells from locus coeruleus in senile dementia of Alzheimer's type. Neurosci. Lett. **39:** 95–100.
59. JAMADA, M. & P. MEHRAEIN. 1968. Vertielungsmuster der senilen Veranderungen im Gehirn. Die Beteiligung des limbischen Systems bei hirnatrophischen Prozessen des Seniums und bei Morbus Alzheimer. Arch. Psychiatr. Z. Neurol. **211:** 308–324.
60. JAVOY-AGID, F., H. TAQUET, A. PLOSKA, C. CHERIF-ZAHAR, M. RUBERG & Y. AGID. 1981. Distribution of catecholamines in the ventral mesencephalon of human brain, with special reference to Parkinson's disease. J. Neurochem. **36:** 2101–2105.
61. JOHNSON. R. T. & D. L. PRICE. 1980. Chronic neurological diseases: Their societal burdens and potential solutions (editorial). J. Chron. Dis. **33:** 129–133.
62. JONES, E. G., H. BURTON, C. B. SAPER & L. W. SWANSON. 1976. Midbrain, diencephalic and cortical relationships of the basal nucleus of Meynert and associated structures in primates. J. Comp. Neurol. **167:** 385–420.
63. KATZMAN, R. & R. TERRY. 1983. Normal aging of the nervous system. *In* The Neurology of Aging. R. Katzman & R. Terry, Eds.: 15–50. F. A. Davis. Philadelphia, PA.
64. KIDD, M. 1963. Paired helical filaments in electron microscopy of Alzheimer's disease. Nature **197:** 192–193.
65. KITT, C. A., D. L. PRICE, M. R. DELONG, R. G. STRUBLE, S. J. Mitchell & J. C. HEDREEN. 1982. The nucleus basalis of Meynert: Projections to the cortex, amygdala, and hippocampus. Soc. Neurosci. Abstr. **8:** 212.
66. LANGSTON, J. W., P. BALLARD, J. W. TETRUD & I. IRWIN. 1983. Chronic parkinsonism in humans due to a product of meperidine-analog synthesis. Science **219:** 979–980.
67. LEHMANN, J. & H. C. FIBIGER. 1979. Acetylcholinesterase and the cholinergic neuron. Life Sci. **25:** 1939–1947.
68. LEHMANN, J., R. G. STRUBLE, P. G. ANTUONO, J. T. COYLE, L. C. CORK & D. L. PRICE. 1984. Regional heterogeneity of choline acetyltransferase activity in primate neocortex. Brain Res. **322:** 361–364.

69. Lieberman, A., M. Dziatolowsky, M. Kupersmith, M. Serby, A. Goodgold, J. Korein & M. Goldstein. 1979. Dementia in Parkinson disease. Ann. Neurol. **6:** 355–359.
70. Lindvall, O. & A. Bjorklund. 1983. Dopamine- and norepinephrine-containing neuron systems: Their anatomy in the rat brain. *In* Chemical Neuroanatomy. P. C. Emson, Ed.: 229–255. Raven Press. New York, NY.
71. Low, W. C., P. R. Lewis, S. T. Bunch, S. B. Dunnett, S. R. Thomas, S. D. Iversen, A. Björklund & U. Stenevi. 1982. Function recovery following neural transplantation of embryonic septal nuclei in adult rats with septohippocampal lesions. Nature **300:** 260–262.
72. Mayeux, R., Y. Stern, J. Rosen & J. Leventhal. 1981. Depression, intellectual impairment, and Parkinson disease. Neurology **31:** 645–650.
73. McGeer, E. G. 1978. Aging and neurotransmitter metabolism in the human brain. *In* Alzheimer's Disease: Senile Dementia and Related Disorders (Aging). R. Katzman, R. D. Terry & K. L. Bick, Eds. Vol. **7:** 427–440. Raven Press, New York, NY.
74. McKinney, M., R. G. Struble, D. L. Price & J. T. Coyle. 1982. Monkey nucleus basalis is enriched with choline acetyltransferase. J. Neurosci. **7:** 2363–2368.
75. Mesulam, M.-M. & M. Dichter. 1981. Concurrent acetylcholinesterase staining and gamma-aminobutyric acid uptake of cortical neurons in culture. J. Histochem. Cytochem. **29:** 306–308.
76. Mesulam, M.-M., E. J. Mufson, A. I. Levey & B. H. Wainer. 1983. Alzheimer's disease and the cholinergic innervation of neocortex by the nucleus basalis of Meynert (Ch4). Biological aspects of Alzheimer's disease. Banbury Rep. **15:** 79–93.
77. Mesulam, M-.M., E. J. Mufson, B. H. Wainer & A. I. Levey. 1983. Central cholinergic pathways in the rat: an overview based on an alternative nomenclature (Ch1—Ch6). Neuroscience **10:** 1185–1201.
78. Molliver, M. E., R. Grzanna, H. G. W. Lidov, J. H. Morrison J. A. Olschowka. 1982. Monoamine systems in the cerebral cortex. *In* Cytochemical Methods in Neuroanatomy. Neurology and Neurobiology. V. Chan-Palay & S. L. Palay, Eds. Vol. **1:** 255–277. Alan R. Liss. New York, NY.
79. Moore, R. Y. & F. E. Bloom. 1978. Central catecholamine neuron systems: Anatomy and physiology of the dopamine systems. Annu. Rev. Neurosci. **1:** 129–169.
80. Moore, R. Y. & F. E. Bloom. 1979. Central catecholamine neuron systems: Anatomy and physiology of the norepinephrine and epinephrine systems. Annu. Rev. Neurosci. **2:** 113–168.
81. Morrison, J. H. & P. J. Magistretti. 1983. Monoamines and peptides in cerebral cortex. Contrasting principles of cortical organization. Trends Neurosci. **6:** 146–150.
82. Mountjoy, C. Q., M. Roth, N. J. R. Evans & H. M. Evans. 1983. Cortical neuronal counts in normal elderly controls and demented patients. Neurobiol. Aging **4:** 1–11.
83. Mufson, E. J., A. Levey, B. Wainer & M.-M. Mesulam. 1982. Cholinergic projections from the mesencephalic tegmentum to neocortex in rhesus monkey. Soc. Neurosci. Abstr. **8:** 135.
84. Nagai, T., P. L. McGeer, J. H. Peng, E. G. McGeer & C. E. Dolman. 1983. Choline acetyltransferase immunohistochemistry in brains of Alzheimer's disease patients and controls. Neurosci. Lett. **36:** 195–199.
85. Nemeroff, C. B., G. Bissette, W. H. Busby, Jr., W. W. Youngblood, M. Rossor, M. Roth & J. S. Kizer. 1983. Regional brain concentrations of neurotensin, thyrotropin-releasing hormone and somatostatin in Alzheimer's disease. Soc. Neurosci. Abstr. **9:** 1052.
86. Ojika, K. & S. H. Appel. 1983. Neurotrophic factors and Alzheimer's disease. Biological Aspects of Alzheimer's Disease. Banbury Rep. **15:** 285–295.
87. Olpe, H.-R., V. J. Balcar, H. Bittiger, H. Rink & P. Sieber. 1980. Central actions of somatostatin. Eur. J. Pharmacol. **63:** 127–133.
88. Palkovits, M., M. J. Brownstein, L. E. Eiden, M. C. Beinfeld, J. Russell, A. Arimura & S. Szabo. 1982. Selective depletion of somatostatin in rat brain by cysteamine. Brain Res. **240:** 178–180.

89. PARNAVELAS, J. G. & J. K. McDONALD. 1983. The cerebral cortex. *In* Chemical Neuroanatomy. P. C. Emson, Ed.: 505–549. Raven Press. New York, NY.
90. PEARSON, R. C. A., K. C. GATTER, P. BRODAL & T. P. S. POWELL. 1983. The projection of the basal nucleus of Meynert upon the neocortex in the monkey. Brain Res. **259:** 132–136.
91. PEARSON, J., M. GOLDSTEIN, K. MARKEY & L. BRANDEIS. 1983. Human brainstem catecholamine neuronal anatomy as indicated by immunocytochemistry with antibodies to tyrosine hydroxylase. Neuroscience **8:** 3–32.
92. PEARSON, R. C. A., M. V. SOFRONIEW, A. C. CUELLO, T. P. S. POWELL, F. ECKENSTEIN, M. M. ESIRI & G. K. WILCOCK. 1983. Persistence of cholinergic neurons in the basal nucleus in a brain with senile dementia of the Alzheimer's type demonstrated by immunohistochemical staining for choline acetyltransferase. Brain Res. **289:** 375–379.
93. PERLOW, M. J., W. J. FREED, B. J. HOFFER, A. SEIGER, L. OLSON & R. J. WYATT. 1979. Brain grafts reduce motor abnormalities produced by destruction of nigrostriatal dopamine system. Science **204:** 643–646.
94. PERRY, E. K., B. E. TOMLINSON, G. BLESSED, K. BERGMANN, P. H. GIBSON & R. H. PERRY. 1978. Correlation of cholinergic abnormalities with senile plaques and mental test scores in senile dementia. Br. Med. J. **2:** 1457–1459.
95. PERRY, E. K., B. E. TOMLINSON, G. BLESSED, R. H. PERRY, A. J. CROSS & T. J. CROW. 1981. Neuropathological and biochemical observations on the noradrenergic system in Alzheimer's disease. J. Neurol. Sci. **51:** 279–287.
96. PERRY, R. H., G. BLESSED, E. K. PERRY & B. E. TOMLINSON. 1980. Histochemical observations on the cholinesterase activities in the brains of elderly normal and demented (Alzheimer-type) patients. Age Ageing **9:** 9–16.
97. PERRY, R. H., J. M. CANDY, E. K. PERRY, D. IRVING, G. BLESSED, A. F. FAIRBAIRN & B. E. TOMLINSON. 1982. Extensive loss of choline acetyltransferase activity is not reflected by neuronal loss in the nucleus of Meynert in Alzheimer's disease. Neurosci. Lett. **33:** 311–315.
98. PRESTY, S. K., L. C. CORK, D. L. PRICE, R. G. STRUBLE, L. C. WALKER, J. BACHEVALIER & M. MISHKIN. 1984. Aged rhesus monkeys (*Macaca mulatta*) are moderately impaired in visual recognition. Soc. Neurosci. Abstr. **10:** 774.
99. PRICE, D. L., P. J. WHITEHOUSE, R. G. STRUBLE, A. W. CLARK, J. T. COYLE, M. R. DELONG & J. C. HEDREEN. 1982. Basal forebrain cholinergic systems in Alzheimer's disease and related dementias. Neurosci. Comment. **1:** 84–92.
100. PRICE, D. L., P. J. WHITEHOUSE, R. G. STRUBLE, D. L. PRICE, JR., L. C. CORK, J. C. HEDREEN & C. A. KITT. 1983. Basal forebrain cholinergic neurons and neuritic plaques in primate brain. Biological Aspects of Alzheimer's Disease. Banbury Rep. **15:** 65–77.
101. PROBST, A., V. BASLER, B. BRON & J. ULRICH. 1983. Neuritic plaques in senile dementia of Alzheimer type: A Golgi analysis in the hippocampal region. Brain Res. **268:** 249–254.
102. REUBI, J.-C., M. H. PERRIN, J. E. RIVIER & W. VALE. 1981. High affinity binding sites for a somatostatin-28 analog in rat brain. Life Sci. **28:** 2191–2198.
103. ROSSOR, M. N., P. C. EMSON, C. Q. MOUNTJOY, M. ROTH & L. L. IVERSEN. 1980. Reduced amounts of immunoreactive somatostatin in the temporal cortex in senile dementia of Alzheimer type. Neurosci. Lett. **20:** 373–377.
104. ROSSOR, M. N., P. C. EMSON, L. L. IVERSEN, C. Q. MOUNTJOY, M. ROTH, J. FAHRENKRUG & J. F. REHFELD. 1982. Neuropeptides and neurotransmitters in cerebral cortex in Alzheimer's disease. *In* Alzheimer's Disease: A Report of Progress in Research (Aging). S. Corkin, K. L. Davis, J. H. Growdon, E. Usdin & R. J. Wurtman, Eds. Vol. **19:** 15–24. Raven Press. New York, NY.
105. ROSSOR, M. N., N. J. GARRETT, A. L. JOHNSON, C. Q. MOUNTJOY, M. ROTH & L. L. IVERSEN. 1982. A post-mortem study of the cholinergic and GABA systems in senile dementia. Brain **105:** 313–330.
106. ROSSOR, M. N., P. C. EMSON, L. L. IVERSEN, C. Q. MOUNTJOY & M. ROTH. 1984. Patterns of neuropeptide deficits in Alzheimer's disease. *In* Alzheimer's Disease: Advances in Basic Research and Therapies. Proceedings of the Third Meeting of the International

Study Group on the Treatment of Memory Disorders Associated with Aging. R. J. Wurtman, S. H. Corkin & J. H. Growdon, Eds.: 29–37. Zurich.
107. Ruberg, M., A. Ploska, F. Javoy-Agid & Y. Agid. 1982. Muscarinic binding and choline acetyltransferase activity in parkinsonian subjects with reference to dementia. Brain Res. **232:** 129–139.
108. Sagar, S. M. & J. B. Martin. 1982. The effect of cysteamine on immunoreactive somatostatin in the rabbit retina. Neurosci. Lett. **34**: 265–269.
109. Saper, C. B. & A. D. Loewy. 1982. Projections of the pedunculopontine tegmental nucleus in the rat: Evidence for additional extrapyramidal circuitry. Brain Res. **252:** 367–372.
110. Saper, C. B. & C. K. Petito. 1982. Correspondence of melanin-pigmented neurons in human brain with A1–A14 catecholamine cell groups. Brain **105:** 87–101.
111. Scatton, B., F. Javoy-Agid, L. Rouquier, B. Dubois & Y. Agid. 1983. Reduction of cortical dopamine, noradrenaline, serotonin and their metabolites in Parkinson's disease. Brain Res. **275:** 321–328.
112. Schwab, M. E., U. Otten, Y. Agid & H. Thoenen. 1979. Nerve growth factor (NGF) in the rat CNS: Absence of specific retrograde axonal transport and tyrosine hydroxylase induction in locus coeruleus and substantia nigra. Brain Res. **168:** 473–483.
113. Selkoe, D. J., Y. Ihara & F. J. Salazar. 1982. Alzheimer's disease: Insolubility of partially purified paired helical filaments in sodium dodecyl sulfate and urea. Science **215:** 1243–1245.
114. Sims, N. R., K. L. Marek, D. M. Bowen & A. N. Davison. 1982. Production of [^{14}C]acetylcholine and [^{14}C]carbon dioxide from [U-^{14}C]glucose in tissue prisms from aging rat brain. J. Neurochem. **38:** 488–492.
115. Struble, R. G., L. C. Cork, P. J. Whitehouse & D. L. Price. 1982. Cholinergic innervation in neuritic plaques. Science **216:** 413–415.
116. Struble, R. G., C. L. White, A. W. Clark, P. J. Whitehouse, L. C. Cork & D. L. Price. 1982. Acetylcholinesterase and amyloid in neuritic plaques in primate brain: evolution of the plaque. J. Neuropathol. Exp. Neurol. **41:** 364.
117. Struble, R. G., L. C. Cork, D. L. Price, Jr., D. L. Price & R. T. Davis. 1983. Distribution of neuritic plaques in the cortex of aged rhesus monkeys. Soc. Neurosci. Abstr. **9:** 927.
118. Struble, R. G., J. Lehmann, S. J. Mitchell, L. C. Cork, J. T. Coyle, D. L. Price, M. R. DeLong & P. G. Antuono. Cortical cholinergic innervation: distribution and source in monkeys. *In* Dynamics of Cholinergic Function. I. Hanin, Ed. Plenum Press. New York, NY.
119. Struble, R. G., J. C. Hedreen, L. C. Cork & D. L. Price. 1984. Acetylcholinesterase activity in senile plaques of aged macaques. Neurobiol. Aging **5:** 191–198.
120. Struble, R. G., D. L. Price, Jr., L. C. Cork & D. L. Price. Senile plaques in cortex of aged normal monkeys. Brain Res. In press.
121. Tagliavini, F. & G. Pilleri. 1983. Neuronal counts in basal nucleus of Meynert in Alzheimer disease and in simple senile dementia. Lancet **1:** 469–470.
122. Tapia-Arancibia, L., J. Epelbaum, A. Enjalbert & C. Kordon. 1981. Somatostatin binding sites in various structures of the rat brain. Eur. J. Pharmacol. **71:** 523–525.
123. Terry, R. D., A. Peck, R. DeTeresa, R. Schechter & D. S. Horoupian. 1981. Some morphometric aspects of the brain in senile dementia of the Alzheimer type. Ann. Neurol. **10:** 184–192.
124. Tomlinson, B. E. 1977. The pathology of dementia. *In* Dementia (Contemporary Neurology Series). C. E. Wells, Ed., Ed. Vol. **2:** 113–153. F. A. Davis. Philadelphia, PA.
125. Tomlinson, B. E., G. Blessed & M. Roth. 1968. Observations on the brains of non-demented old people. J. Neurol. Sci. **7:** 331–356.
126. Tomlinson, B. E., G. Blessed & M. Roth. 1970. Observations on the brains of demented old people. J. Neurol. Sci. **11:** 205–242.
127. Tomlinson, B. E., D. Irving & G. Blessed. 1981. Cell loss in the locus coeruleus in senile dementia of Alzheimer type. J. Neurol. Sci. **49:** 419–428.

128. UHL, G. R., J. C. HEDREEN & D. L. PRICE. 1985. Parkinson's disease: Loss of pigmented cells from the ventral tegmental area. Neurology **35:** 1215–1218.
129. VIJAYASHANKAR, N. & H. BRODY. 1979. A quantitative study of the pigmented neurons in the nuclei locus coeruleus and subcoeruleus in man as related to aging. J. Comp. Neurol. **38:** 490–497.
130. WAGNER, H. N., JR., H. D. BURNS, R. F. DANNALS, D. F. WONG, B. LANGSTROM, T. DUELFER, J. J. FROST, H. T. RAVERT, J. M. LINKS, S. B. ROSENBLOOM, S. E. LUKAS, A. V. KRAMER & M. J. KUHAR. 1983. Imaging dopamine receptors in the human brain by positron tomography. Science **221:** 1264–1266.
131. WHITEHOUSE, P. J., D. L. PRICE, A. W. CLARK, J. T. COYLE & M. R. DELONG. 1981. Alzheimer disease: Evidence for selective loss of cholinergic neurons in the nucleus basalis. Ann. Neurol. **10:** 122–126.
132. WHITEHOUSE, P. J., D. L. PRICE, R. G. STRUBLE, A. W. CLARK, J. T. COYLE & M. R. DELONG. 1982. Alzheimer's disease and senile dementia: Loss of neurons in the basal forebrain. Science **215:** 1237–1239.
133. WHITEHOUSE, P. J., J. C. HEDREEN, B. E. JONES & D. L. PRICE. 1983. A computer analysis of neuronal size in the nucleus basalis of Meynert in patients with Alzheimer's disease. Ann. Neurol. **14:** 149–150.
134. WHITEHOUSE, P. J., J. C. HEDREEN, C. L. WHITE, III & D. L. PRICE. 1983. Basal forebrain neurons in the dementia of Parkinson disease. Ann. Neurol. **13:** 243–248.
135. WILCOCK, G. K. & M. M. ESIRI. 1982. Plaques, tangles and dementia. A quantitative study. J. Neurol. Sci. **56:** 343–356.
136. WILCOCK, G. K., M. M. ESIRI, D. M. BOWEN & C. C. T. SMITH. 1982. Alzheimer's disease. Correlation of cortical choline acetyltransferase activity with the severity of dementia and histological abnormalities. J. Neurol. Sci. **57:** 407–417.
137. WISNIEWSKI, H. M. & R. D. TERRY. 1973. Reexamination of the pathogenesis of the senile plaque. *In* Progress in Neuropathology. H. M. Zimmerman, Ed. Vol. **II:** 1–26. Grune and Stratton. New York, NY.
138. WISNIEWSKI, H. M., H. K. NARANG & R. D. TERRY. 1976. Neurofibrillary tangles of paired helical filaments. J. Neurol. Sci. **27:** 173–181.
139. WISNIEWSKI, K., G. A. JERVIS, R. C. MORETZ & H. M. WISNIEWSKI. 1979. Alzheimer neurofibrillary tangles in diseases other than senile and presenile dementia. Ann. Neurol. **5:** 288–294.
140. KITT, C. A., L. C. CORK, E. EIDELBERG, T. H. JOH, & D. L. PRICE. Injury of nigral neurons with 1-methyl-4-phenyl-1,2,3,6, tetrahydropyridine (MPTP): A tyrosine hydroxylase immunocytochemical study in monkey. Neuroscience. In press.

Neural Grafting in Animal Models of Neurodegenerative Diseases

ANDERS BJÖRKLUND[a] AND FRED H. GAGE

Department of Histology
University of Lund
Lund, Sweden

INTRODUCTION

Work in amphibians and fish was the first to demonstrate the possibilities for neuronal replacement after damage in the central nervous system. In such species, above all in the visual system, it has been shown that grafted neurons can substitute both structurally and functionally for damaged axonal connections, and that afferent and efferent connections can be established with a high degree of specificity between the grafted neurons and the host. As originally reported by Matthey,[69] Stone,[89] and Sperry,[87] vision can be restored in enucleated adult newts or salamanders, or developing frogs, by transplanted or reimplanted whole eye bulbs. These grafts reestablish a new retinotectal pathway with a topographically ordered projection over the contralateral tectum. Similarly, in adult goldfish or developing frogs, grafted or reimplanted tectal tissue can reestablish functional and topographically ordered connections with the regenerating retinotectal axons of the host.[64,85,97,98]

For a long time it was thought that the remarkable regenerative and functional potential of CNS tissue grafts in cold-blooded vertebrates reflected a fundamental difference in the regenerative properties of central nervous tissue between cold-blooded vertebrates and mammals. During the last few years it has become evident, however, that at least certain types of intracerebral neural grafts can perform just as well in developing and adult mammals as in developing or adult submammalian vertebrates. Evidence has accumulated that fetal monoaminergic and cholinergic neurons, in particular, implanted into the depth of the brain in adult rats, can reestablish damaged connections in the host brain and substitute functionally for elements lost or damaged as a result of a preceding lesion. This recent work has led to the realization that, contrary to traditional views, the adult mammalian CNS has a potential to incorporate new neuronal elements into already established neuronal circuitry and that such implanted neurons can modify the function and behavior of the recipient.

Intracerebral grafting of monoaminergic and cholinergic neurons has particular relevance in the context of neurodegenerative diseases. In two

[a] Address for correspondence: Prof. A. Björklund, Department of Histology, Biskopsgatan 5, S-223 62 Lund, Sweden.

neurodegenerative disease syndromes, Parkinson's and Alzheimer's diseases, in particular, the progressive and substantial losses of such types of neurons are likely to underlie some of the major clinical symptoms of the disease. Thus, in Parkinson's disease the severe motor disturbances can be related to a loss of some 80–90% of the neurons in the nigrostriatal dopamine (DA) system. And in both Alzheimer's and Parkinson's diseases there is a strong correlation between the degree of dementia and the loss (or possibly atrophy) of cholinergic neurons in the basal forebrain projection systems, which is the source for the cholinergic afferents to the hippocampal formation and the neocortical mantle. There is experimental evidence in rats to support these relationships. Thus, interference with DA transmission (e.g., by administration of the DA-depleting drug, reserpine) or selective lesioning of the nigrostriatal DA neurons (by the toxins 6-hydroxydopamine, 6-OH-DA, or 1-methyl-4-phenyl-tetrahydropyridine [MPTP]) induces sensorimotor impairments in rats or monkeys which can be said to be analogous to the dysfunctions seen in parkinsonian patients.[21,23,68,95] Interference with cholinergic transmission, on the other hand (e.g., by cholinergic receptor blockade), or surgical lesions to the septohippocampal or basal forebrain–neocortical pathways carrying the cholinergic projection systems causes severe learning and memory impairments in rats (see Refs. 3 and 26 for review). The analogies between such experimentally induced conditions and the clinical disease states with respect to neuropathologic, neurochemical and behavioral changes have justified the use of animals with 6-OH-DA-induced lesions of the nigrostriatal DA pathway, on one hand, and surgical lesions of the septohippocampal or basal forebrain–neocortical cholinergic pathways, on the other, as experimental models for study of at least some aspects of the pathology involved in Parkinson's and Alzheimer's diseases.

In the first part of this paper we will review briefly the results obtained by implantation of dopaminergic and cholinergic neurons in animals with lesions of the nigrostriatal or septohippocampal systems, i.e., in conditions that can be said to represent *analogous* models of Parkinson's and Alzheimer's diseases. Parallel to this work we have taken an interest in the aged rat as an experimental model for age-dependent impairments in brain function and behavior. To the extent that aging affects the brain similarly in rodents and in man, the aged rat can be viewed as a *homologous* model of neurologic impairment associated with aging in man. As we argue in the second part of this paper, neural grafting in aged rats may offer new opportunities to study both the factors underlying the age-related decrements in motor and cognitive function and the possibilities of improving the performance of selected brain systems in the aged brain.

GRAFTING IN RATS WITH LESIONS OF THE NIGROSTRIATAL OR SEPTOHIPPOCAMPAL SYSTEMS

Characteristics of the Lesions

The nigrostriatal DA pathway was lesioned unilaterally, or in a serial bilateral paradigm, by local injection of 6-OH-DA (8 μg in 4μl) into the axon bundle. This lesion causes a >98% depletion of DA in the entire caudate-putamen on the lesion side, and in addition there is in most areas a profound denervation also of limbic forebrain regions, such as nucleus accumbens, olfactory tubercle, and bed nucleus of the stria terminal is.[6,17,80,81] The completeness of the lesion was routinely assessed by measurements of the magnitude of the turning response induced by an intraperitoneal injection of amphetamine, according to the technique of Ungerstedt and Arbuthnott.[94] Only rats that had the criterion for a complete lesion (>7 turns/min over 90 min) have been included in the grafting studies.

The septohippocampal cholinergic pathway has been lesioned uni- or bilaterally with an aspirative lesion of the fornix-fimbria and the overlying cingulate cortex. This so-called fimbria-fornix lesion transects all dorsal routes of cholinergic axons from the septal-diagonal band area innervating the hippocampal formation (as well as the posterior cingulate cortex), running in the fimbria, the dorsal fornix, and the supracallosal striae. The lesion removes about 90% of the cholinergic innervation of the entire hippocampal formation. The residual innervation reaches the hippocampus via the so-called ventral route (through the amygdaloid-piriform lobe); it is confined entirely to the ventral (temporal) tip of the hippocampal formation.[13,44–46] In contrast to the 6-OH-DA lesion, the aspirative fimbria–fornix lesion is nonselective and removes, in addition to the cholinergic afferents, a range of other afferent and efferent connections of the hippocampus and the medial neocortex as well. The fimbria-fornix lesion is made under visual control and thus the completeness of the lesion with respect to its cholinergic denervating effect can reliably be assessed under the operating microscope.

Grafting Procedures

Two principal techniques have been used to graft fetal CNS tissue to the previously denervated striatal or hippocampal regions. The first one involves the transplantation of solid pieces of tissue to a surgically prepared transplantation cavity in which the graft is placed in direct contact with the denervated striatum or hippocampus. In this procedure good graft survival is ensured by preparing the cavity in such a way that the graft can be placed on a richly vascularized surface (e.g., the pia in the choroidal fissure) that can serve as a "culturing bed" for the grafts.[88] The vessel-rich ventral surface of the fimbria-fornix lesion provides such a "culturing bed." This cavity is in direct communication with the lateral ventricle, which may allow the CSF to circulate through the graft cavity and thus probably help the graft to survive, particularly during the early postoperative period. In the case of the striatum, we have adopted a two-stage surgical procedure.[6,14] A cavity is first made in the dorsal parietal cortex to expose the dorsal surface of the head of the caudate-putamen. After a few weeks, when a new vessel-rich pia has grown over the surfaces of the cavity, the cavity is reopened and a graft is placed onto the exposed striatal surface.

The second technique we have used involves injection of dissociated cell suspensions into the depth of the brain.[11,16,79] In this technique pieces of fetal CNS tissue are trypsinized and mechanically dissociated into a milky cell suspension. Small volumes of the suspension can then be stereotaxically injected into the desired site using a microsyringe. A major advantage of this technique is that it allows precise and multiple placements of the cells. The technique also makes possible accurate monitoring of the number of cells injected by counting the density of cells in the suspension.[20] For the remainder of this chapter the first technique will be referred to as the "solid graft" technique and the second technique will be referred to as the "cell suspension" technique.

Reinnervation of the Denervated Host Brain by Monoaminergic and Cholinergic Neurons

In a first series of experiments[4,9,12,13,18] we studied the growth of *monoaminergic and cholinergic neurons in the hippocampal formation* in solid grafts taken from different embryonic brainstem regions. The idea behind these experiments was to test to what extent, and with what degree of precision, neural transplants are able to establish normal cholinergic and monoaminergic terminal innervation patterns in a previously denervated brain region. The hippocampal formation is ideally suited for such studies for two reasons: First, the terminal fields of the afferent inputs are, for the most part, discretely laminated; this gives each afferent system a characteristic termination pattern. Second, the major afferent fiber inputs to the hippocampal formation are readily accessible to surgical transection, and this makes possible fairly selective denervations of this region of the brain.

The transplants, obtained from 16- to 17-day-old rat fetuses, comprised (a) the septal-diagonal band area (which contains an extensive system of cholinergic neurons normally innervating the hippocampus and parts of the neocortex), (b) the locus coeruleus region of the pons (which contains the nucleus of origin of the hippocampal noradrenergic innervation), (c) the pontine and mesencephalic raphe region (with major serotonergic cell groups, including those that innervate the hippocampus), or (d) the dopamine-rich ventral mesencephalon (which does not normally innervate the hippocampus). These different transplants were grafted into the fimbria-fornix cavity in such a way as to allow the grafted neurons to grow toward the denervated hippocampus along the normal routes of the cholinergic and monoaminergic hippocampal afferents. The grafts approximately doubled their initial volume, and axons from the grafted neurons were found to invade large parts of the hippocampal formation. The mode of growth and the patterning of the ingrowing axons in the hippocampus differed markedly, however, among the different grafted neuron types, suggesting that the axonal ingrowth is very precisely regulated in the denervated hippocampal target. FIGURE 1 illustrates camera lucida drawings of the extent and patterning of acetyl cholinesterase (AChE)-positive fibers from a solid septal graft (A) and

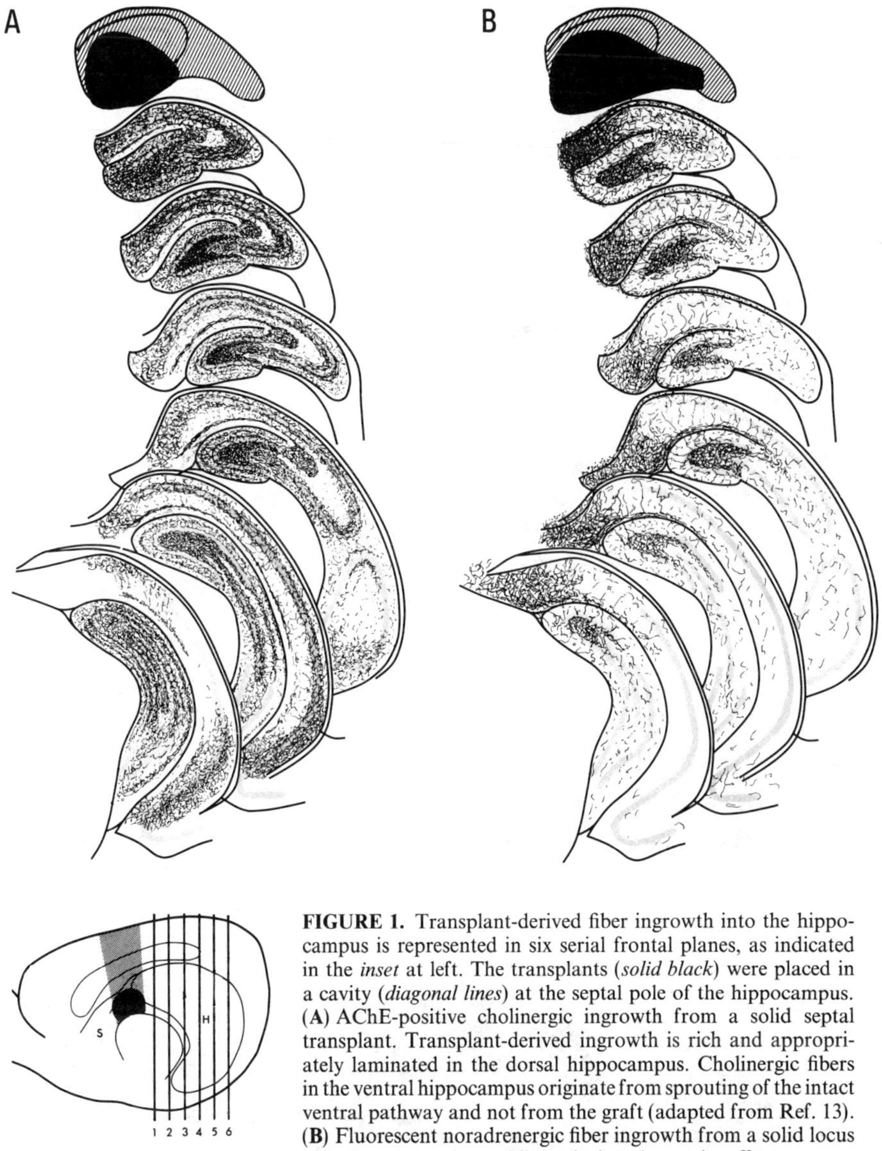

FIGURE 1. Transplant-derived fiber ingrowth into the hippocampus is represented in six serial frontal planes, as indicated in the *inset* at left. The transplants (*solid black*) were placed in a cavity (*diagonal lines*) at the septal pole of the hippocampus. (**A**) AChE-positive cholinergic ingrowth from a solid septal transplant. Transplant-derived ingrowth is rich and appropriately laminated in the dorsal hippocampus. Cholinergic fibers in the ventral hippocampus originate from sprouting of the intact ventral pathway and not from the graft (adapted from Ref. 13). (**B**) Fluorescent noradrenergic fiber ingrowth from a solid locus coeruleus transplant. All intrinsic adrenergic afferents were removed prior to transplantation by an intraventricular injection of 6-OH-DA. (Adapted from Björklund *et al.*[12])

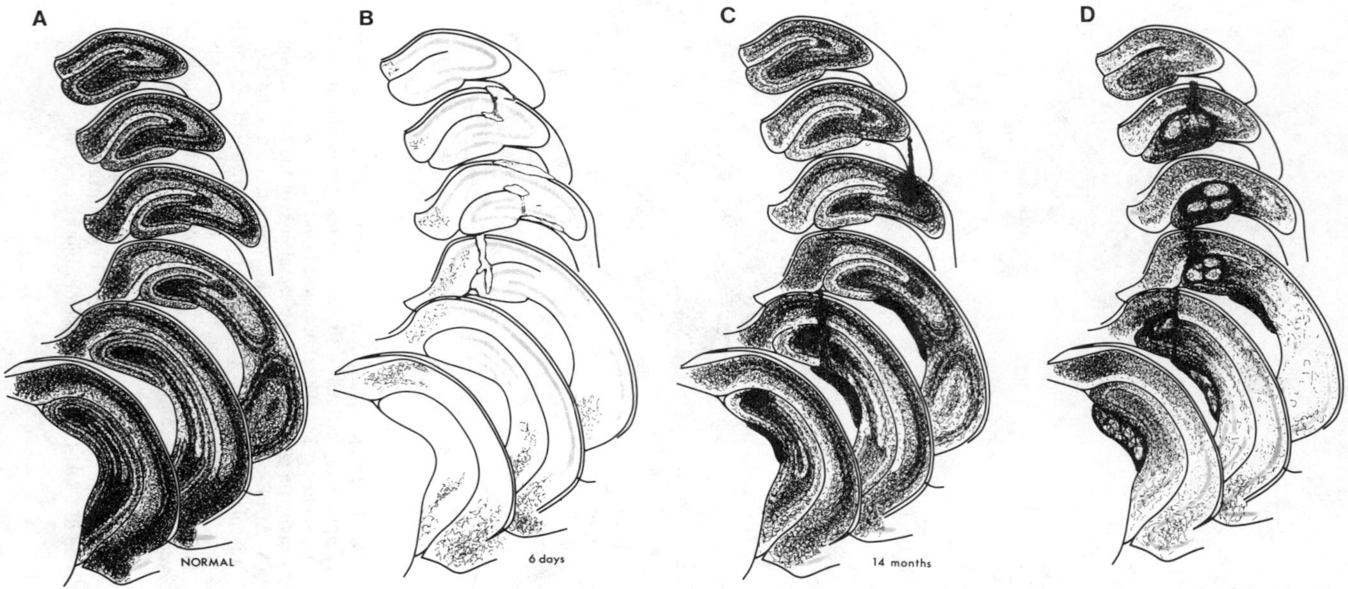

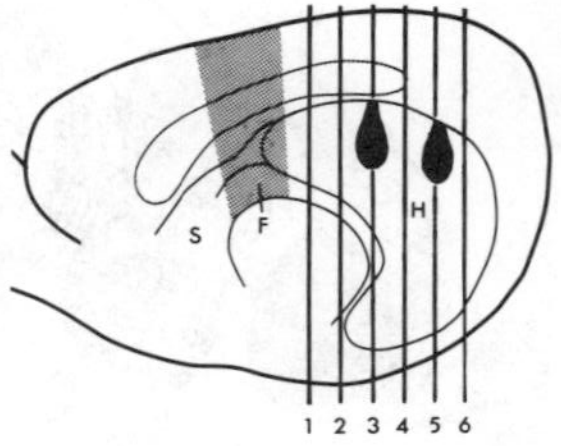

FIGURE 2. Six frontal planes in normal rats (**A**) and those with septal suspension grafts (**B, C and D**), as indicated in the *inset* at *right* (the graft sites are indicated by *solid black areas*). (**B** and **C**) Septal grafts in young rats with fimbria-fornix lesions at 6 days (**B**) and 14 months (**C**) after combined grafting and fimbria-fornix lesioning. By 6 days (**B**) the hippocampus is virtually completely denervated of its AChE-positive septal innervation, and the grafts (*white areas*) have not yet expressed any AChE staining. By 14 months (**C**) the host hippocampus is completely reinnervated from the graft and the patterning of the new AChE-positive fiber plexus is close to normal (cf. **A**). (**D**) Graft-derived AChE-positive fiber outgrowth from three septal suspension grafts in an intact aged rat (4 months post transplantation). The host hippocampus was denervated of its intrinsic AChE-positive innervation by a fimbria-fornix lesion 10 days before sacrifice. Note that the extent of reinnervation in this situation is markedly less than that seen in a denervated hippocampus of a young rat, and that the laminar patterning is more diffuse (cf. **C**). (Adapted from Björklund *et al.*[8] and Gage *et al.*[47])

noradrenalin-containing fibers from a solid locus coeruleus graft (B) from identical positions within the fimbria-fornix cavity. As can be seen from these drawings, there are clear-cut differences in the laminar patterning of the two fiber types within the different hippocampal subfields. On the other hand, the patterning of the graft-derived cholinergic and adrenergic innervations closely mimicked those of the normal cholinergic and adrenergic innervations, respectively, and in successful cases the entire hippocampus and dentate gyrus were reached by the ingrowing axons. The newly formed innervations have been observed in remain unchanged for more than a year after the operation and are thus probably permanent.

Subsequent experiments have shown that suspension grafts of septal cholinergic neurons[8] or pontine noradrenergic neurons,[10] injected directly into the hippocampus, are capable of reinnervating large parts of the previously deafferented hippocampus in a manner closely resembling that seen with solid grafts of the same neuron types (FIG. 2).

Grafts of mesencephalic DA-rich tissue to the denervated striatum in 6-OH-DA-lesioned rats have been studied by catecholamine fluorescence histochemistry and by tyrosine hydroxylase immunohistochemistry.[6,14,17,31,40,83]

With the delayed transplantation procedure, the survival rate of solid nigral grafts is greater than 95%, and they show on the average a $1\frac{1}{2}$–3-fold increase in volume.[6,14] FIGURE 3A shows an example of a solid nigral graft positioned in a dorsal cortical cavity and reinnervating the dorsal third of the denervated caudate-putamen. The fluorescent DA cells are frequently seen to cluster with dendritic arborization perpendicular to the layer of aggregated DA cells, in an arrangement reminiscent of the normal pars compacta–pars reticulata organization of the intact substantia nigra. Bundles of axons are seen to course through the graft and to ramify into a dense terminal plexus in the gray matter of the host neostriatum. Occasionally, ingrowth is seen into cortical areas medial, rostral, and lateral to the graft, but the preferential direction of growth of the ingrowing DA axons is into the proximal portions of the striatum, reinnervating from 1/10 to a maximum of 1/2 of the nucleus's volume at the longest survival times (6 months or longer). A similar pattern of graft survival and growth is seen when solid grafts are placed into a lateral cortical cavity, which results in an equivalent rich ingrowth into proximal (ventrolateral) regions of the striatum.[31]

The survival and growth of DA-rich suspension grafts have been studied in different brain sites.[17,33] The implanted DA neurons survive in clusters or aggregates at the injection site. Some cells have apparently migrated up to about 0.5 mm into the seemingly intact host tissue. Although the DA neurons have been seen to survive quite well in several different brain sites, their fiber outgrowth into the surrounding host tissue varies markedly from one area to another.[17] Rich fiber outgrowth is thus seen only into areas normally richly innervated by DA fibers, such as the caudate-putamen and nucleus accumbens, whereas DA cells implanted into normally poorly innervated areas, such as parietal cortex, globus pallidus, lateral hypothalamus and substantia nigra, demonstrate very little fiber growth into the surrounding host tissue. In the striatum, the DA fibers radiate out in a halo with a radius

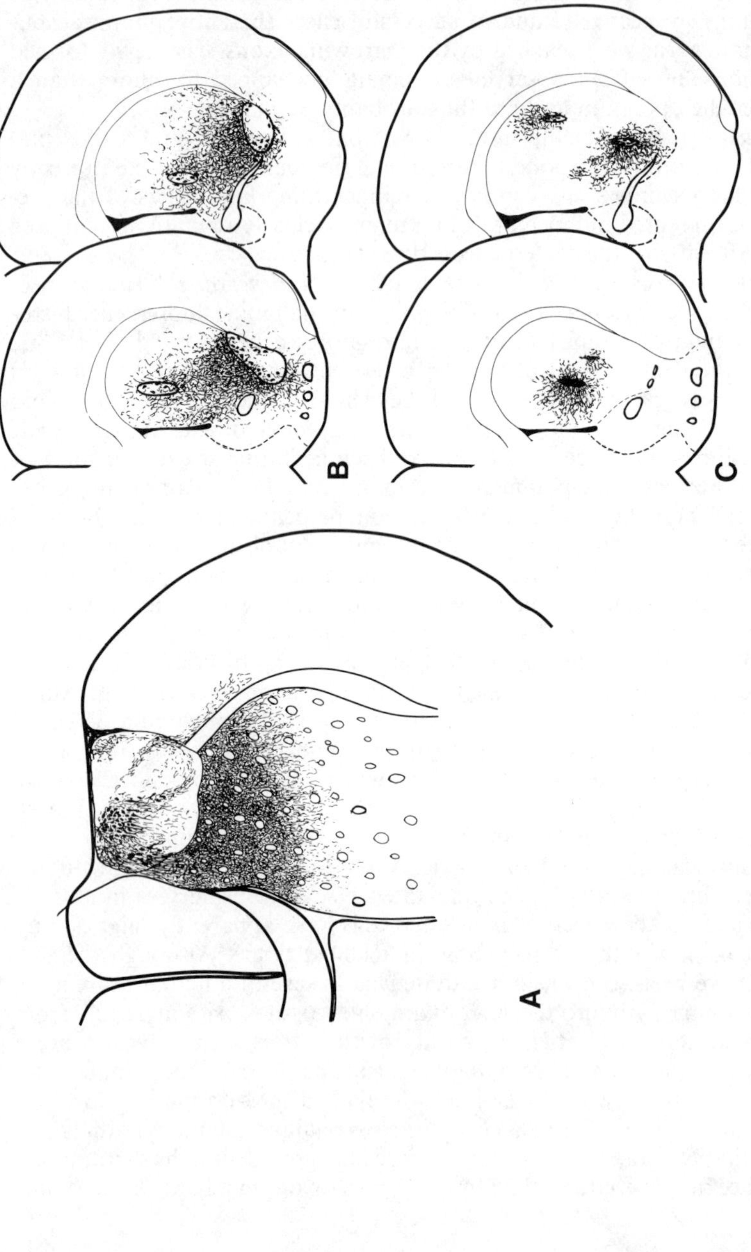

FIGURE 3. Nigral graft survival and associated DA fiber outgrowth in three cases. **(A)** A solid nigral graft placed in a dorsal cortical cavity of a 6-OH-DA-denervated young rat (7 months survival). **(B)** Two nigral suspension grafts (in the dorsal and ventrolateral neostriatum) in a 6-OH-DA-denervated young rat (4 months survival). **(C)** Three nigral suspension grafts in the neostriatum (3 months after grafting) of an aged rat whose intrinsic nigrostriatal DA pathway had been lesioned 1 week before sacrifice. (Adapted from Björklund *et al.*[17] and Gage *et al.*[47])

of about $1\frac{1}{2}$–2 mm around the implant, as seen in FIGURE 3B, which illustrates the DA fiber outgrowth in a 6-OH-DA-denervated animal with two nigral cell suspension deposits in the head of the caudate putamen. Each DA cell deposit reaches only a subportion of the striatum, and extensive reinnervation of the striatum will require several implants in different sites. The regionally restricted fiber outgrowth from each implant will, on the other hand, allow observations of regionally confined effects on behavior, a feature that will be dealt with later in this section.

Reinnervation of the denervated target is only efficient if the DA neurons are placed into or immediately adjacent to the target. Dopamine implants placed along the course of the nigrostriatal pathway (i.e., into the lateral hypothalamus, internal capsule, or globus pallidus) have not been seen to grow any axons into the striatum.[17] This does not necessarily mean that grafted mesencephalic DA neurons are unable to extend their axons over longer distances. Thus, Aguayo *et al.*[1] have recently shown that DA axons growing from solid nigral grafts, placed over the tectum, can reach the caudate-putamen along a piece of sciatic nerve placed as a bridge (running over the parietal cortex) between the nigral graft and the denervated striatum, a distance of about 2 cm.

Experiments with septal grafts in the hippocampal formation have provided evidence that the ingrowth from the grafted neurons into the surrounding host tissue is markedly modified by the presence or absence of the homologous intrinsic innervation. Thus, the extension of AChE-positive, presumably cholinergic, fibers into the hippocampal formation is considerably greater in animals denervated of their hippocampal cholinergic afferents by a fimbria-fornix lesion than in animals with intact cholinergic inputs.[13,43] With intrahippocampal septal suspension grafts, the choline acetyltransferase (ChAT) level in the host hippocampus reached about 75% of normal in animals with lesioned fimbria at the time of transplantation, as compared to about 25% in rats whose cholinergic inputs were left intact until 1 week before sacrifice. The parallel AChE histochemistry suggested that the denervating fimbrial lesion, made at the time of transplantation, made the cholinergic axons from the graft grow over greater distances within the host hippocampus and ramify more extensively in some of the normal terminal zones of the intrinsic septohippocampal cholinergic projection. Interestingly, McLoon and Lund[70] have reported a similar effect of removal of the normal retinal input on the ingrowth of axons from retinal grafts into the superior colliculus in neonatal rats.

These various observations suggest that the ingrowth and patterning of axons from implanted neurons are greatly influenced by the target tissue, and that this regulatory influence exhibits a relative specificity with respect to different types of neurons within the graft. The effects of denervating lesions suggest moreover that the proliferation and terminal patterning of the reinnervating axons may in some way be related to the filling of vacated terminal space in the denervated target, analogous to what has been described for lesion-induced collateral sprouting in the septohippocampal system (see

Refs. 25 and 77 for reviews). The monoaminergic and cholinergic neurons in the implants can also reinnervate the adult host hippocampus or striatum in a reproducible and orderly manner, even if the fibers are made to enter from abnormal directions and along routes that are inconspicuous in normal animals. The extension, proliferation, and patterning of the ingrowing fibers can be drastically modified by the removal of intrinsic afferents of both homologous and heterologous kinds.[9,13,18] As in the experiments of McLoon and Lund[70] in the visual system of neonatal recipients, the ingrowing axons in the adult hippocampus thus exhibit in some respects a considerable degree of specificity, while being at the same time markedly flexible and modifiable to the extent that abnormal zones of termination can be induced (see Ref. 9 for discussion).

Ultrastructural and Electrophysiological Evidence of Synaptic Graft–Host Connections

The question of whether ingrowing monoaminergic and cholinergic axons from the grafts can establish functional synaptic contacts with neuronal elements in the host target tissue has been addressed by both electrophysiological and ultrastructural techniques.

As mentioned above, fetal locus coeruleus grafts implanted in the denervated hippocampus have been shown to grow new noradrenergic axons from the implant to the appropriate denervated hippocampal terminal fields. In electrophysiological experiments,[12] stimulation of solid locus coeruleus implants was found to cause an inhibition of the spontaneous activity of neurons in the host hippocampus, similar to the long-latency, long-duration inhibition observed after stimulation of the intrinsic locus coeruleus in the intact rat. Likewise, as in the intact rat, the evoked inhibitory responses were blocked by local or systemic application of the beta-adrenergic receptor blockers, propranolol or sotalol. In another experiment[66] stimulation of solid septal grafts evoked characteristic field potentials in the dentate gyrus, and the depth profile revealed a relatively diffuse innervation characteristic of the normal septal afferents. Furthermore, prepulse stimulation of the septal grafts was found to potentiate the field potentials evoked by perforant path stimulation. This latter effect is a characteristic response to septal cholinergic stimulation also in the intact hippocampus.

Recently, Segal *et al.*[84] analyzed the connections of septal suspension implants by intracellular recordings in hippocampal slices. Stimulation of the septal graft, contained within the slice, produced voltage-dependent depolarization in some host CA1 neurons located up to about 2 mm away from the graft. This was associated with an increase in spontaneous action potential discharges and in spontaneous postsynaptic potentials. These responses were similar to those seen after topical application of acetylcholine. Since topical application of atropine attenuated, and physostigmine potentiated, the graft-induced depolarizing responses, these results are consistent with the formation of functional excitatory cholinergic synapses by the grafted septal neurons onto the host pyramidal neurons.

Ultrastructural support for the formation of true synaptic connections of ingrowing monoaminergic axons in the host comes from the study of Beebe *et al.*[4] and Clarke *et al.*[24a] in the hippocampus and of Freund *et al.*[41] in the neostriatum. In the first study, solid grafts of the mesencephalic raphe region were lesioned electrolytically, and degenerating synapses were identified in the host dentate. In the study of Clarke *et al.*,[24a] using ChAT immunocytochemistry, grafted septal cholinergic neurons were seen to form abundant synapses with neuronal targets in the dentate gyrus and CA1 area of the host.

Freund *et al.*[41] used tyrosine hydroxylase (TH) immunocytochemistry to trace DA synapses in the neostriatum reinnervated by solid nigral grafts. They identified abundant graft-derived TH-positive synapses on neuronal elements in the host neostriatum. As in normal animals,[42] the principal target was the dendrites of the spiny neurons, the majority of which are likely to be the striatal projection neurons. In addition, there was a clearly abnormal pericellular innervation of the cholinergic interneurons.

From these various studies it thus seems safe to conclude that grafted monoaminergic and cholinergic neurons are capable of forming relatively normal and functional synaptic inputs to their normal principal target neurons in the previously denervated host brain.

Biochemical Measures of Graft Function

Intrahippocampal Septal Grafts

The activity of the cholinergic innervation of the denervated hippocampus, derived from solid or suspension grafts of the septal-diagonal band area, has been monitored biochemically by measurements of the acetylcholine-synthesizing enzyme, ChAT, and of acetylcholine synthesis rates *in vitro*. Although AChE is a useful anatomic marker of the septohippocampal projection system, the AChE enzyme is not a specific marker for cholinergic neurons. The synthetic enzyme, ChAT, by contrast, is an enzyme specifically localized in cholinergic neurons and is therefore a better marker of cholinergic neurotransmission. This enzyme has been used to measure the time course and magnitude of fiber outgrowth from both solid and suspended septal grafts.[7,9,13] Graft-derived ChAT activity was barely detectable 10 days after cell suspension grafting, but sharply increased between 10 days and 1 month in the region of the host hippocampus close to the graft. By 6 months, ChAT activity was restored to near-normal levels in all segments of the previously denervated hippocampal formation. When the total amount of ChAT activity derived from the solid grafts is compared with that of the cell suspension grafts, the cell suspension grafts appeared to be about twice as effective as the solid grafts, although the amount of tissue grafted was about the same in each case.

The functional activity of the septal grafts was further assessed by measurements of [^{14}C]acetylcholine synthesis from [^{14}C]glucose *in vitro* in fimbria-fornix lesioned rats with septal suspensions implanted into the depth of the denervated hippocampus. The overall hippocampal [^{14}C]acetylcholine synthesis was restored to normal levels in the receiving grafts, and estimates of acetylcholine turnover rate suggested that the transmitter machinery of the newly established septohippocampal connections operated at a rate similar to that of the intrinsic septohippocampal pathway. Thus, these septal cell suspensions seem capable of maintaining function at a relatively "physiological" level despite their abnormal position.

In a more recent study, Kelly *et al.*[59] investigated the magnitude of lesion-induced alterations in the hippocampal formation, as reflected in the local rates of [^{14}C]2-deoxyglucose (2-DG) utilization and the degree to which this index of functional activity could be normalized after reinnervation by solid septal grafts. Six months after transection of the septohippocampal pathway by a unilateral fimbria-fornix lesion, the 2-DG utilization was reduced by 30–50% throughout the ipsilateral hippocampal formation of the animals without grafts. Fimbria-fornix-lesioned rats that had received septal grafts displayed a significant recovery in hippocampal 2-DG use, to within the normal range, as compared to the rats with lesion alone. In addition, the changes in 2-DG utilization were significantly correlated with the density of AChE staining in adjacent sections from the same brains ($r = 0.75$; $p < 0.01$), thus suggesting a relationship between the cholinergic reinnervation from the septal grafts and the restoration of functional glucose utilization. Together with the electrophysiological data quoted above, these results strongly suggest that the cholinergic component of the grafts is functioning at the biochemical level and influencing, or normalizing, the function of the deafferented hippocampal formation.

Intrastriatal Nigral Grafts

For grafted DA neurons also, measurements of DA turnover and synthesis rates *in vivo* indicate that the implanted DA neurons are capable of restoring DA neurotransmission in the initially denervated target.[80,81]

With solid nigral grafts placed on the dorsal striatal surface, as described above, the DA concentrations were restored from less than 0.5% in the 6-OHDA-lesioned neostriatum to a mean of 13.6% (maximum = 36%) in the reinnervated neostriatum. Moreover, measurements of the rate of DOPA accumulation after DOPA decarboxylase inhibition and measurements of the DA metabolite, DOPAC, indicated a restitution of normal (or even above normal) DA synthesis and release rates in the new "nigrostriatal" connections established by the grafted DA neurons.

Nigral suspension implants restored neostriatal DA levels to an average of 13–18%, with the highest individual values reaching about 50% of control. DOPAC was restored from about 5% of control (in the 6-OH-DA-denervated rats) to an average of about 20% of normal in the animals with grafts. The DOPAC: DA ratio and the DOPA accumulation rates indicated that the DA turnover and synthesis in the grafted neurons were on the average some 50–100% higher than in the intrinsic nigrostriatal pathway.

Behavioral Recovery

Sensorimotor Impairments after 6-OH-DA-Induced Lesions of the Nigrostriatal Pathway

6-OH-DA-induced lesions of the nigrostriatal DA pathway currently represent the most widely used experimental model of the principal neuropathology in Parkinson's disease, and the behavioral syndrome induced by such lesions has been thoroughly characterized in rats. A unilateral 6-OH-DA-induced lesion (FIG. 4A, left panel) causes *asymmetric motor behavior* (both spontaneously and in response to DA-releasing drugs, such as amphetamine, and DA-receptor-activating drugs, such as apomorphine), *asymmetric posture*, and *sensory inattention* (or *sensory neglect*) towards stimuli applied to the side of the body contralateral to the lesion (FIG. 4B, left panel). Bilateral lesions result in a state of profound behavioral unresponsiveness, including *akinesia*, *bilateral sensory inattention*, *catalepsy*, *hunched posture*, and *aphagia* and *adipsia* (see Refs. 68, 90, and 95 for reviews).

In unilaterally 6-OH-DA-lesioned rats, solid nigral grafts, placed in a dorsal cortical cavity or in the lateral ventricle, have been shown to reduce or completely abolish both spontaneous and drug-induced motor asymmetries,[6,14,30,40,76] but have no effect on the sensory neglect.[6,30] As more extensive testing has been conducted on rats with nigrostriatal grafts after unilateral or bilateral 6-OHDA lesions,[15,28–33] it has become apparent that graft-derived recovery is dependent upon graft placement, in parallel with the known topographic organization of striatal function.[35,58,60]

Thus, to summarize a range of observations in animals with both solid and suspended nigral grafts (FIG. 4): reinnervation of the dorsal caudate-putamen is a requirement for alleviation of both spontaneous and drug-induced rotation[6,15,30]; reinnervation of ventral and lateral caudate-putamen is required for reinstatement of sensorimotor attention and responsiveness on the contralateral side of the body[28,29,31]; and reinnervation of nucleus accumbens and/or prefrontal cortex is required for alleviation of the akinesia in bilaterally lesioned rats and normalization of the locomotor response to dopaminergic drugs.[29,33,73] The only behavioral deficit that has so far not been influenced in any substantial way is the severe aphagia and adipsia seen in bilaterally 6-OH-DA-lesioned rats.[29,32]

The compensation of motor asymmetry induced by solid nigral grafts has been shown to be correlated with the degree of striatal reinnervation. Interestingly, restoration of as little as 3–5% of the normal striatal DA content is sufficient for complete compensation of amphetamine-induced turning

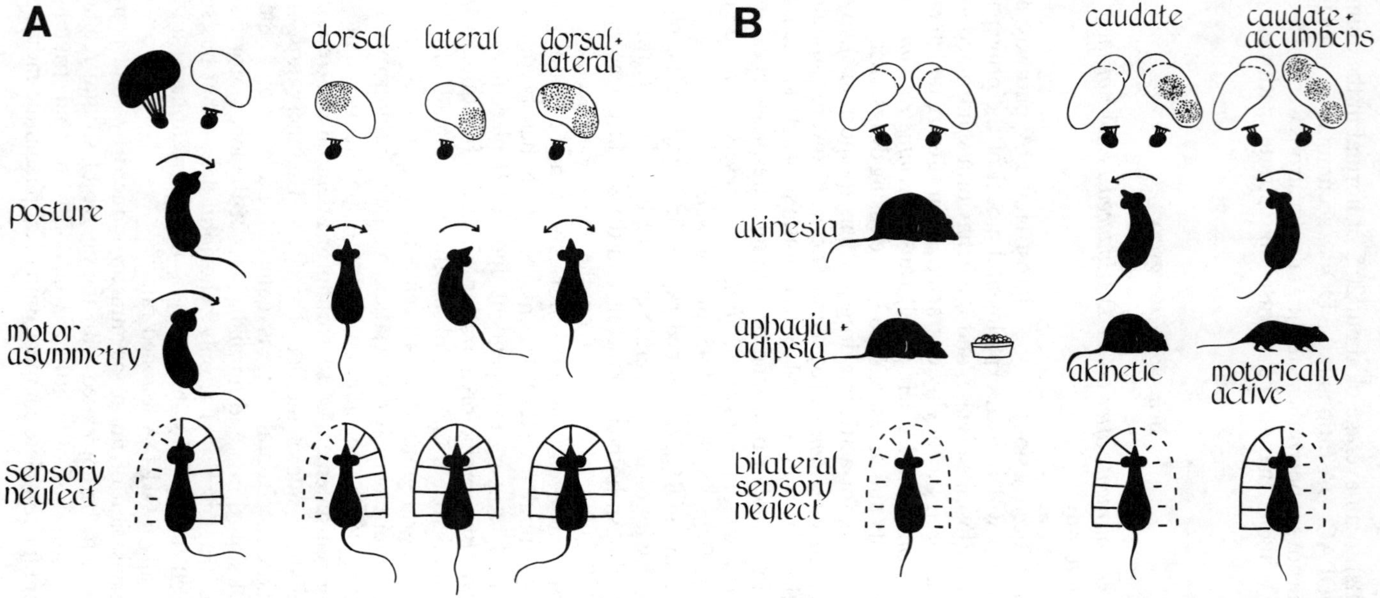

FIGURE 4. Main behavioral deficits in unilaterally (**A**) and bilaterally (**B**) 6-OH-DA-lesioned rats. The *right panels* in **A** and **B** illustrate the effects of grafts reinnervating the dorsal or lateral caudate-putamen or the nucleus accumbens. For further explanation, see text.

behavior,[6,80,81] and it has been estimated that some 120 surviving DA neurons (i.e., about 2% of the number present in the normal substantia nigra) are sufficient to produce a substantial compensatory effect on this behavior.[20]

Cognitive Impairments after Fimbria-Fornix Damage

The hippocampus has a special role in learning and memory, and bilateral fimbria-fornix lesions in rats are known to result in severe impairments in both working memory[75] and spatial memory.[74] This lesion disrupts several major afferent and efferent connection systems of the hippocampal formation. Nevertheless, since similar effects are obtained by pharmacologic blockade of cholinergic transmission,[37,91] it appears that lesioning of the cholinergic septohippocampal pathway contributes importantly to the memory impairments seen after fimbria-fornix transection.

The ability of the fetal septal grafts to reverse these impairments has been studied with tests of spatial learning and memory in different types of radial mazes. In the eight-arm radial maze,[66] rats with solid septal grafts showed a positive linear trend in maze performance over days of testing, but did not differ significantly from those of lesioned rats without grafts. However, potentiation of cholinergic transmission by pretreatment with the cholinesterase inhibitor, physostigmine, produced a significant enhancement of maze performance in the group with grafts, but not in the lesioned control group, and in some cases the rats with grafts performed as well as the nonlesioned control animals. In another study[36] using a T-maze forced-choice alternation test, seven of nine rats with solid septal grafts and four of five rats with septal cell suspensions learned the task, some of them up to the level of the control rats. The remaining rats with septal grafts, and a separate group of rats with locus coeruleus grafts, performed at chance level, similar to the rats that only received the fimbria-fornix lesion. In this study there was a positive and significant correlation between performance of the rats with grafts and the amount of graft-derived AChE-positive staining in the previously denervated hippocampal formation. This result has subsequently been replicated by Low *et al.*[65] in experiments with cross-species (mouse to rat) septal suspension grafts in fimbria-fornix-lesioned rats.

Together these three studies strongly suggest not only that the grafts can partially lessen lesion-induced deficits in maze learning tasks in fimbria-fornix-lesioned animals, but also that the behavioral recovery shows some specificity for the septal grafts, which provide a cholinergic reinnervation of the deafferented hippocampus. Interestingly, the effect of the septal grafts seems specific also with respect to different components of the lesion-induced behavioral syndrome. Thus, it has been found that those animals with septal grafts that showed improvement in spatial learning remained impaired with respect to the marked hyperactivity and hypoexploration which is characteristic of the fimbria-fornix-lesioned animals. Locus coeruleus grafts (rich in noradrenergic neurons), on the other hand, had a significant normalizing effect on activity and exploration, but did not influence the spatial learning deficit.[34]

GRAFTING IN BRAINS OF AGED RATS

Aging can result in naturally occurring brain damage, with anatomic, biochemical, and behavioral changes that appear to be substantial yet selective (see Refs. 3, 26, 72, and 92 for reviews). Such age-dependent decline in brain function is seen also in aged rodents, particularly in variables of sensorimotor coordination, learning, and memory, which has justified the use of the aged rat as a homologous model for age-related impairments in man.[22,49,51,67,96] Recent experiments have attempted to correlate these deficits with age-dependent impairments in specific neurotransmitter pathways. In our own grafting experiments in aged rats, we have focused our attention on the cholinergic innervation of the hippocampus and on the dopaminergic innervation of the striatum for the following reasons: (1) Age-related anatomic, biochemical, and functional changes have been repeatedly documented for both of these neurochemical systems[2,27,53,57,78,86]; (2) deficits in sensorimotor coordination and swimming abilities in aging rats are similar to those seen after DA-depleting brain lesions, and they may be reduced by the administration of DA-receptor agonists[57,67,96]; (3) age-related declines in learning and memory are reminiscent of the deficits seen after lesions to the septohippocampal system or after administration of anticholinergic drugs [3,37,49,75,91]; (4) as summarized above, intracerebral grafts of suspensions of embryonic tissue rich in dopaminergic and cholinergic neurons are known to grow and survive successfully for long periods in the striatum and hippocampus of young adult rats and they have been demonstrated to restore functional deficits associated with damage to either the cholinergic septohippocampal system or the dopaminergic nigrostriatal system. On the basis of these considerations we have undertaken a series of experiments to explore the potential of intracerebral implants of embryonic dopaminergic and cholinergic neurons to alleviate sensorimotor and learning deficits appearing with advancing age in nonlesioned animals.

Graft Survival and Fiber Outgrowth

The first stage in our study of neural implants in the aged rat brain was to demonstrate that such transplants could survive well in the aged brain and that they were able to provide appropriate reinnervation of the host.[47] To this end, neuronal cell suspensions prepared from the ventral mesencephalon and septal-diagonal band of rat embryos were implanted into the depth of the intact neostriatum or hippocampus of 21- to 23-month-old female rats of the same strain. Graft survival assessed 3–4 months after grafting was comparable to that seen in our previous studies of young adult recipients. Fiber outgrowth into the host brain was evaluated in animals that were subjected to lesions of the intrinsic nigrostriatal or septohippocampal system 6–10 days before killing. As illustrated in FIGURE 3C, dense dopaminergic fiber outgrowth was seen within a zone of up to about 1 mm radius around the nigral implants, and dense outgrowth of AChE-positive fibers occurred up to about 2 mm away from the septal implants (FIG. 2D). The overall magnitude of fiber outgrowth was less than that generally seen in previously denervated targets in young adult recipients (compare FIGURE 2C and D, and FIGURE 3B and C). However, the outgrowth seen in the aged rats with intact afferent inputs appeared to be as extensive as in young recipients when the grafts are placed in nondenervated targets.[43] The distribution of the AChE-positive fibers from the septal implants in the host hippocampus suggested that the pattern found in the nondenervated target of the aged recipients was more diffuse, and partly different, from the normal pattern. It is an interesting possibility, therefore, that synapse loss in intrinsic connections [53,56] may influence the patterning of the graft-derived innervation, and, in fact, improve the implants' ability to terminate in the otherwise intact target of the aged host brain.

Behavioral Effects

The next step in the study was to determine whether and to what extent the grafts could lessen any of the motor coordination or learning deficits seen in the aged animals prior to grafting.[48,50]

Motor coordination skills were assessed on four measures adapted from the battery described by Campbell *et al.*[22]: (*a*) the ability to maintain balance on and successfully reach a safety platform at either end of a narrow bridge of square cross section; (*b*) the ability to maintain balance on a similar bridge of round cross section; (*c*) the period of time that the animal could sustain its own weight clinging suspended from a taut wire; and (*d*) the ability to descend in a coordinated manner on a vertical pole covered with wire mesh. Prior to transplantation, the aged rats were significantly impaired on the four measures compared to the young control animals. On the square and round bridges, young rats had no difficulty walking and exploring along the rod, and they generally reached the platform within 30–60 seconds. By contrast, before transplantation, the aged rats had greater difficulties maintaining balance. Most animals fell off the bridges or alternatively lay on the bridges without attempting to walk, and clung tightly with all four paws or with the forepaws while the hind paws hung freely. Twelve weeks after transplantation the aged rats with nigral grafts, but not the aged controls or the rats with septal grafts, showed marked and significant improvement in their balance and limb coordination on both the square and round bridges. Typically they could walk along the bridge without falling, displayed gait posture similar to that of the young rats, and fell less frequently than did the other aged rats. On the wire-mesh-covered pole the aged rats descended more rapidly before transplantation than did the young controls, frequently falling, slipping or sliding down backwards. Although the aged rats with nigral transplants had a tendency to descend in a more controlled and coordinated manner, with the head-down orientation that was seen in the young controls, the differences from the other aged rats did not reach significance on this measure. The aged rats showed no difference between groups in either body weight or in latency to fall from the taut wire; this suggests that enhanced motor coordination in the aged rats with nigral grafts was not attributable to nonspecific differences in weight or strength of these animals.

Spatial learning was assessed in the Morris' water-maze task 1 week prior to transplantation and $2\frac{1}{2}$–3 months after transplantation.[71] This test requires that the rat use spatial cues in the environment to find a platform hidden below the surface of a pool of opaque water. Normal young rats have no trouble learning this task with speed and accuracy (FIG. 5A and open triangles in FIG. 5D). Since our previous studies using this task[49,51] showed that only a portion (1/4 to 1/3) of our rats were markedly impaired, a pretransplant test served to identify those impaired individuals in the aged rat group. On the basis of performance of the young control animals, we set

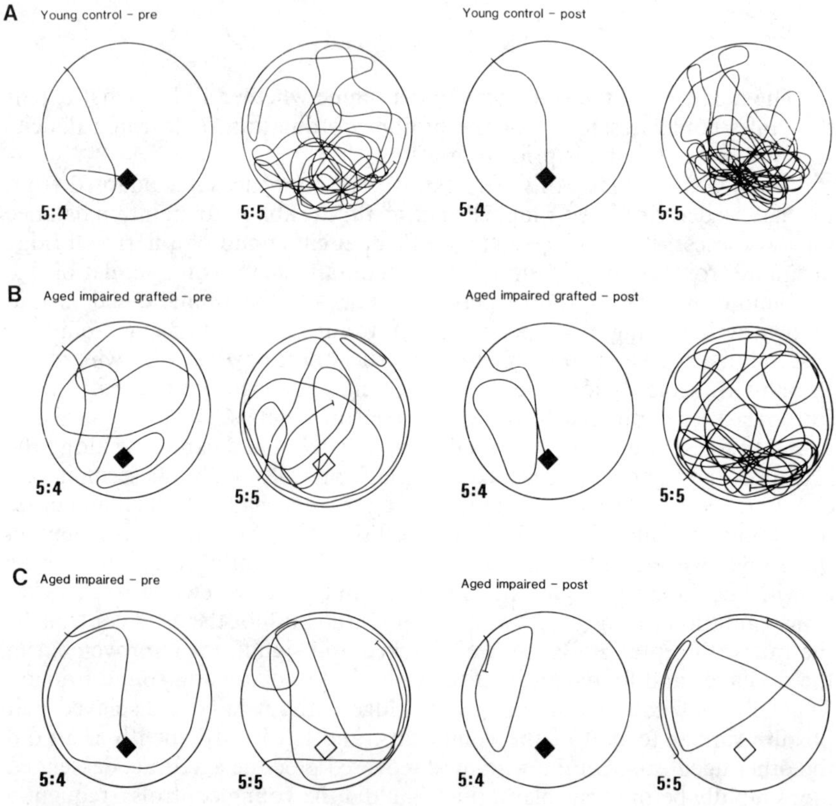

FIGURE 5. A, B and C. Actual swim paths showing spatial learning in the Morris' water-maze task in normal young rat (**A**), an impaired aged rat that received septal suspension implants (**B**), and an aged-impaired control rat (**C**). The two *left panels* in each figure illustrate the performance on the fifth day (before and after platform removal) of the first (pretransplant) test, and the two *right panels* show the performance on the fifth day (before and after platform removal) of the second (post-transplant) test 3 months later.

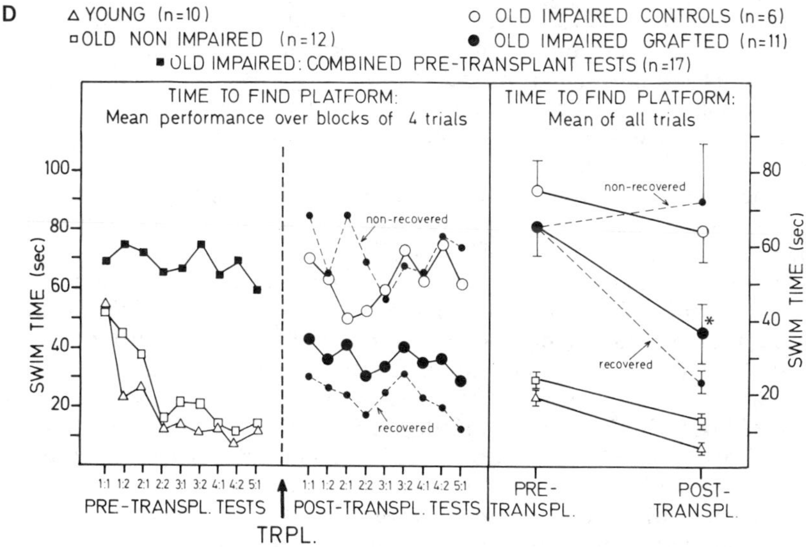

FIGURE 5D. Escape latency in the water-maze task plotted as 9 blocks of four trials, with eight trials presented each day. **Left panel:** *Solid squares* represent the performance of all old impaired rats prior to transplantation. **Middle panel:** post transplant performance of old impaired rats with or without grafts. "Recovered" refers to 8 of the 11 old impaired rats with grafts that on the post-transplant trials had recovered to within the 99% confidence interval values of the pre-transplant young control group. "Non-recovered" refers to the remaining 3 old impaired rats with grafts that showed no improvement post transplant. **Right panel:** Total mean escape latency summed over all 36 trials. The *asterisk* (*) indicates a significant decrease in escape latency by the old impaired rats with grafts as compared with their pretransplant performance and as compared with the old impaired control rats post transplant (error bars indicate SEM). (Adapted from Gage *et al.*[48])

the criterion for impaired performance in the aged rats such that the mean escape latency (i.e., swim time to find the submerged platform) should be above an upper 99% confidence limit of the escape latencies recorded in the young control group.[48] A subgroup of old rats showed mean swim times greater than the criterion and were thus allocated to the "old impaired" group, which was used for subsequent transplantation (FIG. 5B and C and *solid squares* in FIG. 5D). The remaining subgroup of aged rats constituted the "old nonimpaired" group (*open squares* in FIG. 5D). This latter group together with a young control group served as reference groups. A portion of the "old impaired" group received bilateral suspension grafts prepared from the septal-diagonal band area obtained from 14- to 16-day-old embryos of the same rat strain. Three implant deposits were made stereotaxically into the hippocampal formation on each side, as shown in FIGURE 2D. The remaining "old impaired" rats were not operated upon and served as the "old impaired" control group. On the post-transplantation test, $2\frac{1}{2}$–3 months after grafting, the groups without grafting remained impaired (FIG. 5C [post] and *solid circles* in FIG. 5D), while the animals with grafts, as a group, showed a significant improvement in performance, as indicated by escape latency. This improvement in group with the grafts was demonstrated by comparisons with its pretransplantation performance as well as with the performance of the old controls without grafts in the second test (FIG. 5B [post] and *open circles* in FIG. 5D).

The ability of the rats to use spatial cues for the location of the platform in the pool was assessed by analyzing their search behavior after removal of the platform on the fifth day of testing. While the young rats and rats in the old nonimpaired groups focused their search on the fourth quadrant, where the platform had previously been placed, the "old impaired" rats failed to do so in the pretransplantation test (compare the "5:5" test in FIGS. 5A, B and C). In the post-transplantation test the rats with grafts, but not the "old impaired" group without grafts, showed significantly improved performance. Swim distance in the fourth quadrant was increased 83% and the animals swam significantly more in the fourth quadrant than in other quadrants of the pool (compare the "5:5" test in the pre- and post-transplantation tests in FIG. 5B). By contrast the control animals without grafts showed no significant change over their pre-transplant performance.

These results[48,50] demonstrate, for the first time, the ability of intracerebral grafts to lessen age-related impairments in motor and complex cognitive behaviors. To what extent this effect is dependent on the dopaminergic and cholinergic neurons in the nigral and septal grafts, respectively, is not clear at present. It is interesting to note, however, that intrahippocampal septal grafts, identical to the ones used here, had no effect on the motor coordination disabilities described above, while the fetal substantia nigra implanted into the striatum was effective in reducing these motor-related disabilities. This suggests that the behavioral effects of the grafts are regionally specific and may be mediated through a direct action on elements in the surrounding region of the host brain. These various initial findings indicate that the intracerebral neural grafting technique should provide a new powerful tool for the analysis of the neurologic deficits underlying functional and behavioral decline in the aged rat brain and for the analysis of mechanisms of functional recovery of such age-dependent neurologic impairments.

MECHANISM OF ACTION OF INTRACEREBRAL NEURAL IMPLANTS: A WORKING MODEL

The combined morphologic, biochemical, electrophysiological, and behavioral data summarized above show that implanted embryonic nerve cells in some cases can substitute quite well for a lost intrinsic neuronal system in mammals. The intracerebral implants probably exert their effects in several ways. The functional effects seen with grafts placed into one of the cerebral ventricles, such as those described in the studies of Perlow *et al.*,[76] Freed *et al.*,[39,40] and Gash *et al.*,[52] are thus probably explained on the basis of a diffuse release of an active amine or peptide into the host CSF and adjacent brain tissue. In other instances, as in animals with DA-rich grafts reinnervating the neostriatum of acetylcholine-rich grafts reinnervating the hippocampus, we believe that the available data provide quite substantial evidence that the behavioral recovery is caused by the ability of the grafted neurons to reinnervate relevant parts of the host brain. This is illustrated by the studies mentioned above that show that the degree of functional recovery in 6-OH-DA-lesioned rats with nigral transplants is directly correlated with the extent of striatal DA reinnervation, and that the "profile" of functional recovery is dependent on which area of the striatal complex is reinnervated by the graft. This point is particularly well illustrated in a further study[38] in which rats with electrodes implanted into the center of intracortical nigral grafts were allowed to "self-stimulate" via the graft. The results show that the graft can indeed sustain self-stimulation behavior, and that the rate of lever-pressing is related to the proximity between the electrode tip and the dopamine-containing neurons in the graft. This strongly supports the notion that the implanted DA neurons can transmit behaviorally meaningful and temporally organized information to the host brain via their efferent connections.

To what extent the intracerebral implants can be functionally integrated with the host brain is still poorly known, however, and therefore remains an interesting question for further investigation. The chances for extensive integration may be greatest for neuronal suspension grafts implanted as deposits directly into the depth of the brain, but even solid grafts inserted as whole pieces into the brain have in several cases been seen to become reinnervated from the host brain in adult and developing recipients. Nevertheless, a recent HRP study[41] failed to detect any host afferents to intracortical solid nigral grafts, despite the fact that these grafts had themselves formed extensive DA connections in the host striatum and had produced behavioral recovery. This suggests that implanted neurons can also function well in the absence of some, or perhaps even all, of their normal afferent inputs.

Available data, derived primarily from studies on monoaminergic and cholinergic systems, indicate that implanted embryonic central neurons can substitute to some degree for a lost set of afferents to a denervated brain region in adult rats and can replace a lost intrinsic neuronal system in normalizing the rat's behavior. This indicates a remarkable plasticity of the mature rat CNS in incorporating new neuronal elements into its already established circuitries. There is now abundant evidence that the adult CNS can reorganize and rebuild itself in response to damage (see Refs. 25 and 93 for review), and in some cases continued neurogenesis and incorporation of newly-formed neurons are likely to play a normal physiological role, such as in the continuous replacement of damaged olfactory neurons (see the papers by Graziadei and Monti-Graziadei and by Bayer in this volume) or in the replacement of HVc neurons in the vocal control system of songbirds (see the paper by Nottebohm in this volume).

Neuronal replacement by neural implants is a striking further example of how the brain can allow new elements to be inserted and linked into its own functional subsystems. Obviously there must be definite limitations as to which types of neurons or functional subsystems can successfully be manipulated in this way. Neural implants would seem most likely to have behaviorally meaningful functional effects with types of neurons that normally do not convey, or link, specific or patterned messages, e.g., in sensory or motor input and output systems. Indeed, functional or behavioral recovery in the neuronal replacement paradigm has so far been demonstrated primarily for neurons of the types that normally appear to act as tonic regulatory of level-setting systems.

Both the mesencephalic DA neurons and the basal forebrain acetylcholine neurons are commonly conceived of as modulatory or level-setting systems which tonically regulate the activity of the neostriatal and hippocampal neuronal machineries.[62,90] Removal of the dopaminergic or cholinergic control mechanisms results in severe inhibition or impairment of neostriatal and hippocampal functions, respectively. Functional recovery seen after reinstatement of dopaminergic or cholinergic transmission by drugs or by neural implants can thus be interpreted as a reactivation of an inhibited, but otherwise intact, neuronal machinery.

The diagrams in FIGURE 6 provide a simple model for how such graft-induced activation may operate in the nigrostriatal system (A) and in the septohippocampal system, (B). *In the striatum*, the nigral DA neurons are normally proposed to act by regulating, or gating, the response of the striatal output neurons to the excitatory (probably glutaminergic) cortical input (*upper panel* in FIG. 6A). This could be achieved either as a result of an interaction of the dopaminergic and cortical inputs on the same dendrites or dendritic spines (as suggested, for example, by Herrling and Hull,[55] Brown and Arbuthnott,[19] and Freund *et al.*[40,41]), or through a presynaptic dopaminergic regulation of glutamate release from the corticostriatal terminals (as suggested, for example, by Schwarcz *et al.*,[83] Brown and Arbuthnott,[19] and Godukhin *et al.*[54]). Removal of the nigrostriatal DA input, as in the "DA-lesioned" animal (*middle panel* in FIG. 6A), results in inhibition of neostriatal function and an increase in the threshold for initiation of motor acts from the cortex. In the *lower panel* in FIGURE 6A, the grafted DA neurons act by reducing, or normalizing, the threshold for behavioral responding to cortical (or other) inputs.

In the hippocampus, the septal cholinergic neurons are supposed to regulate the transmission through the entorhinal-dentate-CA3-CA1-subicular relay circuit. In electrophysiological studies the cholinergic afferents have been shown to facilitate pyramidal cell firing, probably via both direct excitatory action as well as a disinhibitory mechanism.[5,61] This modulatory effect most likely serves to potentiate hippocampal responses to diverse excitatory inputs.[61,62,66] In the normal hippocampus (*upper panel* in FIG. 6B), the septal cholinergic afferents are thus presumed to have a permissive or activating action on the hippocampal responses to its principal cortical input system, which is the entorhinal perforant path. Cholinergic deafferentation (induced by the fimbria-fornix lesion) would then result in impaired transmission across the dentato-hippocampo-subicular synapse chain (as shown in the middle panel in FIG. 6B), leaving the hippocampus in a nonresponsive or

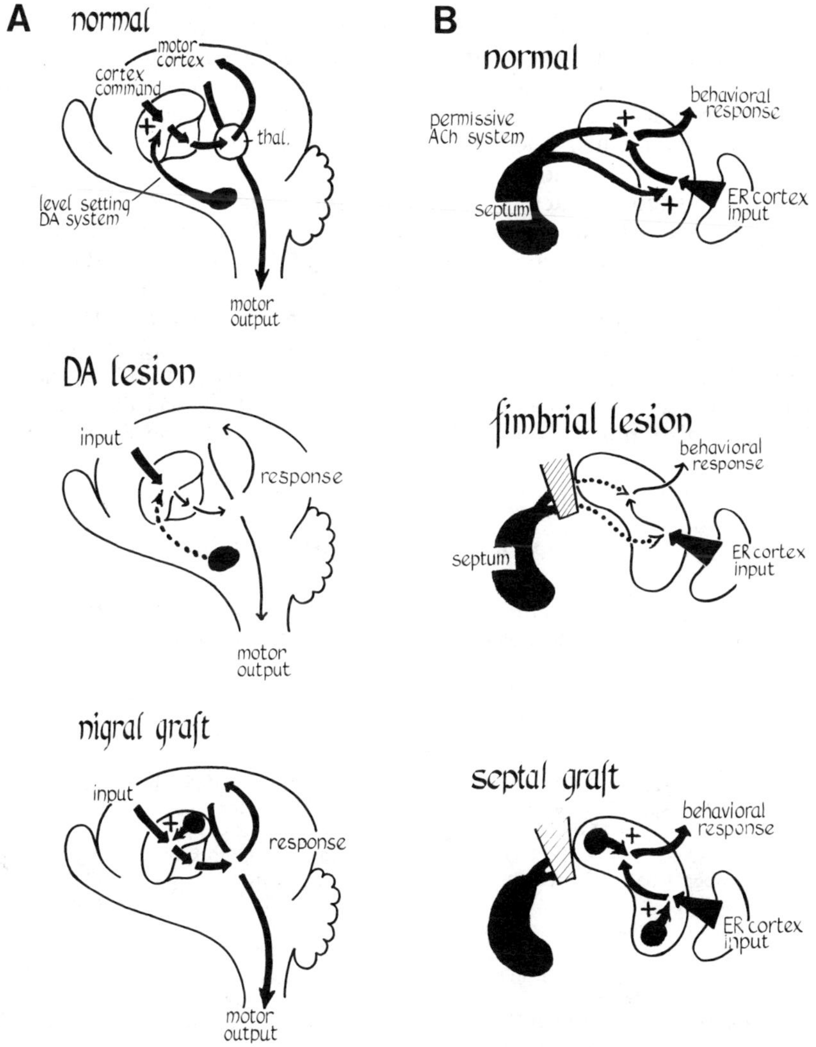

FIGURE 6. Proposed mode of action of the nigral and septal grafts as "level-setting" or permissive systems which reactivate the nonfunctioning or dysfunctioning striatal and hippocampal targets, respectively. For further discussion, see text.

dysfunctioning state. As with the intrastriatal nigral grafts, the behavioral effects of the septal grafts can then be explained by a restoration of hippocampal responsiveness to cortical inputs (FIG. 6B, *lower panel*). This has indeed been observed in electrophysiological recordings from dentate granule cells in rats with septal grafts reinnervating the hippocampus.[66]

An interesting implication of this model is that it may be sufficient for the nigral and septal grafts to reinstate dopaminergic and cholinergic transmission in the reinnervated target in a tonic and relatively nonspecific manner in order to compensate for at least some of the lesion-induced behavioral impairments. Since temporally or spatially patterned inputs to the grafted neurons may not be necessary for the maintenance of such tonic activity, this mode of action would allow for behavioral recovery to occur even in the absence of afferent connections from the host. Indeed, our biochemical studies on nigral grafts reinnervating the neostriatum indicate that the grafted DA neurons can maintain a sufficiently high spontaneous activity even in the absence of any major afferents from the host brain. The reason for this may be that even in the intact situation local regulation at the terminal level (e.g., through local transmitter interactions or presynaptic autoreceptors) may play an important role in the maintenance of tonic, baseline transmission in the aminergic systems (see Refs. 24 and 63 for further discussion).

ACKNOWLEDGMENTS

We thank Eva Björklund for drawing the illustrations in FIGURES 4 and 6, and Siv Carlson for generous assistance in the preparation of the manuscript.

REFERENCES

1. AGUAYO, A. J., A. BJÖRKLUND, U. STENEVI & T. CARLSTEDT. 1984. Fetal mesencephalic neurons survive and extend long axons across peripheral nervous system grafts inserted into the adult rat striatum. Neurosci. Lett. **43:** 53–58.
2. BARNES, C. A., B. L. MCNAUGHTON & J. O'KEEFE. 1983. Loss of place specificity in hippocampal complex spike cells of senescent rat. Neurobiol. Aging **4:** 113–119.
3. BARTUS, R. T., R. L. DEAN, B. BEER & A. S. LIPPA. 1982. The cholinergic hypotheses of geriatric memory dysfunction. Science **217:** 408–417.
4. BEEBE, B. K., K. MØLLGÅRD, A. BJÖRKLUND & U. STENEVI. 1979. Ultrastructural evidence of synaptogenesis in the adult rat dentate gyrus from brain stem implants. Brain Res. **167:** 391–395.
5. BEN-ARI, Y., K. KRNJEVIC, W. REINHARDT & N. ROPERT. 1981. Intracellular observations on the disinhibitory action of acetylcholine in the hippocampus. Neuroscience **6:** 2475–2484.
6. BJÖRKLUND, A., S. B. DUNNETT, U. STENEVI, M. E. LEWIS & S. D. IVERSEN. 1980. Reinnervation of the denervated striatum by substantia nigra transplants: Functional consequences as revealed by pharmacological and sensorimotor testing. Brain Res. **199:** 307–333.
7. BJÖRKLUND, A., F. H. GAGE, R. H. SCHMIDT, U. STENEVI & S. B. DUNNETT. 1983. Intracerebral grafting of neuronal cell suspensions. VII. Recovery of choline acetyltransferase activity and acetylcholine synthesis in the denervated hippocampus reinnervated by septal suspension implants. Acta Physiol. Scand. (Suppl.) **522:** 59–66.
8. BJÖRKLUND, A., F. H. GAGE, U. STENEVI & S. B. DUNNETT. 1983. Intracerebral grafting of neuronal cell suspensions. VI. Survival and growth of intrahippocampal implants of septal cell suspensions. Acta Physiol. Scand. (Suppl.) **522:** 49–58.

9. BJÖRKLUND, A., L. F. KROMER & U. STENEVI. 1979. Cholinergic reinnervation of the rat hippocampus by septal implants is stimulated by perforant path lesion. Brain Res. **173:** 57–64.
10. BJÖRKLUND, A., H. NORNES, S. B. DUNNETT, F. H. GAGE & U. STENEVI. 1983. Intracerebral and intraspinal implants of locus coeruleus cell suspensions: Deleterious effect of trypsin in the suspension medium. Soc. Neurosci. Abstr. **9:**101.
11. BJÖRKLUND, A., R. H. SCHMIDT & U. STENEVI. 1980. Functional reinnervation of the neostriatum in the adult rat by use of intraparenchymal grafting of dissociated cell suspensions from the substantia nigra. Cell Tissue Res. **212:** 39–45.
12. BJÖRKLUND, A., M. SEGAL & U. STENEVI. 1979. Functional reinnervation of rat hippocampus by locus coeruleus implants. Brain Res. **170:** 409–426.
13. BJÖRKLUND, A. & U. STENEVI. 1977. Reformation of the severed septohippocampal cholinergic pathway in the adult rat by transplanted septal neurones. Cell Tissue Res. **185:** 289–302.
14. BJÖRKLUND, A. & U. STENEVI. 1979. Reconstruction of the nigrostriatal dopamine pathway by intracerebral nigral transplants. Brain Res. **177:** 555–560.
15. BJÖRKLUND, A., U. STENEVI, S. B. DUNNETT, & S. D. IVERSEN. 1981. Functional reactivation of the deafferented neostriatum by nigral transplants. Nature **289:** 497–499.
16. BJÖRKLUND, A., U. STENEVI, R. H. SCHMIDT, S. B. DUNNETT & F. H. GAGE. 1983. Intracerebral grafting of neuronal cell suspensions. I. Introduction and general methods of preparation. Acta Physiol. Scand. Suppl. **522:** 1–10.
17. BJÖRKLUND, A., U. STENEVI, R. H. SCHMIDT, S. B. DUNNETT & F. H. GAGE. 1983. Intracerebral grafting of neuronal cell suspensions. II. Survival and growth of nigral cells implanted in different brain sites. Acta Physiol. Scand. Suppl. **522:** 11–22.
18. BJÖRKLUND, A., U. STENEVI, & N.-A. SVENDGAARD. 1976. Growth of transplanted monoaminergic neurones into the adult hippocampus along the perforant path. Nature **262:** 787–790.
19. BROWN, J. R. & G. W. ARBUTHNOTT. 1983. The electrophysiology of dopamine (D_2) receptors: A study of the actions of dopamine on corticostriatal transmission. Neuroscience **10:** 349–355.
20. BRUNDIN, P., O. ISACSON & A. BJÖRKLUND. 1985. Monitoring of cell viability in suspensions of embryonic CNS tissue and its criterion for intracerebral graft survival. Brain Res. **331:** 251–259.
21. BURNS, R. S., C. C. CHIUCH, S. P. MARKEY, M. H. EBERT, D. M. JACOBOWITZ & I. J. KOPIN. 1983. A primate model of parkinsonism: Selective destruction of dopaminergic neurons in the pars compacta of the substantia nigra by *N*-methyl-4-phenyl-1,2,3,6-tetrahydropyridine. Proc. Natl. Acad. Sci. USA **80:** 4546–4550.
22. CAMPBELL, B. A., E. E. KRAUTER & J. E. WALLACE. 1980. Animal models of aging: Sensory-motor and cognitive function in the aging rat. *In* Psychology of Aging: Problems and Perspectives, D. G. Stein, Ed.: 201–226. Elsevier North Holland. Amsterdam.
23. CARLSSON, A. 1959. The occurrence, distribution and physiological role of catecholamines in the nervous system. Pharm. Rev. **11:** 490–493.
24. CHESSELET, M.-F. 1984. Presynaptic regulation of neurotransmitter release in the brain: Facts and hypothesis. Neuroscience **12:** 347–375.
24a. CLARKE, D. J., F. H. GAGE & A. BJÖRKLUND. 1985. Formation of cholinergic synapses by intra-hippocampal septal grafts as revealed by choline acetyltransferase immunocytochemistry. Brain Res. In press.
25. COTMAN, C. W., & G. S. LYNCH. 1976. Reactive synaptogenesis in the adult nervous system. *In* Neuronal Recognition. S. H. Barondes, Ed.: 69–108. Plenum. New York, NY.
26. COYLE, J., D. PRICE & M. DELONG. 1983. Alzheimer's disease: A disorder of cortical cholineric innervation. Science **219:** 1184–1190.
27. CUBELLS, J. F. & J. A. JOSEPH. 1981. Neostriatal dopamine receptor loss and behavioural deficits in the senescent rat. Life Sci. **28:** 1215–1218.
28. DUNNETT, S. B., A. BJÖRKLUND, R. H. SCHMIDT, U. STENEVI & S. D. IVERSEN. 1983. Intracerebral grafting of neuronal cell suspensions. IV. Behavioural recovery in rats with

unilateral 6-OHDA lesions following implantation of nigral cell suspensions in different brain sites. Acta Physiol. Scand. Suppl. **522:** 29–37.

29. DUNNETT, S. B., A. BJÖRKLUND, R. H. SCHMIDT, U. STENEVI & S. D. IVERSEN. 1983. Intracerebral grafting of neuronal cell suspensions. V. Behavioural recovery in rats with bilateral 6-OHDA lesions following implantation of nigral cell suspensions. Acta Physiol. Scand. Suppl. **522:** 39–47.
30. DUNNETT, S. B., A. BJÖRKLUND, U. STENEVI & S. D. IVERSEN. 1981. Behavioural recovery following transplantation of substantia nigra in rats subjected to 6-OHDA lesions of the nigrostriatal pathway. I. Unilateral lesions. Brain Res. **215:** 147–161.
31. DUNNETT, S. B., A. BJÖRKLUND, U. STENEVI & S. D. IVERSEN. 1981. Grafts of embryonic substantia nigra reinnervating the ventrolateral striatum ameliorate sensorimotor impairments and akinesia rats with 6-OHDA lesions of the nigrostriatal pathway. Brain Res. **229:** 209–217.
32. DUNNETT, S. B., A. BJÖRKLUND, U. STENEVI & S. D. IVERSEN. 1981. Behavioural recovery following transplantation of substantia nigra in rats subjected to 6-OHDA lesions of the nigrostriatal pathway. II. Bilateral lesions. Brain Res. **229:** 457–470.
33. DUNNETT, S. B., S. T. BUNCH, F. H. GAGE & A. BJÖRKLUND. 1984. Transplantation of dopamine-rich tissue into rats with 6-OHDA lesions of the ventral tegmental area. I. Effects on spontaneous and drug-induced activity. Behav. Brain Res. **13:** 71–82.
34. DUNNETT, S. B., F. H. GAGE, A. BJÖRKLUND, U. STENEVI, W. C. LOW & S. D. IVERSEN. 1982. Hippocampal deafferentation: transplant-derived reinnervation and functional recovery. Scand. J. Physchol. (Suppl.) **I:** 104–111.
35. DUNNETT, S. B. & S. D. IVERSEN. 1982. Sensorimotor impairments following localized kainic acid and 6-hydroxydopamine lesions of the neostriatum. Brain Res. **248:** 121–127.
36. DUNNETT, S. B., W. C. LOW, S. D. IVERSEN, U. STENEVI & A. BJÖRKLUND. 1982. Septal transplants restore maze learning in rats with fornix-fimbria lesions. Brain Res. **251:** 335–348.
37. ECKERMAN, D. A., W. A. GORDON, J. D. EDWARDS, R. C. MACPHAIL & M. I. GAGE. 1980. Effects of scopolamine, pentobarbital and amphetamine on radial arm maze performance in the rat. Pharm. Biochem. Behav. **12:** 595–602.
38. FRAY, P. J., S. B. DUNNETT, S. D. IVERSEN, A. BJÖRKLUND U. STENEVI. 1983. Nigral transplants reinnervating the dopamine-depleted neostriatum can sustain intracranial self-stimulation. Science **219:** 416–419.
39. FREED, W. J., J. M. MORISHISA, E. SPOOR, B. J. HOFFER, L. OLSON, A. SEIGER & R. J. WYATT. 1981. Transplanted adrenal chromaffin cells in the rat brain reduce lesion-induced rotational behavior. Nature **292:** 351–352.
40. FREED, W. J., M. J. PERLOW, F. KAROUM, A. SEIGER, L. OLSON, B. J. HOFFER & R. J. WYATT. 1980. Restoration of dopaminergic function by grafting of fetal rat substantia nigra to the caudate nucleus: Long-term behavioural, biochemical and histochemical studies. Ann. Neurol. **8:** 510–519.
41. FREUND, T., P. BOLAM, A. BJÖRKLUND, U. STENEVI, S. B. DUNNETT & A. D. SMITH. 1985. Synaptic connections of nigral transplants reinnervating the host neostriatum: A TH-immunocytochemical study. J. Neurosci. **5:** 603–616.
42. FREUND, T. F., J. F. POWELL & A. D. SMITH. 1984. Tyrosine hydroxylase-immunoreactive synaptic boutons in contact with identified striatonigral neurons. with particular reference to dendritic spines. Neuroscience **13:** 1189–1215.
43. GAGE, F. H. & A. BJÖRKLUND. 1985. Enhanced graft survival in the hippocampus following selective denervation. Neuroscience. In press.
44. GAGE, F. H., A. BJÖRKLUND & U. STENEVI. 1983. Reinnervation of the partially deafferented hippocampus by compensatory collateral sprouting from spared cholinergic and noradrenergic afferents. Brain Res. **268:** 27–37.
45. GAGE, F. H., A. BJÖRKLUND & U. STENEVI. 1984. Cells of origin of the ventral cholinergic septohippocampal pathway undergoing compensatory collateral sprouting following fimbria-fornix transection. Neurosci. Lett. **44:** 211–216.
46. GAGE, F. H., A. BJÖRKLUND, U. STENEVI & S. B. DUNNETT. 1983. Functional correlates

of compensatory collateral sprouting by aminergic and cholinergic afferents in the hippocampal formation. Brain Res. **268:** 39–47.

47. GAGE, F. H., A. BJÖRKLUND, U. STENEVI & S. B. DUNNETT. 1983. Intracerebral grafting of neuronal cell suspensions. VIII. Cell survival and axonal outgrowth of dopaminergic and cholinergic cells in the aged brain. Acta Physiol. Scand. Suppl. **522:** 67–75.
48. GAGE, F. H., A. BJÖRKLUND, U. STENEVI, S. B. DUNNETT & P. A. T. KELLY. 1984. Intrahippocampal septal grafts ameliorate learning impairments in aged rats. Science **225:** 533–535.
49. GAGE, F. H., S. B. DUNNETT & A. BJÖRKLUND. 1984. Spatial learning and motor deficits in aged rats. Neurobiol. Aging **5:** 43–48.
50. GAGE, F. H., S. B. DUNNETT, A. BJÖRKLUND & U. STENEVI. 1983. Aged rats: Recovery of motor coordination impairments by intrastriatal nigral grafts. Science **221:** 966–969.
51. GAGE, F. H., P. A. T. KELLY & A. BJÖRKLUND. 1984. Regional changes in brain glucose metabolism reflect cognitive impairments in aged rats. J. Neurosci. **4:** 2856–2866.
52. GASH, D., J. R. SLADEK, & C. D. SLADEK. 1980. Functional development of grafted vasopressin neurons. Science **210:** 1367–1369.
53. GEINISMAN, Y., W. BONDAREFF & J. T. DODGE. 1977. Partial deafferentation of neurons in the dentate gyrus of the senescent rat. Brain Res. **134:** 541–545.
54. GODUKHIN, O. V., A. D. ZHARIKOVA & A. YU. BUDANTSEV. 1984. Role of presynaptic dopamine receptors in regulation of the glutamatergic neurotransmission in rat neostriatum. Neuroscience **12:** 377–383.
55. HERRLING, P. L., & C. D. HULL. 1980. Iontophoretically applied dopamine depolarizes and hyperpolarizes the membrane of cat caudate neurons. Brain Res. **192:** 441–462.
56. HOFF, S. F., S. W. SCHEFF, L. S. BERNARDO & C. W. COTMAN. 1982. Lesion-induced synaptogenesis in the dentate gyrus of aged rats: I. Loss and reacquisition of normal synaptic density. J. Comp. Neurol. **205:** 246–252.
57. JOSEPH, J. A., R. T. BARTUS, D. CLODY, D. MORGAN, C. FINCH, B. BEER & S. SESACK. 1983. Psychomotor performance in the senescent rodent: Reduction of deficits via striatal dopamine receptor up-regulation. Neurobiol. Aging **4:** 313–319.
58. KELLEY, A. E., V. B. DOMESICK & W. J. H. NAUTA. 1982. The amygdalostriatal projection in the rat—an anatomical study of anterograde and retrograde tracing methods. Neuroscience **7:** 615–630.
59. KELLY, P. A. T., F. H. GAGE, M. INGVAR, O. LINDVALL, U. STENEVI, A. BJÖRKLUND. 1985. Functional reactivation of the deafferented hippocampus by embryonic septal grafts as assessed by measurements of local glucose utilization. Exp. Brain Res. **58:** 570–579.
60. KELLY, P. H., P. W. SEVIOUR & S. D. IVERSEN. 1975. Amphetamine and apomorphine responses in the rat following 6-OHDA lesions of the nucleus accumbens septi and corpus striatum. Brain Res. **94:** 507–522.
61. KRNJEVIC, K., R. J. REIFFENSTEIN & N. ROPERT. 1981. Disinhibitory action of acetylcholine in the rat's hippocampus: extracellular observations. Neuroscience **6:** 2465–2474.
62. KRNJEVIC, K. & N. ROPERT. 1982. Electrophysiological and pharmacological characteristics of facilitation of hippocampal population spikes by stimulation of the medial septum. Neuroscience **7:** 2165–2183.
63. LEHMANN, J. & S. Z. LANGER. 1983. The striatal cholinergic interneuron: Synaptic target of dopaminergic terminals? Neuroscience **10:** 1105–1120.
64. LEVINE, R. & M. JACOBSON. 1974. Deployment of optic nerve fibers is determined by positional markers in the frog's tectum. Exp. Neurol. **43:** 527–538.
65. LOW, W. C., J. K. DANILOFF, R. P. BODONY & J. WELLS. 1985. Cross-species transplants of cholinergic neurons and the recovery of function. *In* Neural Grafting in the Mammalian CNS. A. Björklund & U. Stenevi, Eds.: 575–584. Elsevier. Amsterdam.
66. LOW, W. C., P. R. LEWIS, S. T. BUNCH, S. B. DUNNETT, S. R. THOMAS, S. D. IVERSEN, A. BJÖRKLUND & U. STENEVI. 1982. Functional recovery following neural transplantation of embryonic septal nuclei in adult rats with septohippocampal lesions. Nature **300:** 260–262.
67. MARSHALL, J. F., & N. BERRIOS. 1979. Movement disorders of aged rats: Reversal by dopamine receptor stimulation. Science **206:** 477–479.

68. MARSHALL, J. F. & P. TEITELBAUM. 1977. New considerations in the neuropsychology of motivated behaviours. *In* Handbook of Psychopharmacology, Vol. 7. L. L. Iversen, S. D. Iversen & S. H. Snyder, Eds.: 201–229. Plenum Press. New York, NY.
69. MATTHEY, R. 1926. La greffe de l'oeil. Étude experimental de la greffe de l'oeil chez le Triton (Triton cristatur). Arch. Entwicklungsmech. Org. **109:** 326–341.
70. MCLOON, S. C. & R. D. LUND. 1980. Specific projections of retina transplanted to rat brain. Exp. Brain Res. **40:** 273–282.
71. MORRIS, R. G. M. 1981. Spatial localization does not require the presence of locus cues. Learn. Motiv. **12:** 239–260.
72. MONTJOY, C., M. ROTH, N. EVANS & H. EVANS. 1983. Cortical neuronal counts in normal elderly control and demented patients. Neurobiol. Aging **4:** 1–11.
73. NADAUD, D., J. P. HERMAN, H. SIMON & M. LEMOAL. 1984. Functional recovery following transplantation of ventral mesencephalic cells in rats subjected to 6-OHDA lesions of the mesolimbic dopaminergic neurons. Brain Res. **304:** 137–141.
74. O'KEEFE, J. & L. NADEL. 1978. The Hippocampus as a Cognitive Map. Clarendon Press. Oxford.
75. OLTON, D. S., J. T. BECKER & G. E. HANDELMAN. 1979. Hippocampus, space and memory. Behav. Brain Sci. **2:** 313–365.
76. PERLOW, M. J., W. J. FREED, B. J. HOFFER, A. SEIGER, L. OLSON & R. J. WYATT. 1979. Brain grafts reduce motor abnormalities produced by destruction of nigrostriatal dopamine system. Science **204:** 643–647.
77. RAISMAN, G. & P. M. FIELD. 1973. A quatitative investigation of the development of collateral reinnervation after partial deafferentation of the septal nuclei. Brain Res. **50:** 241–264.
78. SABEL, B. A. & D. G. STEIN. 1981. Extensive loss of subcortical neurons in the aging rat brain. Exp. Neurol. **73:** 507–516.
79. SCHMIDT, R. A., A. BJÖRKLUND & U. STENEVI. 1981. Intracerebral grafting of dissociated CNS tissue suspensions: A new approach for neuronal transplantation to deep brain sites. Brain Res. **218:** 347–356.
80. SCHMIDT, R. H., A. BJÖRKLUND, U. STENEVI, S. B. DUNNETT & F. H. GAGE. 1983. Intracerebral grafting of neuronal cell suspension. III. Activity of intrastriatal nigral suspension implants as assessed by measurements of dopamine synthesis and metabolism. Acta Physiol. Scand. (Suppl.) **522:** 23–32.
81. SCHMIDT, R. H., M. INGVAR, O. LINDVALL, U. STENEVI & A. BJÖRKLUND. 1982. Functional activity of substantia nigra grafts reinnervating the striatum: Neurotransmitter metabolism and (^{14}C)-2-deoxy-D-glucose autoradiography. J. Neurochem. **38:** 737–748.
82. SCHULTZBERG, M., S. B. DUNNETT, A. BJÖRKLUND & STENEVI. 1984. Dopamine and cholecystokinin immunoreactive neurones in mesencephalic grafts reinnervating the neostriatum: evidence for selective growth regulation. Neuroscience **12:**17–32.
83. SCHWARCZ, R., J. CREESE, J. T. COYLE & S. H. SNYDER. 1978. Dopamine receptors localized on cerebral cortical afferents to rat corpus striatum. Nature **271:** 766–768.
84. SEGAL, M., A. BJÖRKLUND & F. H. GAGE. 1985. Transplanted septal neurons make viable cholinergic synapses with a host hippocampus. Brain Res. **336:** 302–307.
85. SHARMA, S. C. & R. M. GAZE. 1971. The retinotopic organization of visual responses from tectal reimplants in adult goldfish. Arch. Ital. Biol. **109:** 357–366.
86. SIMS, N. R., K. L. MAREK, D. M. BOWEN & A. N. DAVISON. 1982. Production of (^{14}C) acetylcholine and (^{14}C)carbon dioxide from (U^{14}C)glucose in tissue prisms from aging rat brain. J. Neurochem. **38:** 488–492.
87. SPERRY, R. W. 1945. Restoration of vision after uncrossing of optic nerves and after contralateral transposition of the eye. J. Neurophysiol. **8:** 15–28.
88. STENEVI, U., A. BJÖRKLUND & N.-AA. SVENDGAARD. 1976. Transplantation of central and peripheral monoamine neurons to the adult rat brain: Techniques and conditions for survival. Brain Res. **114:** 1–20.
89. STONE, L. S. 1944. Functional polarization in retinal development and its reestablishment in regenerated retinae of rotated eyes. Proc. Soc. Exp. Biol. Med. **57:** 13–14.
90. STRICKER, E. M. & M. J. ZIGMOND. 1976. Recovery of function after damage to central catecholamine-containing neurons: a neurochemical model for the lateral hypothalamic

syndrome. *In* Progress in Physiological Psychology and Psychobiology. J. M. Sprague & A. E. Epstein, Eds.: 121–188. Academic Press. New York, NY.

91. Sutherland, R. J., I. Q. Whishaw & J. C. Regeher. 1982. Cholinergic receptor blockade impairs spatial localization using distal cues in the rat. J. Comp. Physiol. Psychol. **96:** 563–573.
92. Terry R. & R. Katzman. 1983. Senile dementia of the Alzheimer type. Ann. Neurol. **5:** 497–506.
93. Tsukahara, N. 1981. Synaptic plasticity in the mammalian central nervous system. Ann. Rev. Neurosci. **4:** 351–379.
94. Ungerstedt, U. & G. W. Arbuthnott. 1970. Quantitative recording of rotational behavior in rats after 6-hydroxydopamine lesions of the nigrostriatal dopamine system. Brain Res. **24:** 485–493.
95. Ungerstedt, U., T. Ljungberg, & C. Ranje. 1977. Dopamine neurotransmission and the control of behaviour. *In* Psychobiology of the Striatum. A. R. Cools, A. H. M. Lohman & J. H. L. van den Bercken, Eds.: 85–97. Pergamon Press. New York, NY.
96. Wallace, J. E., E. E. Krauter & B. A. Campbell. 1980. Animal models of declining memory in the aged: short-term and spatial memory in the aged rat. J. Gerontol. **35:** 355–363.
97. Yoon, M. G. 1973. Retention of the original topographic polarity by the 180° rotated tectal reimplant in young adult goldfish. J. Physiol. **233:** 275–288.
98. Yoon, M. 1979. Reciprocal transplantation between the optic tectum and the cerebellum in adult goldfish. J. Physiol. **288:** 211–225.

Progress in Facilitating the Recovery of Function after Central Nervous System Trauma

CARL W. COTMAN AND MANUEL NIETO-SAMPEDRO

Department of Psychobiology
University of California, Irvine
Irvine, California 92717

INTRODUCTION

Basic studies during the last quarter of the century on the response of the central nervous system (CNS) to injury have made it increasingly clear that, given the proper stimulus, most events necessary for the reconstruction of injured circuits in the CNS can take place in the mature adult. However, clinical evidence shows that most injuries to the mature CNS are not spontaneously repaired. Thus, we are faced with the paradox of a CNS where individual molecular and cellular events leading to injury repair can take place, but where regeneration or repair of interrupted pathways nevertheless does not occur.

We believe that a key to this paradox is the lack of temporal organization of the events in adult synaptogenesis. Perhaps the most distinctive feature of development is the strict temporal order of cellular and molecular events. The development of the nervous system depends on a complex series of steps, each of which must occur in the right place and at the right time. In our opinion, regeneration and reactive synaptogenesis, that is, synaptogenesis triggered by injury, could repair the damaged CNS in most cases if the various responses would take place in the proper ordered sequence, as they do in development. From this point of view, the role of the neurologist is to learn how to initiate and guide the steps of the repair process so as to allow each of them to occur at the appropriate moment. Interventive treatments need to be inserted into the natural repair process, complementing it when natural repair is, as in the case of neuronal cell loss, clearly insufficient.

In this article we will show that a conceptual framework is beginning to emerge on how to combine interventive treatments with the natural response to injury, although all the mechanisms are by no means yet completely clear and many processes are still unexplored at the molecular level. We will begin by generally describing the cellular events that occur after CNS injury. We will then briefly examine several natural events which are mobilized after injury that can and probably do participate in the regrowth of injured circuitry. We will describe how brain transplantation is proving to be a powerful interventive technique both for revealing the inherent restorative capacities of the CNS after injury and for replacing lost neurons that can lead to the recovery of function. Given the present data, we propose a model in which the temporal order of natural events may restrict those mechanisms induced by injury from reaching their potential restorative capacities. We will show that ways of preventing the deleterious effects of these essentially beneficial processes are beginning to emerge.

GENERAL CELLULAR EVENTS AFTER CNS INJURY

Immediately after severe CNS trauma (FIG. 1), neuronal death occurs at the site of injury accompanied by local breakdown of the blood–CNS barrier. Generally, local vasculature is disrupted and blood cells and serum proteins massively invade the zone of injury. About 24 hours postlesion, CNS edema is patent. Edema probably results from both extracellular fluid accumulation, particularly in white matter, and astrocytic swelling.[1,2] Accumulations of blood-derived macrophages are observed 48 hours after a stab wound to the brain, and these proceed to engulf degenerating myelin and other cell debris.

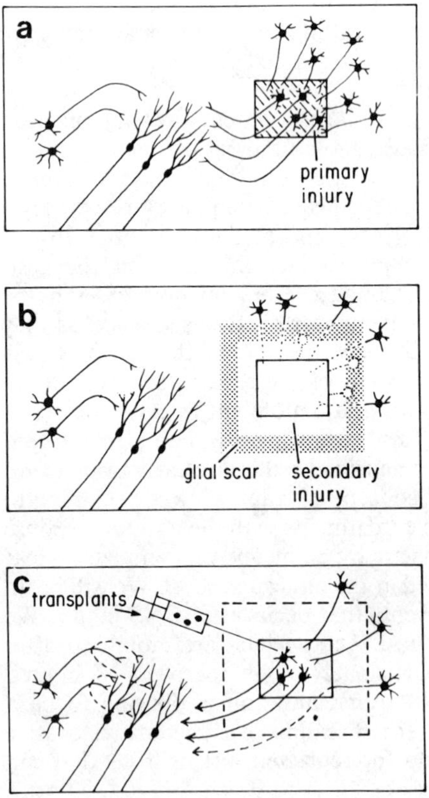

FIGURE 1. Schematic diagram illustrating the various events after injury and the cellular processes that can facilitate the restoration of circuitry. (**a**) Hypothetical circuit is shown with major neuronal elements. (**b**) Loss of one cluster of neurons results in secondary neuronal death around the primary injury site. (**c**) Denervation stimulates undamaged axons to sprout new synapses. Transplantation of fetal neurons can restore lost neurons and at least partially repair the injured circuitry.

Astrocytes also appear to participate in this process.[3] Neurons not directly affected by injury begin to die, and gradually enlarging cysts develop and coalesce to form cavities within the CNS parenchyma[4] that progressively increase the distance between the ends of a transected pathway. This wave of secondary neuronal death after the primary injury (FIG. 1b) is probably responsible for a larger proportion of neuronal death than the initial injury itself. While phagocytosis is going on, astrocytes adjacent to the lesion proliferate and their enlarged fibrous processes form a web that isolates the surfaces of the injury from the surrounding tissue.[5,6] At about the same time, fibroblasts from proximal connective tissue invade the injury site overlaying the CNS surfaces with a dense layer of collagen.[7,8] The so-called glial "scar" (FIG. 1b) is thus formed. Complete clearing of degenerative debris may take many months, but in the adult the bulk of it has been removed 4 to 5 days postlesion, and sprouts from undamaged axons and regenerative sprouts begin to appear.[9]

Denervation or other disturbances in the synaptic environment elicit the growth of sprouts from nearby undamaged axons (FIG. 1c). These fibers grow new terminals and effectively repopulate the temporarily vacated fields. At about the same time, cut axons near the injury site begin to regenerate, but unless aided they die back. Recently such interventions as the use of transplants and exogenous chemical agents point toward new directions in the restoration of CNS circuitry, although such approaches are still in their early stages.

SECONDARY NEURONAL LOSS

Since neurons do not divide after they are formed, it is necessary to either prevent their loss in the first place or to replace them once they are lost. It is critical to determine the causes of cell death and to derive treatments that restore traumatized neurons. Neuronal death after injury probably arises from multiple causes such as ischemia, traumatic insult, absence of nutrients, and metabolic imbalances. One well-known metabolic requirement of neurons is the need for their appropriate target-derived trophic factor.[10,11] In peripheral sympathetic neurons, for example, the loss of their trophic factor, nerve growth factor (NGF), results in chromatolytic reactions and in many cases cell death. The health of sympathethic neurons deprived of NGF by axotomy or immunosympathectomy can be restored by providing exogenous NGF. It is relevant, therefore, to investigate the consequences of injury on trophic factors in the CNS.

Do such factors exist in the CNS and how are their levels affected by injury? We can expect that neurons whose axons project into an area of injury and are severed will be deprived of target-derived trophic factors and will be affected much like peripheral neurons. Some cells near an injured site may die because of the loss of trophic factor available or because of other mechanisms such as the presence of toxic factors. In order to better understand such injury-induced cell loss, we have recently studied the levels and

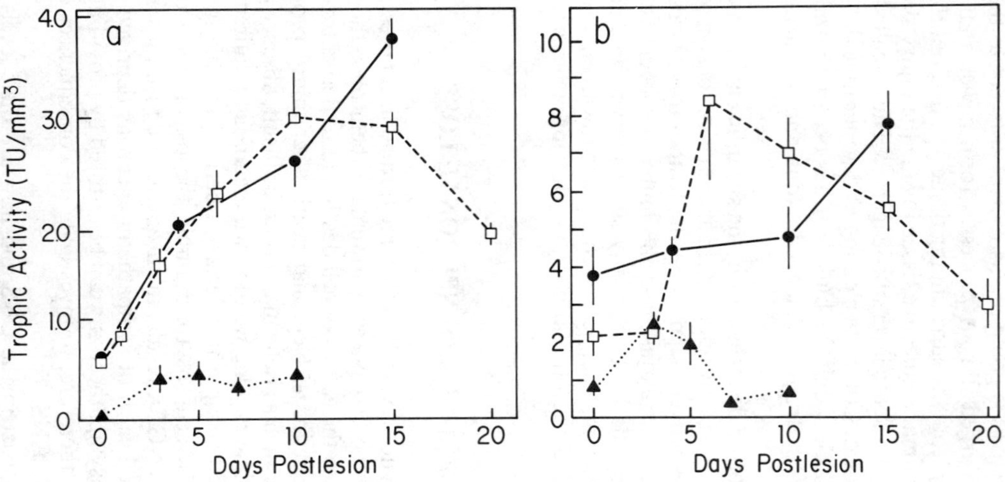

FIGURE 2. Levels of neurotrophic activity in tissue adjacent to a lesion of the entorhinal cortex as a function of time after the lesion was made using ciliary ganglion neurons (**a**) or striatal neurons (**b**).[17,18] The age of the experimental animals (Sprague-Dawley rats) was 3 days (▲), 2 months (□), and 24 months (●).

properties of neurotrophic factors at and around the site of injury. Previously it had been reported that factors that promote neuron survival (neurotrophic factors) increase after peripheral nerve injury.[12,13]

Our studies have shown that injury to the CNS causes an increase in the activity of neurotrophic factors in injured parts of the CNS. In the developing, mature, or aged rodent brain, injury causes a time-dependent rise in the activity of neurotrophic factors as assayed with cultured peripheral or central neurons. A wound was made in the entorhinal cortex of neonatal, adult, and aged rats and the lesion cavity was filled with a fragment of Gelfoam moistened with saline solution. At various times after the lesion was created (the "postlesion" time), the animals were sacrificed and both the Gelfoam fragment and the tissue surrounding the wound cavity were separately analyzed for amount of neurotrophic activity. Initially, ciliary ganglia, sympathetic ganglia, and dorsal root ganglia neurons in low-density culture were used as test cells.[14–16] After brain injury, extracts of both tissue and Gelfoam had increased amounts of neurotrophic activity. In the tissue surrounding the wound, the maximal levels of trophic activity were successively higher in neonatal, adult, and aged animals, and they were reached at 3, 10, and 15 days postlesion, respectively[17] (FIG. 2a). The activity was highest on sympathetic ganglion neurons and one order of magnitude lower on dorsal root and ciliary ganglion cells. Injury-enhancement of neurotrophic activity occurred in all regions of the CNS parenchyma, but not in the corpus callosum.[15] Accumulation of neurotrophic activity in the Gelfoam placed into the wound cavities in neonatal and adult animals lagged behind the levels in tissue by 4–5 days, suggesting that either the neurotrophic factors or the cells that produce them are transferred from the tissue into the Gelfoam. The activity of neurotrophic factors was highest near the injured site and decayed with distance (FIG. 3).

We have also examined injury induction of neurotrophic factors on dissociated cultures of neurons from embryonic rat brain corpus striatum, thalamus, hippocampus and septum.[18] The normal (basal) levels of central neurotrophic activity in extracts of neonatal, adult, and aged rat brain tissue were lowest in the neonatal brain and two-fold and four-fold higher in the adult and the aged rat brain, respectively. Ablation of the occipital/entorhinal cortex caused an increase in neurotrophic activity in the tissue surrounding the wound with respect to basal noninjured levels of three-fold in neonates and four-fold in adult and aged brain. Maximal activities occurred at 3 days, 6 days, and 15 days postlesion in neonatal, adult, and aged tissue, respectively, and subsequently returned to basal levels (FIG. 2b). The slower neurotrophic response to injury in the brain of older animals may be one of the determinants of the slower recovery from brain damage observed with aging.

The specificity of neurotrophic factors present in adult brain tissue 10 days postlesion was examined using neurons from various brain regions. Injured brain extract supported the survival of the neurons from all the regions examined, but the highest trophic activity was on hippocampal neu-

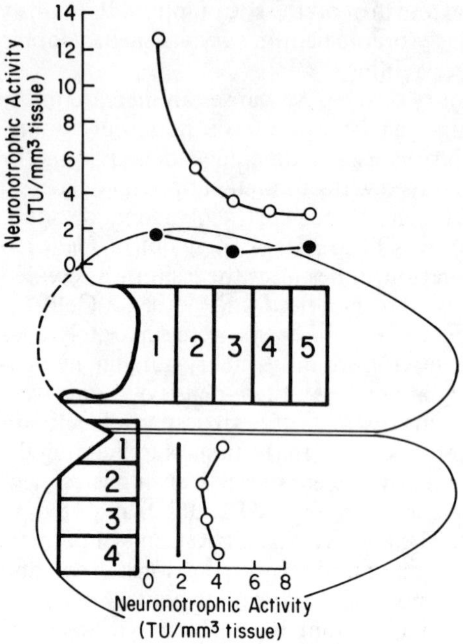

FIGURE 3. Levels of neurotrophic factors as a function of distance from an entorhinal/occipital lesion. The neurotrophic factors were assayed by means of ciliary ganglion neurons and tissue extracts prepared from animals 15 days postlesion.[15]

rons, followed by septum, striatum, and thalamus (TABLE 1). This is consistent with the hypothesis that injury-induced growth factors act preferentially on neurons connected to the injured area. Rat serum at dilutions similar to those of brain extract had little trophic activity on striatal neurons, making it extremely unlikely that injury-induced neurotrophic activity originated in blood released at the site of injury. This is supported by the finding that the tissue had higher levels of trophic acitivity than did Gelfoam extracts and that the levels rose over several days rather than immediately after the lesion was created. These observations suggest that serum or other blood-derived factors are not the sole sources of the neurotrophic activities.

TABLE 1. Neurotrophic Factors in Various Brain Regions

Region	Trophic Activity (TU/ml)
Hippocampus	7920 ± 1162 (3)
Septum	5610 ± 1373 (3)
Striatum	3115 ± 0531 (10)
Thalamus	1843 ± 0366 (8)

Neurotoxic activity was also present in noninjured brain tissue at all ages and was four-fold greater in adult and aged brain than in neonatal tissue. Toxic activity did not change in either tissue or Gelfoam after injury. It is unlikely that neurotoxic activity is due to intracellular proteolytic substances released during preparation of the extracts because leupeptin, α-macroglobulin, aprotonin, pepstatin and a mixture of all four protease inhibitors were ineffective in reducing the neuronal death caused by high concentrations of brain extract.

Thus, injury is accompanied by a time-dependent increase in the activity of neurotrophic factors effective on several neuronal types. The induction of trophic factors seems contradictory to the observed secondary loss of neurons surrounding the injury. We believe that the induction is not sufficiently rapid to provide adequate trophic factors to injured neurons so that some neurons, particularly those with very short residual axons, die in the interim. This hypothesis predicts that neurotrophic factors may prove useful in preventing secondary cell death, if provided sufficiently early. However, at present, a direct test of this hypothesis has not been carried out.

TRANSPLANTATION CAN BE ENHANCED BY TAKING ADVANTAGE OF THE NATURAL HEALING PROCESS

The requirements for neuronal survival can be further studied by transplantation techniques. Neurons introduced into the brain must first survive in order to integrate effectively into the circuitry. It seemed that the natural response of the brain might be used to facilitate the survival and integration of transplanted neurons into the host CNS. Recently, therefore, we have studied the survival and integration characteristics of transplants introduced into the host brain at various times after injury. Our results suggest that survival of neurons, particularly those that transplant with difficulty, is greatly enhanced and that their integration with the host is also improved.

Fetal rat septal, raphe, or entorhinal neurons placed into a freshly made cavity in the entorhinal cortex of a host animal survive adequately and innervate the host hippocampus.[19–22] Acetylcholinesterase (AChE)-positive neurons from embryonic corpus striatum cells show very poor survival, however, when grafted immediately after the cavity was made. In neonatal rats a delay of 3 or 6 days in the placement of the implants into the wound cavity improves their viability to 36% and 76%, respectively.[14,16,23] The delay in implantation also increases the ability of the transplant to innervate the host hippocampus and to form a lamination pattern there similar to that of the normal septal input. The differences in survival between septal and striatal AChE-positive neurons were also observed for implants into adult host rats.[15] Striatal tissues placed in a fresh cortical cavity in an adult host do not survive to any significant degree. Delaying transplantation improved the grafts' survival and, depending on the length of the delay, a range of survival scores

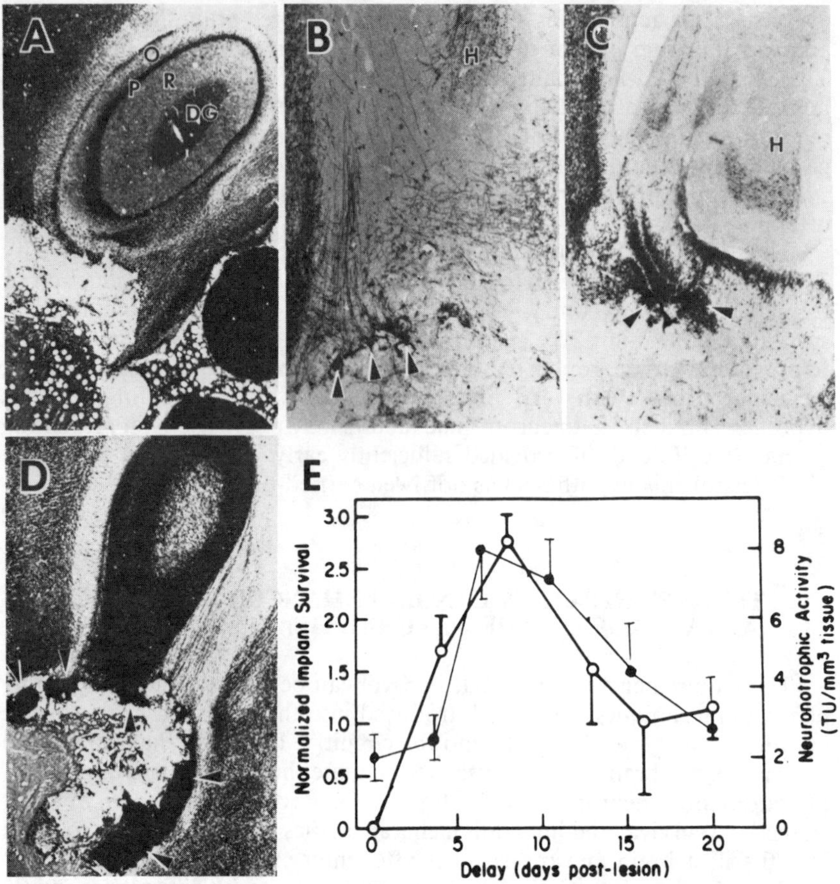

FIGURE 4. Survival of embryonic rat corpus striatum implanted into wound cavities in the entorhinal cortex of adult hosts at various times after operation. Animals were sacrificed 30 days after implantation and implant survival was graded on serial sections stained for acetylcholine esterase activity. (**A**) score 0: implanted cell survival. (**B**) score +1: a few isolated cells were observed. (**C**) score +2: groups of cells (up to 0.05 mm^3) were observed. (**D**) score +3: large clumps of cells were present. (**E**) graph of relative implant survival (○) versus delay after implantation. Also plotted on the graph is the level of neurotrophic activity in the tissue adjacent to the injury assayed *in vitro* using dissociated striatal neurons (●). Note the correlation between survival *in vivo* and *in vitro*.[15,18]

was observed (FIG. 4). Survival is optimal when implantation is delayed by about 8 days after the initial wound is made. However, significant improvement is evident as long as 20 days after surgery, the longest time point examined.[15] Survival of fetal sympathetic ganglion neurons also is greatly enhanced if transplanted several days after the lesion is made.[24]

The hypothesis that an increased concentration of trophic factors promotes the survival and growth of transplanted tissue into CNS predicts that exogenously added neurotrophic factors should enhance the survival of CNS tissue transplanted into freshly made wound cavities. Accordingly, an implant cavity was filled with injured brain extract and the implant placed in it covered either with Gelfoam soaked in wound fluid or with Gelfoam transferred directly from an animal that had received a lesion 8 days earlier. As shown in FIGURE 5, survival of transplanted striatal neurons is improved in animals supplied with extracts from injured brain.[25] It is likely that neurotrophic factors are at least in part responsible for the enhanced survival. Clearly, however, neuronal survival is also dependent on vascularization, and substances such as angiogenesis factors may be present in the extracts and contribute to their effect.

Death of transplanted neurons as well as secondary cell death may also arise from perturbation of the blood flow in the injured area, together with breakdown in the CNS–brain barrier. This results in the accumulation of many CNS and non-CNS components near the primary site of injury, including abnormal ionic concentrations and free radicals as well as many potential neurotoxins.[26] The presence of potential excitotoxins together with the ionic imbalance and the hyperexcitability attending neuronal deafferentation could also lead to neuronal death. Significantly, however, neurotrophic factors can effectively retard the deteriorative effects of many such events.[10,11]

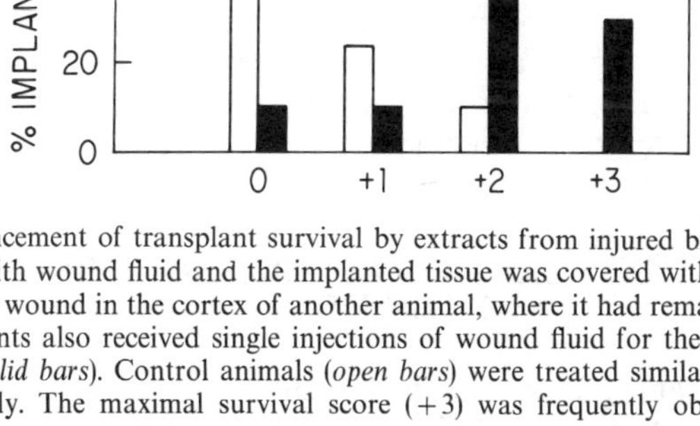

FIGURE 5. Enhancement of transplant survival by extracts from injured brain. The implant cavity was filled with wound fluid and the implanted tissue was covered with a Gelfoam fragment taken from a wound in the cortex of another animal, where it had remained the previous 8 days. The implants also received single injections of wound fluid for the first 3 days after transplantation (*solid bars*). Control animals (*open bars*) were treated similarly with balanced saline solution only. The maximal survival score (+3) was frequently observed in treated animals.[25]

PARTIAL DENERVATION PROMOTES NEW SYNAPSE FORMATION

An essential requisite for the restoration of damaged circuitry is the ability to reform new synapses. It was once believed that new synapses could not form in the mature CNS. It is now clear, however, that injury as well as other factors can stimulate new synapse formation. Neuronal death elicits a cascade of events that extend far beyond the injury site into the related circuitry. Axons disconnected from the cell body degenerate, resulting in partial denervation and causing the remaining undamaged axons to sprout and form new synapses. Reactive synaptogenesis has been extensively documented in many regions of the CNS. Almost any type of injury resulting in partial denervation triggers a reaction that culminates in the emergence of new circuitry.

Reactive synaptogenesis is robust, selective and follows a stereotyped time course. The essential features can be illustrated by briefly describing the effects of unilateral entorhinal lesion on reactive synaptogenesis in the hippocampus. One day postlesion, 90% of the synapses in the outer two-thirds of the dendritic tree of the granule cells on the side of the lesion are lost. A massive growth response begins at 3 days postlesion in which all of the residual fiber systems in the dentate gyrus, except for the raphe, participate. New synapses are formed by sprouting fibers originating in the contralateral entorhinal cortex,[27–30] the septum,[31–34] and the CA4 area (commissural/associational system).[35–38] Synapse replacement is complete by about 60 days postlesion. This results in a new mixture of synaptic inputs within the denervated zone. The newly formed synapses made by CA4 and contralateral entorhinal neurons are functional[39–42] and the homologous entorhinal fibers probably mediate the same function as the entorhinal path they replace.[43,44] Replacement occurs initially very quickly, but the full time course extends over several weeks.[45–47] Thus, it is clear that new synapses can indeed grow in the mature CNS and replace those lost by injury.[48–52]

Reactive synaptogenesis, however, cannot replace the original circuitry and, in fact, in the dentate gyrus, it results in an increase of the residual inputs proportional to their normal abundance. Thus, while reactive synaptogenesis may participate in the recovery of function in some cases, it may also compete with the process of restoration by introducing aberrant connections. Similarly, transplant fibers must compete with synapses formed by host sprouts as well as regenerating axons. Ironically, it is thus likely that reactive synaptogenesis retards regeneration in some cases, particularly in multi-innervated targets. Other natural growth responses may also retard regeneration.

INTEGRATION OF TRANSPLANTS INTO THE HOST BRAIN

Reactive synaptogenesis is limited to short-range growth occurring maximally over tens of microns.[53] Can fibers grow over long distances into the mature CNS? Studies on the outgrowth of fibers from transplanted neurons into the mature CNS have clearly shown that fibers can extend through the mature CNS over relatively long distances. The fibers from transplants are usually very successful in recreating the terminal fields of the homologous normal cell if placed in reasonable proximity to their targets. Thus, for example, septal fibers form the same trilaminar synaptic pattern on granule cell dendrites as that of the normal septal projection (FIG. 6), even if placed in the entorhinal cortex rather than in the fimbria. In growing to their proper zones they must bypass denervated fields and apparently available synaptic sites. Septal fibers from a transplant respond to an entorhinal lesion as native axons do, creating a pattern typical of the sprouted septal system. Striatal neurons placed into an entorhinal cavity can also form a projection pattern similar to that of septal fibers, even though normally they do not project to the hippocampus.[23] Transplants of monoaminergic cells also establish their own distinctive nerve-ending fields.[54,55] Therefore, the specificity of synapse formation resides in both the transplant and the host target cells.

Can fibers from transplanted neurons effectively compete with native synapses or those formed by reactive synaptogenesis? If native septal fibers or entorhinal fibers are left intact, they compete with their own native fiber type but not with heterologous fiber populations,[56,57] indicating that a strict hierarchy of synaptic regrowth exists. Fibers from septal transplants, for example, do not grow effectively if the native septal input is intact. As noted above, after an entorhinal lesion is made, reactive synaptogenesis results in the replacement and rearrangement of the synaptic fields. Can transplanted entorhinal cortex reverse reactive synaptogenesis? If the entorhinal cortex is replaced by transplantation of another entorhinal cortex, some animals display a partial reversal of the rearranged fiber systems, particularly it seems in cases where the innervation is very strong (Gibbs and Cotman, in preparation). In many cases, however, local synapse formation cannot be reversed. Thus, it seems that initiating growth is inadequate for ensuring that the initial circuitry can be restored. Apparently several other constraints exist within the terminal fields.

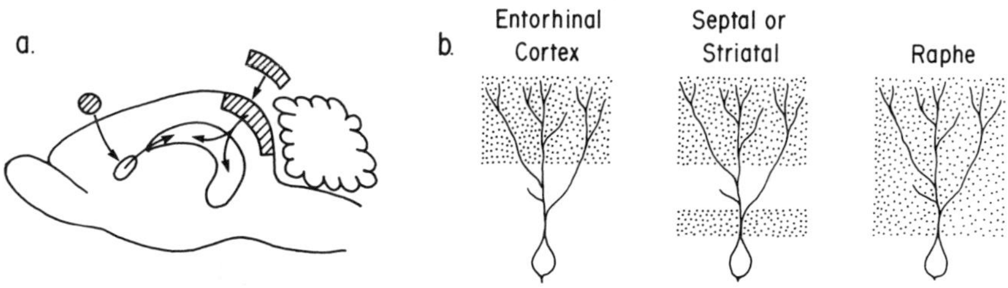

FIGURE 6. (**a**) Transplant (*crosshatched*) of embryonic cortex, septum, corpus striatum or raphe when placed either in their normal position or in a cavity of the occipital/entorhinal cortex project (*arrows*) to the dentate gyrus and form their correct synaptic fields.[53] (**b**) A dentate granule cell showing the nerve-ending fields of the various transplanted neurons.

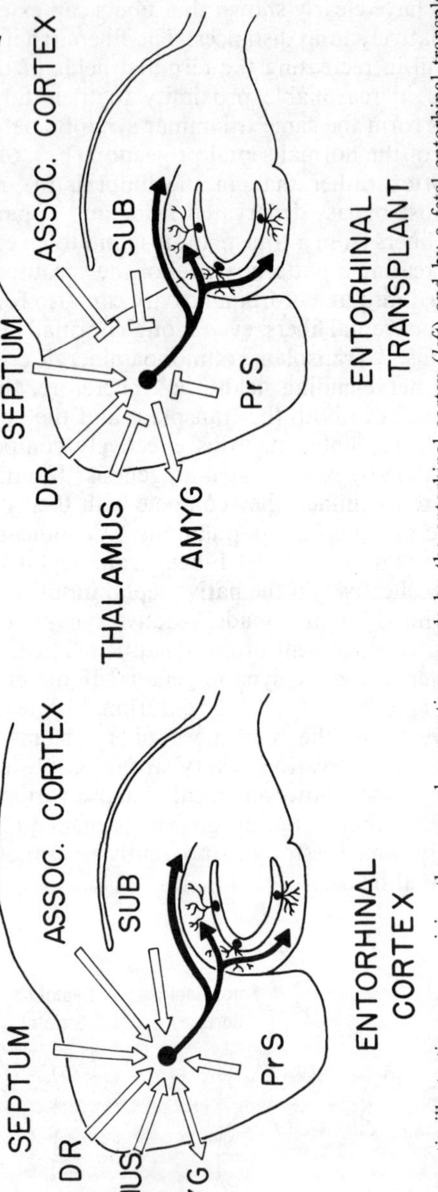

FIGURE 7. Schematic illustration summarizing the normal connections made by the entorhinal cortex (*left*) and by a fetal entorhinal transplant made in the mature rat (*right*). Axons from the entorhinal transplant relocate their proper targets (*solid arrows*), but the transplant only receives part of the inputs characteristic of the entorhinal cortex (*open arrows*). LC, locus coeruleus; DR, dorsal raphe; AMYG, amygdala; PrS, presubiculum; SUB, subiculum; ASSOC. CORTEX, associational cortex.

Very little is known at present about the nature of the inputs from the host onto transplanted neurons, though transplants probably receive synaptic input from local neurons, including those in the transplant itself. We have recently examined in detail the connectivity of embryonic entorhinal cortex implanted into adult hosts because this area contains a mixture of neuronal types that both form and receive myelinated and unmyelinated axons. The major output of the entorhinal cortex is to the hippocampal formation (perforant path) and most perforant path fibers are myelinated. The entorhinal cortex receives inputs primarily from eight other brain areas, several of which are myelinated (FIG. 7). Nearly all entorhinal transplants were found to receive three of their normal eight inputs. These are generally unmyelinated fiber systems (e.g., septal or raphe inputs). Fibers from mature myelinated neurons, however, only rarely regenerate into transplants. After partial removal of entorhinal cortex and transplantation of fetal entorhinal neurons, we have observed in select cases regeneration of fibers from the contralateral entorhinal cortex into remaining entorhinal cortex and into the transplant itself.

Thus, transplanted neurons apparently serve to stimulate incoming axons from the host as well as to innervate the host brain. If placed in the injury cavity at the right time, transplants provide appropriate growth cues to host axons that stimulate their growth and overcome the misguiding effect of the glial scar. It is also clear that peripheral nerve segments have the ability to sustain long-distance axonal growth.[58] Clearly, mature brain neurons have the capacity to grow and the brain can support such growth. However, these axons fail to penetrate long distances into the neuropile.[53]

In a sense then, transplants are incompletely integrated relay stations in injured networks since they usually do not receive their complete inputs. The terrain that axons have to cross on their way to the target presents a problem primarily for mature long-tract myelinated fibers. The reason why this occurs only in select cases and innervation is incomplete is not clear, but we suspect that it involves glial cells and the nature of the temporal organization of events resulting in the integration of host and transplant tissues.

MULTI-INNERVATED NEURONS: COMPETITIVE GROWTH AND INAPPROPRIATE TIMING HINDERS THE RESTORATION OF CIRCUITRY

Ultimately the molecular mechanism guiding the cellular responses potentially involved in repair must be elucidated. We believe that the discovery of injury-induced neurotrophic factors is a start towards developing an appropriate conceptual framework. A working hypothesis is that the source of growth and guidance factors is produced in partially denervated target areas and that the production of factors is restricted by innervation. Production decreases in the fully innervated state and increases after partial denervation. Denervation activates cells to produce neurotrophic factors and substrates, and, as reinnervation occurs, their production subsides.

The hypothesis that the production of growth factors is regulated by the extent of innervation sheds some light on why fibers may grow only over short distances in the CNS or, when induced to grow over long distances, why they fail to penetrate extensively into the target area. After injury, local sprouting reactions occur very rapidly, reinnervating the denervated target cells and arresting the production of growth and guidance factors. This may be a unique property of multi-innervated neurons and constitutes an important distinction between peripheral and central neurons. The hypothesis predicts that partial denervation at the time of arrival of regenerating fibers should result in further regenerative growth, but the prediction has not yet been tested.

THE PIVOTAL ROLE OF GLIAL CELLS

Glial cells play a critical role in the development of the nervous system; for example, they guide fibers to their appropriate places and maintain a proper ionic and trophic environment. It would also be expected that they play a critical role in renewed synapse growth in the mature brain, and indeed this is becoming increasingly evident. Glial cells also, however, present a paradox, since they potentially have both beneficial and harmful effects simultaneously.

Glial cells probably aid in providing an appropriate substrate environment for growing axons. Astrocytes produce laminin early during development, and they again secrete laminin after injury to the mature CNS.[59–61] Laminin promotes neurite formation from central as well as peripheral neurons.[62,63]

Reactive astrocytes may also be the source of most of the increase in trophic factors associated with injury. Astrocytes maintained in cell culture secrete central neurotrophic substances into the culture medium.[18,64,65] Astrocytes hypertrophy and increase in number after brain injury, and these reactive astrocytes may produce an increase in trophic factors. Histologic analysis of the tissue surrounding an injury made in the entorhinal cortex shows an increase in glial cells[66] (Nieto-Sampedro and Cotman, unpublished observations). Perhaps molecules associated with CNS injury activate glial cells, which in turn produce neutrotrophic activity.

On the other hand, astrocytes may provide a boundary to either sprouting axons from undamaged or regenerating cells. Neither undamaged fiber sprouts nor regenerating sprouts appear able to readily cross the glia-fibroblast boundary. They most frequently turn around, making contact on available synaptic sites on the same side of the area of injury. However, the mechanical barrier effect of the glial "scar" cannot be the reason for lack of fiber growth across an injury site such as a transection. Indeed, in fiber path transections in which such scars are not obvious crossing of the injury zone is not observed.[67] Still, the role of an injury area as a barrier cannot be underestimated. Bulbospinal monoamine fibers do not cross a spinal cord transection, but are able to regenerate and innervate all segments of the spinal cord after a selective chemical lesion that minimally perturbs the rest of the tissue.[68,69] The glial "scar" could exert part of its deleterious influence by misguiding axonal sprouts. Injured brain astrocytes secrete laminin,[59-61] which, as already noted, is a neurite promoter for central neurons.[62,63] Neurites tend to grow associated to glial fibers, which in development appear to provide them with guidance. However, after an injury, the formation of a new glia limitans may effectively prevent axons from crossing the transection area and steer them to inappropriate targets on the same side of the injury. This, together with suppression of local trophic factor induction, may further deter growth once it is initiated. The glial response very efficiently isolates the CNS from the outside, but it probably has disastrous effects on regeneration. Glial cells show a peculiar dichotomous role—they are both beneficial and detrimental.

It is necessary to identify the types of factors associated with injury which control glial cell activities. Surprisingly little is known about the types of molecules that are associated with injury that act on glial cell function even though such factors have been identified in the normal developing and adult CNS. Astroglial cells can be readily isolated and maintained in primary cultures consisting of about 95% pure astrocytes.[70] It is thus possible to study the correlation between *in vivo* proliferation of glia after CNS injury and the *in vitro* changes during the same period in the activity of astrocyte mitogens and morphogens.

We have recently carried out such a study.[71] A cavity of about 40–50 mm^3 was aspirated in the occipital cortex of adult rats and the cavity was filled with a fragment of Gelfoam soaked in saline solution. At postlesion intervals ranging from 1 hour to 60 days, the animals were sacrificed and the mitogenic and morphogenic activities in the tissue surrounding the wound (to a depth of 2 mm) and the Gelfoam were determined. The results (FIG. 8) show that mitogenic activity in both the tissue around the injured area and in the Gelfoam that filled that wound cavity increases considerably after injury. The maximum activity observed in the tissue peaks broadly at about 6 and 15 days postlesion, whereas in Gelfoam a sharp peak was observed at about 10 days (FIG. 8a). Simultaneously, the activity of molecules capable of causing a change in astrocyte morphology (morphogens) also increases in the tissue surrounding the wound cavity, reaching maximal values at about 20 days postlesion. Gelfoam morphogenic activity is negligible. The increase in glial mitogens and morphogens correlates with the observed gliosis in the area of injury in the brain (FIG. 8b). Furthermore, brain mitogens also promote fibroblast proliferation and collagen deposition, thereby completing the molecular justification for the formation of a collagen-fibrous glial layer covering injured CNS surfaces.

An interesting question remains concerning the control of glial populations in the CNS. The number of CNS glial cells reaches a maximum soon after birth and then remains practically constant throughout adulthood. Glial cells retain their ability to proliferate,[72] and the normal CNS contains

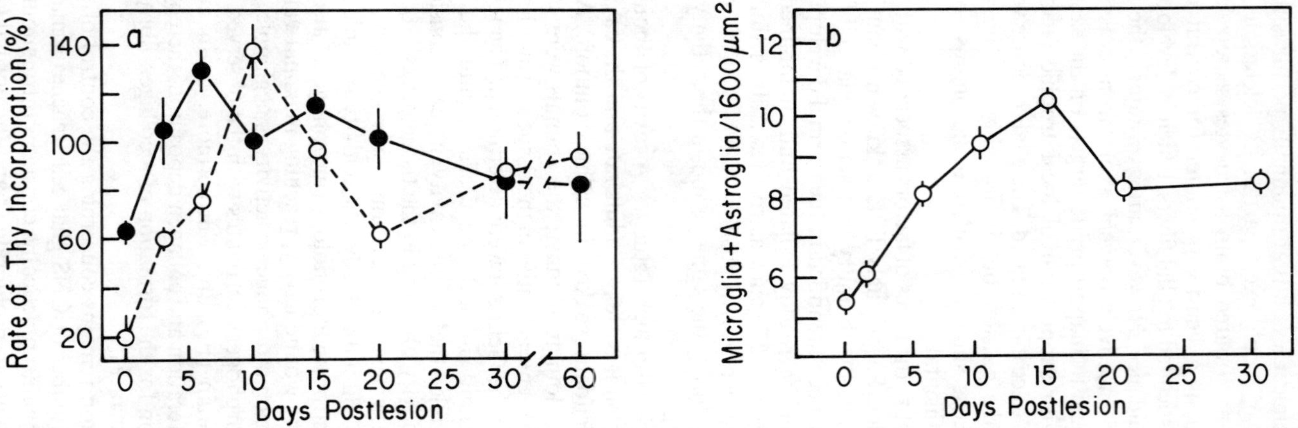

FIGURE 8. Glial cell responses *in vitro* and *in vivo*. (**a**) Changes relative to postlesion time in the mitogenic activities of extracts of brain tissue adjacent to an injury (●) and the Gelfoam that filled the wound cavity (○). Mitogenic activity was measured by the relative rate of [^{3}H] thymidine incorporation in a 6-hr period after a 20-hr exposure to several dilutions of the test extract (tissue at 10 days postlesion, 10,000 to 15,000 cpm/hr, 100%). The values are the mean (±SEM) of 12 independent experiments. (**b**) Glial cell number in the tissue surrounding a cortical wound cavity paralleled the mitogenic activity in that area at various times postlesion (Nieto-Sampedro, Kesslak and Cotman, in preparation).

molecules capable of causing division and differentiation of cultured astrocytes.[73–78] Yet in a healthy adult, glial division is a potentiality rather than a normal event.

What prevents glia from proliferating in the normal CNS? An answer to this question has been provided in two ways (Nieto-Sampedro, in preparation). In one set of experiments, we compared the dose–response curves of the mitogenic activity of extracts from normal brain and brain tissue adjacent to an injury inflicted 10 days before (FIG. 9). Not only did the injured tissue extract promote [^{3}H]thymidine incorporation at a faster rate than did normal brain extract, but also, at high concentrations of injured tissue extract, the presence of an inhibitor of the mitogenic activity in noninjured brain was apparent. Such an inhibitory factor appears to be lost after injury. The presence of an inhibitor in normal brain was confirmed in an independent set of experiments in which normal brain extract was subjected to molecular filtration through Amicon membranes. The total mitogenic activity recovered was always considerably greater than 100%. The inhibitor had an apparent molecular weight lower than 30,000 and in preliminary experiments also filtered through a PM-10 membrane (mol. wt., 10,000). The data of Hatten (1985), using defined mixtures of purified cerebellar neurons and glia, point to a similar conclusion, suggesting, in addition, that neurons may be the source of both mitogen inhibitors and glial morphogens.[79]

Brain glial mitogens seem to be immunologically different from epidermal growth factor and have mitogenic properties that distinguish them from alkaline fibroblast growth factor.[71] Several molecular species are present in both normal and injured brain tissue extracts, ranging in apparent molecular weight from around 10,000 to 36,000. Some of the mitogens share

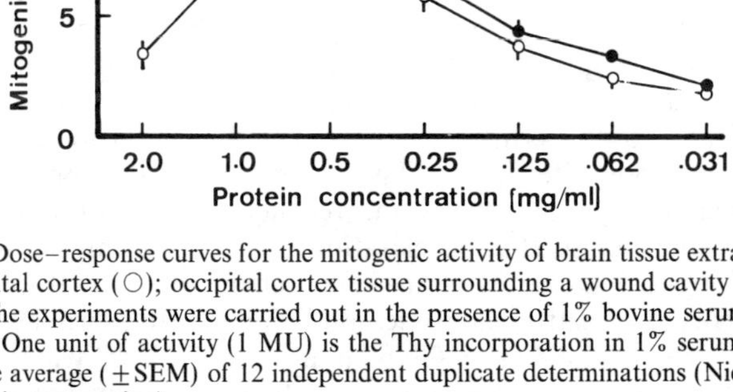

FIGURE 9. Dose–response curves for the mitogenic activity of brain tissue extract from: normal rat occipital cortex (○); occipital cortex tissue surrounding a wound cavity 10 days postlesion (●). The experiments were carried out in the presence of 1% bovine serum (either fetal or newborn). One unit of activity (1 MU) is the Thy incorporation in 1% serum in 1 hr. The results are the average (±SEM) of 12 independent duplicate determinations (Nieto-Sampedro and Cotman, in preparation).

physicochemical properties with interleukin-1 (IL-1), and monoclonal antibodies to purified human IL-1 inhibit 50 to 70% of the brain mitogen activity on astrocytes and almost 100% of it on fibroblasts.[80] Therefore, at least one of the mitogens is an IL-1-like molecule if not IL-1 itself. This point of contact between the CNS and the immune system also helps to understand how the CNS response to injury may be initiated. Injury would make the brain accessible to serum proteins, some of which will enter directly or following endocytosis[81] and act to suppress inhibition of mitogens as well as to induce an increase in the activity of these molecules. The new directions of research point to new clues toward developing appropriate molecular interventions.

CONCLUSION

It is now clear that the CNS can mobilize many of the responses that are necessary for the restoration of its circuitry. Some occur naturally, while others can be induced. In response to injury, factors are produced that stimulate glial cell division and morphogenesis. These cells seal off the injury and also probably give rise to neurotrophic factors which can act on injured neurons. The CNS increases the production of neurotrophic factors that appear to aid in preserving nerve cells and in facilitating their growth. Transplantation can be used to replace lost neurons. These neurons survive and innervate the host brain, although the inputs they receive are limited. Transplant survival and growth are improved if transplantation is carried out several days after the injury, when neurotrophic factors are induced. This suggests that the healing response of the CNS will facilitate successful transplantation and probably also restoration of its normal circuitry. New synapse formation is essential for the reconstruction of injured circuitry. Axons from undamaged neurons will sprout and form new functional synapses. Axons from damaged neurons are normally unsuccessful at regenerating completely, but both peripheral and central nervous system transplants will support their successful regeneration.

Thus, enhanced neuronal synapse survival, regrowth, and regeneration are all within the range of potentialities of the mature CNS. Major steps need to be taken to optimally couple these processes. Progress at the molecular level should eventually make this possible. For example, the purification and cloning of growth and substrate factors should open the way for new therapeutic methods that facilitate natural responses. Secondary neuronal death could perhaps be prevented if neurotrophic factors were made available soon after injury. The inductive period is probably critical. Similarly, reactive synaptogenesis and regenerative growth appear to compete with each other so that accelerating regeneration may result in more successful long-distance growth. In development, the growth of long pathways must occur at particular times and there is also probably a critical interval for regeneration after CNS injury, particularly when similar cell types are competing for synaptic space. There are many unresolved questions concerning the response to injury. Yet in spite of the many unsolved problems, the realization that the CNS has many of the necessary capacities to repair damage represents a major advance toward conceptualizing approaches for the treatment of CNS injury and a new neurology in the foreseeable future.

REFERENCES

1. KLATZO, I. 1967. Neuropathological aspects of brain edema. J. Neuropathol. Exp. Neurol. **26:** 1–14.
2. HIRANO, A. 1969. The fine structure of brain in edema. *In* The Structure and Function of the Nervous Tissue. G. H. Bourne, Ed.: 69–135. Academic Press. New York, NY.
3. ROSE, G., G. LYNCH & C. W. COTMAN. 1976. Hypertrophy and redistribution of astrocytes in the deafferented dentate gyrus. Brain Res. Bull. **1:** 87–92.
4. KAO, C. C. & L. W. CHANG. 1977. The mechanism of spinal cord cavitation following spinal cord transection. Part 1: A correlative histochemical study. J. Neurosurg. **46:** 197–209.
5. CLEMENTE, C. D. 1955. Structural regeneration in the mammalian CNS and the role of neuroglia and connective tissue. *In* Regeneration in the Central Nervous System. W. F. Windle, Ed.: 147–161. Charles C. Thomas. Springfield, IL.
6. ADRIAN, E. K. & M. G. WILLIAMS. 1973. Cell proliferation in injured spinal cord. An electron microscopic study. J. Comp Neurol. **151:** 1–24.
7. WINDLE, W. F. 1956. Regeneration of axons in the vertebrate central nervous system. Physiol. Rev. **36:** 427–440.
8. KRIKORIAN, J. G., L. GUTH & E. DONATI. 1981. The origin of connective tissue scar in the transected rat spinal cord. Exp. Neurol. **72:** 698–707.
9. COTMAN, C. W., M. NIETO-SAMPEDRO & E. HARRIS. 1981. Synapse replacement in the nervous system of adult vertebrates. Physiol. Rev. **61:** 684–784.
10. THOENEN, H. & Y.-A. BARDE. 1980. Physiology of nerve growth factor. Physiol. Rev. **60:** 1284–1335.
11. BERG, D. K. 1984. New neuronal growth factors. Ann. Rev. Neurosci. **7:** 149–170.
12. EBENDAL, T., L. OLSON, A. SEIGER & K. O. HEDLUND. 1980. Nerve growth factors in the rat iris. Nature **286:** 25–28.
13. LUNDBORG, G., F. M. LONGO & S. VARON. 1982. Nerve regeneration model and trophic factors *in vivo*. Brain Res. **232:** 157–161.
14. NIETO-SAMPEDRO, M., E. R. LEWIS, C. W. COTMAN, M. MANTHORPE, S. D. SKAPER, G. BARBIN, F. M. LONGO & S. VARON. Brain injury causes a time-dependent increase in neuronotrophic activity at the lesion site. Science **2217:** 860–861.
15. NIETO-SAMPEDRO, M., M. MANTHORPE, G. BARBIN, S. VARON & C. W. COTMAN. 1983. Injury-induced neuronotrophic activity in adult rat brain: Correlation with survival of delayed implants in the wound cavity. J. Neurosci. **3:** 2219–2229.
16. MANTHORPE, M., M. NIETO-SAMPEDRO, S. D. SKAPER, E. R. LEWIS, G. BARBIN, F. M. LONGO, C. W. COTMAN & S. VARON. 1983. Neuronotrophic activity in brain wounds of the developing rat. Correlation with implant survival in the wound cavity. Brain Res. **267:** 47–56.
17. NEEDELS, D. L., M. NIETO-SAMPEDRO, S. R. WHITTEMORE & C. W. COTMAN. 1985. Neuronotrophic activity for ciliary ganglion neurons. Induction following injury to the brain of neonatal, adult and aged rats. Dev. Brain Res. **18:** 275–284.
18. WHITTEMORE, S. R., M. NIETO-SAMPEDRO, D. L. NEEDELS & C. W. COTMAN. 1985. Neuronotrophic factors for mammalian brain neurons: Injury induction in neonatal, adult and aged rat brain. Dev. Brain Res. **20:** 169–178.
19. BJÖRKLUND, A. & U. STENEVI. 1977. Reformation of severed septohippocampal cholinergic pathways in the adult rat by transplanted septal neurons. Cell Tissue Res. **185:** 289–302.

20. HOLETS, V. T. & C. W. COTMAN. 1984. Postnatal development of the serotonin innervation of the hippocampus and dentate gyrus: Normal development and reinnervation following raphe implants. J. Comp. Neurol. **226:** 457–476.
21. LEWIS, E. R., J. C. MUELLER & C. W. COTMAN. 1980. Neonatal septal implants: Development of afferent lamination in the rat dentate gyrus. Brain Res. Bull. **5:** 217–221.
22. GIBBS, R., E. W. HARRIS & C. W. COTMAN. Replacement of damaged cortical projections by homotypic transplants of entorhinal cortex. Submitted for publication.
23. LEWIS, E. R. & C. W. COTMAN. 1983. Neurotransmitter characteristics of brain grafts: Striatal and septal tissues form the same laminated input to hippocampus. Neuroscience **8:** 57–66.
24. GAGE, F., A. BJÖRKLUND & U. STENEVI. 1984. Denervation releases a neuronal survival factor in adult rat hippocampus. Nature **308:** 637–639.
25. NIETO-SAMPEDRO, M., S. R. WHITTEMORE, D. L. NEEDELS, J. LARSON & C. W. COTMAN. 1984. The survival of brain transplants is enhanced by extracts from injured brain. Proc. Natl. Acad. Sci. USA. **81:** 6250–6254.
26. FADEN, A. I. 1983. Recent pharmacological advances in experimental spinal injury. TINS **6:** 375–377.
27. STEWARD, O., C. W. COTMAN & G. S. LYNCH. 1974. Growth of a new fiber projection in the brain of adult rats: Re-innervation of the dentate gyrus by the contralateral entorhinal cortex following ipsilateral entorhinal lesions. Exp. Brain. Res. **20:** 45–66.
28. ZIMMER, J., & A. HJORTH-SIMONSEN. 1975. Crossed pathways from the entorhinal area to the fascia dentate. II. Provokable in rats. J. Comp. Neurol. **161:** 71–101.
29. STEWARD, O., C. W. COTMAN & G. S. LYNCH. 1976. A quantitative autoradiographic and electrophysiological study of the reinnervation of the dentate gyrus by the contralateral entorhinal cortex following ipsilateral entorhinal lesions. Brain Res. **114:** 181–200.
30. COTMAN, C. W., C. GENTRY & O. STEWARD. 1977. Synaptic replacement in the dentate gyrus after unilateral entorhinal lesion: Electron microscopic analysis of the extent of replacement of synapses by the remaining entorhinal cortex. J. Neurocytol. **6:** 455–464.
31. LYNCH, G. S., D. A. MATTHEWS, S. MOSKO, T. PARKS & C. W. COTMAN. 1972. Induced acetylcholinesterase-rich layer in rat dentate gyrus following entorhinal lesions. Brain Res. **42:** 311–318.
32. COTMAN, C. W., D. A. MATTHEWS, D. TAYLOR & G. S. LYNCH. 1973. Synaptic rearrangement in the dentate gyrus: Histochemical evidence of adjustments after lesions in immature and adult rats. Proc. Natl. Acad. Sci. USA **70:** 3473–3477.
33. STORM-MATHISEN, J. 1974. Choline acetyltransferase and acetylcholinesterase in fascia dentate following lesion of the entorhinal afferents. Brain Res. **80:** 181–197.
34. STEWARD, O. & J. A. MESSENHEIMER. 1978. Histochemical evidence for a postlesion reorganization of cholinergic afferents in the hippocampal formation of the mature cat. J. Comp. Neurol. **178:** 697–710.
35. ZIMMER, J. 1973. Extended commissural and ipsilateral projections in postnatally deentorhinated hippocampus and fascia dentata demonstrated in rats by silver impregnation. Brain Res. **64:** 293–311.
36. WEST, J. R., S. A. DEADWYLER, C. W. COTMAN & G. LYNCH. 1975. Time-dependent changes in commissural field potentials in the dentate gyrus following lesions of the entorhinal cortex in adult rats. Brain Res. **97:** 215–233.
37. LYNCH, G., C. GALL, G. ROSE & C. W. COTMAN. 1976. Changes in the distribution of the dentate gyrus associational system following unilateral or bilateral entorhinal lesions in the adult rat. Brain Res. **110:** 57–71.
38. LEE, K. S., E. J. STANFORD, C. W. COTMAN & G. S. LYNCH. 1977. Ultra-structural evidence for bouton proliferation in the partially deafferented dentate gyrus of the adult rat. Exp. Brain Res. **29:** 475–485.
39. STEWARD, O., C. W. COTMAN & G. S. LYNCH. 1973. Re-establishment of electrophysiologically functional entorhinal cortical input to the dentate gyrus deafferented by ipsilateral entorhinal lesions: Innervation by the contralateral entorhinal cortex. Exp. Brain Res. **18:** 396–414.

40. STEWARD, O., W. F. WHITE, C. W. COTMAN & G. LYNCH. 1976. Potentiation of excitatory synaptic transmission in the normal and in the reinnervated dentate gyrus of the rat. Exp. Brain Res. **26:** 423–441.
41. HARRIS, E. W., S. S. LASHER & O. STEWARD. 1978. Habituation-like decrements along the normal and lesion-indued temporodentate pathways in the rat. Brain Res. **150:** 623–631.
42. WILSON, R. C., W. B. LEVY & O. STEWARD. 1979. Functional effects of lesion-induced plasticity: Long-term potentiation in normal and lesion-induced temporodentate connections. Brain Res. **176:** 65–78.
43. MESSENHEIMER, J. A., E. W. HARRIS & O. STEWARD. 1979. Sprouting fibers gain access to circuitry transynaptically altered by kindling. Exp. Neurol. **64:** 469–481.
44. STEWARD, O. 1982. Assessing the functional significance of lesion-induced neuronal plasticity. Int. Rev. Neurobiol. **23:** 197–254.
45. MATTHEWS, D. A., C. W. COTMAN & G. S. LYNCH. 1976. An electron microscopic study of lesion-induced synaptogenesis in the dentate gyrus of the adult rat. I. Magnitude and time course of degeneration. Brain Res. **115:** 1–21.
46. HOFF, S. F., S. W. SCHEFF & C. W. COTMAN. 1982. Lesion-induced synaptogenesis in the dentate gyrus of aged rats: Demonstration of an impaired clearing response. J. Comp. Neurol. **205:** 253–259.
47. VIJAYAN, V. K. & C. W. COTMAN. 1983. Lysosomal enzyme changes in young and aged control and entorhinal-lesioned rats. Neurobiol. Aging **4:** 13–23.
48. MATTHEWS, D. A., C. W. COTMAN & G. S. LYNCH. 1976. An electron microscopic study of lesion-induced synaptogenesis in the dentate gyrus of the adult rat. II. Reappearance of morphologically normal contacts. Brain Res. **115:** 23–41.
49. RAISMAN, G. & P. M. FIELD. 1973. A quantitative investigation of the development of collateral reinnervation after partial deafferentation of the septal nuclei. Brain Res. **50:** 241–264.
50. MCWILLIAMS, R. & G. LYNCH. 1978. Terminal potentiation and synaptogenesis following partial deafferentation: The reinnervation of the inner molecular layer of the dentate gyrus following removal of its commissural afferents. J. Comp. Neurol. **180:** 581–616.
51. HOFF, S. F., S. W. SCHEFF, L. S. BENARDO & C. W. COTMAN. 1982. Lesion-induced synaptogenesis in the dentate gyrus of aged rats: I. Loss and reacquisition of normal synaptic density. J. Comp. Neurol. **205:** 246–252.
52. MCWILLIAMS, R. & G. LYNCH. 1983. Rate of synaptic replacement in denervated rat hippocampus declines precipitiously from the junvenile period to adulthood. Science **221:** 572–574.
53. COTMAN, C. W. & M. NIETO-SAMPEDRO. 1984. Cell biology of synaptic plasticity. Science **225:** 1287–1294.
54. AZMITIA, E. C., M. J. PERLOW, M. J. BRENNAN & J. M. LAUDER. 1981. Fetal raphe and hippocampal transplants into adult and aged C57BL/6N mice: A preliminary immunocytochemical study. Brain Res. Bull. **7:** 703–710.
55. BJÖRKLUND, A., U. STENEVI & N.-A. SVENDGAARD. 1976. Growth of transplanted monoaminergic neurons into the adult hippocampus along the perforant path. Nature **262:** 787–790
56. LEWIS, E. R. & C. W. COTMAN. 1982. Mechanisms of septal lamination in the developing hippocampus revealed outgrowth of fibers from septal implants. III. Competitive interactions. Brain Res. **233:** 29–44.
57. BJÖRKLUND, A. & U. STENEVI. 1977. Reformation of the severed septohippocampal cholinergic pathway in the adult rat by transplanted septal neurons. Cell Tissue Res. **185:** 289–302.
58. AGUAYO, A. J. 1985. Axonal regeneration from injured neurons in the adult mammalian central nervous system. *In* Synaptic Plasticity and Remodeling. C. W. Cotman, Ed. Guildford Press, New York, NY. In press.
59. LIESI, P., D. DAHL & A. VAHERI. 1983. Laminin is produced by early rat astrocytes in primary culture. J. Cell Biol. **96:** 920–924.
60. LIESI, P., S. KAAKKOLA, D. DAHL & A. VAHERI. 1984. Laminin is induced in astrocytes of adult brain by injury. Embo J. **3:** 683–686.

61. LIESI, P., D. DAHL & A. VAHERI. 1984. Neurons cultured from developing rat brain attach and spread preferentially to laminin. J. Neurosci. Res. **11:** 241–251.
62. MANTHORPE, M., E. ENGVALL, E. RUOSLAHTI, F. M. LONGO, G. E. DAVIS & S. VARON. 1983. Laminin promotes neurite regeneration from cultured peripheral and central neurons. J. Cell Biol. **97:** 1882–1890.
63. ROGERS, S. L., P. C. LETOURNEAU, S. L. PALM, J. MCCARTHY & L. T. FARCHT. 1983. Neurite extension by peripheral and central nervous system neurons in response to substratum-bound fibronectin and laminin. Dev. Biol. **98:** 212–220.
64. BANKER, G. 1980. Trophic interactions between astroglial cells and hippocampal neurons in culture. Science **209:** 809–810.
65. MULLER, H. W. & W. SEIFERT. 1982. A neurotrophic factor (NTF) released from primary glial cultures supports survival and fiber outgrowth of cultured hippocampal neurons. J. Neurosci. Res. **8:** 195–204.
66. AZMITIA, E. C. & P. M. WHITAKER. 1983. Formation of a glial scar following microinjection of fetal neurons into the hippocampus or midbrain of adult rat: An immunocytochemical study. Neurosci. Lett. **38:** 145–150.
67. GUTH, L., C. P. BARRETT, E. J. DONATI, S. S. DASHPANDE & E. ALBUQUERQUE. 1981. Histopathological reactions and axonal regeneration in the transected spinal cord of hibernating squirrels. J. Comp. Neurol. **203:** 297–308.
68. NOBIN, H. G., A. BAUMGARTEN, A. BJÖRKLUND, L. LACHENMAYER & U. STENEVI. 1973. Axonal degeneration and regeneration of the bulbospinal indolamine neurons after 5,6-dihydroxytryptamine treatment. Brain Res. **56:** 1–24.
69. NYGREN, L. G. & L. OLSON. 1977. Intracisternal neurotoxins and monoamine neurons innervating the spinal cord: Acute and chronic effects on cell and axon counts and nerve terminal densities. Histochemistry **52:** 281–306.
70. MCCARTHY, K. D. & J. DE VELLIS. 1980. Preparation of separate astroglial and oligodendroglial cell cultures from rat cerebral tissue. J. Cell Biol. **85:** 890–902.
71. NIETO-SAMPEDRO, M., R. P. SANETO, J. DE VELLIS & C. W. COTMAN. 1985. The control of glial populations in brain: Changes in astrocyte mitogenic and morphogenic factors in response to injury. Brain Res. **343:** 320–328.
72. STURROCK, R. R. 1982. Cell division in the normal central nervous system. Advan. Cell Neurobiol. **3:** 3–33.
73. BROCKES, J. P., G. E. LEMKE & D. R. BALZE. 1980. Purification and preliminary characterization. of a glial growth factor from the bovine pituitary. J. Biol Chem. **255:** 8374–8377.
74. KATO, T., Y. FUKUI, D. E. TURRIFF, S. NAKAGAWA, R. LIM, B. G. W. ARNASON & R. TANAKA. 1981. Glia maturation factor in bovine brain: Partial purification and physicochemical characterization. Brain Res. **212:** 393–402.
75. LIM, R., K. MITSUNOBU & W. K. P. LI. 1973. Maturation-stimulating effect of brain extract and dibutyryl cyclic AMP on dissociated embryonic brain cells in culture. Exp. Cell Res. **79:** 243–247.
76. MORRISON, R. S., R. P. SANETO & J. DE VELLIS. 1982. Developmental expression of rat brain mitogens for cultured astrocytes. Neurosci. Res. **8:** 435–442.
77. PETTMAN, B., M. SENSENBRENNER & G. LABOURDETTE. 1980. Isolation of a glial maturation factor from beef brain. FEBS Lett. **118:** 195–199.
78. PRUSS, R. M., P. F. BARTLETT, J. GAVRILOVIC, R. P. LISAK & S. RATTRAY. 1982. Mitogen for glial cells: A comparison of the response of cultured astrocytes, oligodendrocytes and Schwann cells. Dev. Brain Res. **2:** 19–35.
79. HATTEN, M. B. 1985. Neuronal regulation of astroglial morphology and proliferation *in vitro*. J. Cell Biol. **100:** 384–396.
80. NIETO-SAMPEDRO, M., G. CHANDI, M. BERMAN, S. GUPTA & C. W. COTMAN. Interleukin effects on cultured brain astrocytes. Submitted for publication.
81. TRACHTENBERG, M. C. 1983. Glial endocytosis of protein in the traumatized brain. J. Neurosci. Res. **9:** 413–423.

Transplantation of Monoamine-Producing Cell Systems *in Oculo* and Intracranially: Experiments in Search of a Treatment for Parkinson's Disease[a]

LARS OLSON,[b,c] ERIK-OLOF BACKLUND,[d] WILLIAM FREED,[e] MARIO HERRERA-MARSCHITZ,[f] BARRY HOFFER,[g] ÅKE SEIGER,[c] AND INGRID STRÖMBERG[c]

Departments of [c]Histology and [f]Pharmacology
Karolinska Institute
S-10401 Stockholm, Sweden

[d]Department of Neurosurgery
Haukeland Hospital
Bergen, Norway

[e]Preclinical Neurosciences Section
Adult Psychology Branch
National Institutes of Mental Health
St. Elizabeth's Hospital
Washington, D.C. 20032

[g]Department of Pharmacology
University of Colorado Medical Center
Denver, Colorado 80262

The adult mammalian central nervous system (CNS) is probably the most complex structure known to man. This fact and the irreversibility of most forms of clinical brain damage are the basis for the long-held belief that the adult brain cannot repair itself and cannot be repaired. The permanent disabilities of patients with spinal cord lesions are a constant reminder of the force of this dogma. There are, however, reasons to challenge the view that CNS lesions cannot be repaired.

In order to gain insight into how reparative neuronal growth might occur, it is important to learn more about how the CNS is formed. Studies of mechanisms that control brain development—and particularly of the initiation, direction, selectivity, and cessation of neurite growth—are necessary

[a] This work was supported by Grants 14P-5867, 14X-03185, 14X-06555, and 25P-6326 from the Swedish Medical Research Council, the Expressen Prenatal Research Foundation, and by the Swedish Council for Planning and Coordination of Research (image analysis system), Magnus Bergvalls Stiftelse, and Karolinska Institutets Fonder.

[b] Address for correspondence: Lars Olson, Department of Histology, Karolinska Institute, Box 60400, S-104 01 Stockholm, Sweden.

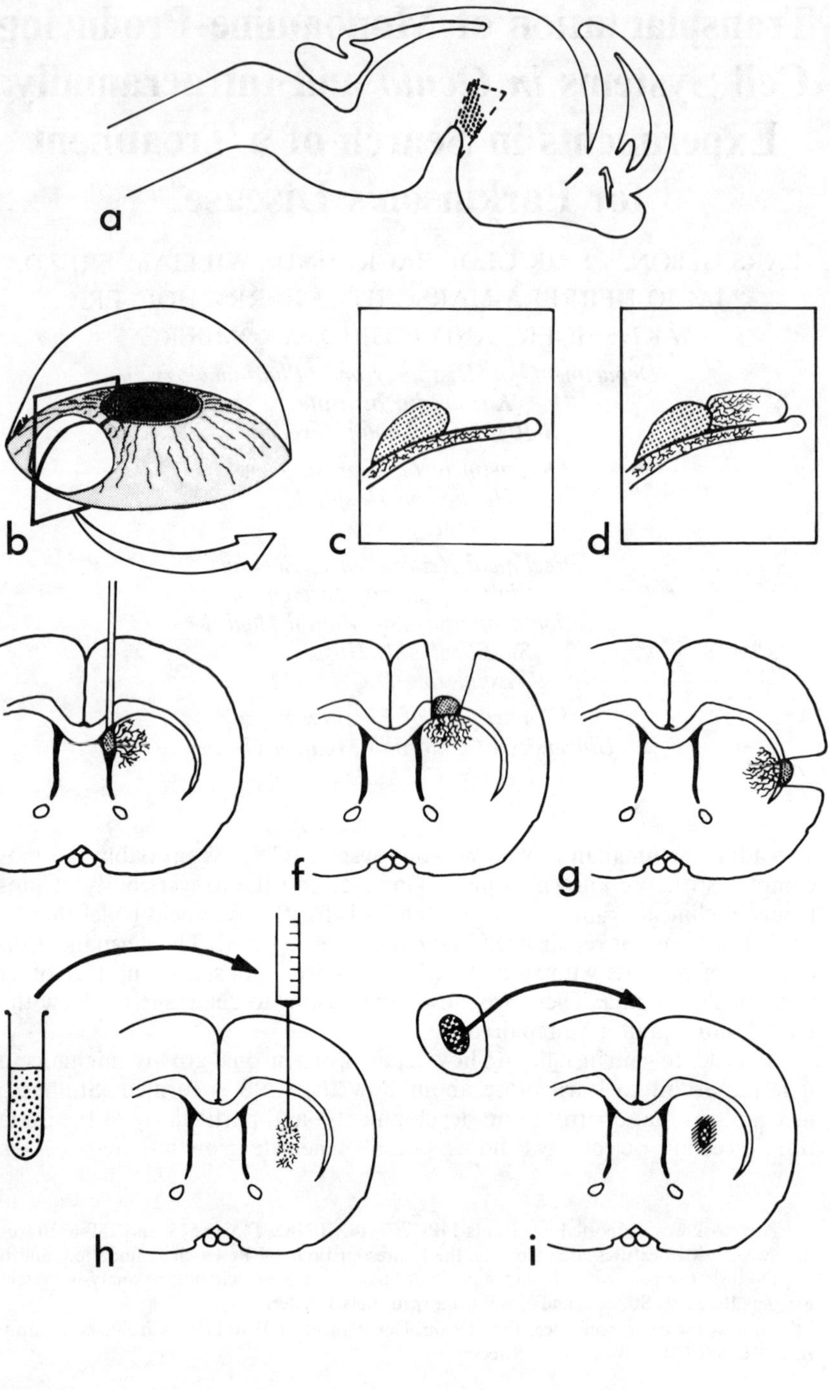
a
b
c
d
e
f
g
h
i

to understand how disturbances of brain development as well as malfunction of the adult brain may come about and how they should be prevented or treated.

There are two principal ways of reducing the degree of complexity when studying the CNS. One is to move along the phylogenetic axis to animals with more simple, and thus more accessible, nervous systems. The other approach, which will be discussed in this paper, is to isolate small defined areas of the developing CNS from the rest of the CNS by grafting to a non-CNS site. In the following, we shall discuss how transplantation of tissues to the anterior chamber of the eye in rodents can be used to learn about nerve growth and development. Experience gathered in this model system will then be used in transplantations to the brain of animals with an experimentally induced parkinsonism. The various transplantation procedures used by us and others are schematically illustrated in FIGURE 1. Finally, our recent attempts at counteracting some of the symptoms of Parkinson's disease in patients using intracranial transplantations will be described.

INTRAOCULAR TRANSPLANTATION: VERSATILE SYSTEM FOR STUDIES OF NERVE GROWTH AND DEVELOPMENT

The anterior chamber of the eye is a classical site for transplantation studies.[27,28,37] It is particularly well suited for grafting fetal brain tissue, and should be looked upon not as an alternative to tissue culture, but as a bridge between tissue culture methods and whole-animal studies. The technique has recently been described in detail.[35] Tissues to be grafted may have

FIGURE 1. Schematic illustration of transplantation procedures involving grafts of catecholamine-producing cell systems to the anterior chamber of the eye and to the brain. (**a**) Sagittal section through the fetal brain at embryonic day 17. The developing substantia nigra area containing dopamine neuroblasts is shown as the *stippled area.* From the area at the mesencephalic flexure, pieces are microdissected and used for the various grafting procedures depicted in (**b–h**). (**b**) Graft of substantia nigra to the anterior chamber of the eye is schematically illustrated after intraocular maturation. The graft has become attached to and vascularized from the host iris. (**c** and **d**) Sections through graft and host iris show that dopamine nerve terminals from the graft are able to innervate the host iris (**c**) and are also able to innervate a co-graft, e.g., of striatum (**d**). (**e–h**) Various types of grafting of fetal central dopamine neurons to the brain. In all cases, the right striatum has been deprived of its dopamine innervation by a 6-hydroxydopamine denervation prior to grafting. (**e**) Fetal substantia nigra was implanted into the lateral ventricle. At this position it attaches to the medial surface of host striatum and reinnervates dorsomedial aspects of host striatum. (**f** and **g**) Use of the delayed cavity approach, in which cortex and corpus callosum are first removed to create a cavity. Substantia nigra grafts are placed at the bottom of the cavities. They will then partially reinnervate either dorsal or lateral aspects of host striatum. (**h**) Use of dissociated cells. Mechanically or enzymatically dissociated cell suspensions containing dopamine neuroblasts and other cells from the dissected region are injected stereotaxically into the desired target in striatum. Cells survive along the injection tract to innervate surrounding areas. (**i**) Use of chromaffin tissue from the adrenal medulla. Pieces of the medulla are dissected free of surrounding cortex and stereotaxically grafted into striatum, as illustrated, or into the lateral ventricle in the way shown in (**e**). From an intrastriatal adrenal medullary graft, catecholamines will spread by diffusion into adjacent areas of host striatum.

a volume of 1–3 mm^3 and are introduced into the anterior chamber through a slit opening in the cornea by means of a modified Pasteur pipet. Once in the eye chamber, grafts can be pushed to the desired position in the lateral angle between the anterior surface of the iris and the inner surface of the cornea by applying gentle pressure to the temporarily collapsed cornea. The whole operation takes but a few minutes; there is no bleeding. The cut in the cornea will heal rapidly and intraocular pressure is regained within hours. Vision is usually preserved. Thus, in all, this is probably one of the least harmful transplantation procedures that can be performed in an experimental animal.

A specific time- and animal-saving feature of the intraocular transplantation site is that the grafts can be inspected repeatedly postoperatively through the cornea (FIG. 2). Thus "taking," vascularization, and growth can be followed for individual grafts. Survival and growth of brain tissue is excellent.[37] The eye is, in essence, a protrusion of the central nervous system, already carrying CNS tissue in the form of the retina, and the aqueous humor

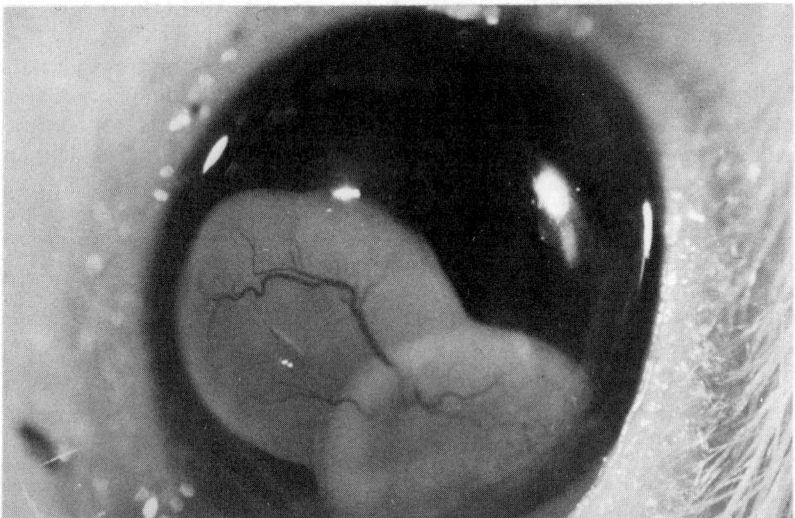

FIGURE 2. In situ appearance of double brain grafts after intraocular maturation. In this case a fetal substantia nigra piece was grafted first (*lower right graft*). After 6 weeks a fetal parietal cortex piece (*upper left graft*) was placed close to the nigral graft. After an additional 6 weeks, the eye contained two rounded, well-demarcated, partly fused mature brain areas. Blood vessels derived from the host eye arborize in the two grafts. The overlying cornea is clear and undisturbed. Original magnification × 12; reduced by 25%. (From Olson *et al.*[36] Reprinted by permission from *Experimental Brain Research.*)

is similar to cerebrospinal fluid. Another advantageous feature is probably that the anterior half of the eye is specialized in maintaining nonvascularized tissues such as the cornea and the lens. It is likely that direct oxygenation through the cornea as well as nutrition from the aqueous humor improve graft survival during the initial nonvascular phase. The anterior surface of the iris has minimal epithelial coverage, and a rapid so-called stromal reaction occurs attaching the graft to the iris. Blood vessels in the iris will connect to proliferating epithelial buds within the graft, and thus vascularization will be established within a few days. The available evidence suggests that blood vessels within the graft are mainly derived from the graft. Thus, graft vessels have pericytes and a blood–brain barrier. Whether this barrier is less developed than the normal blood–brain barrier remains to be investigated.

Grafts will remain viable in the anterior chamber as long as the host animal lives. They will grow and develop largely according to intrinsic, genetically determined programs, after which they will age at a normal rate. In very old grafts accumulations of lipofuscin pigment granules and calcifications can be seen.

Several interesting possibilities to study nerve fiber growth and function are possible in the anterior eye chamber system.[27,28,37] First, it is interesting to study by structural and functional techniques how various defined and isolated areas of the developing central nervous system are able to develop with no connections to the rest of the brain. Such experiments could not be done in tissue culture because of the lack of vascularization, and therefore greatly decreased possibilities of growth and cellular proliferation. This type of analysis of single intraocular grafts becomes a way of differentiating between the relative importance of intrinsic genetically programmed determinants of development versus the importance of influences from the environment. Second, many different types of CNS grafts are able to extend nerve fibers into the host iris. Here, they will form an almost two-dimensional network that can be studied with proper histochemical and immunohistochemical methods in "stretch-prepared" whole mounts of the iris. Thus nerve fibers that normally form complex three-dimensional networks intermingled with many other different types of nerves in the brain, can be isolated and studied in more detail.

The intrinsic innervation of the iris offers several interesting possibilities for studies of interaction between various types of growing nerve fibers. Adrenergic nerves from the superior cervical ganglion and cholinergic nerves from the ciliary ganglion as well as several different types of sensory nerves, many of which are derived from the trigeminal ganglion, may interact with nerve fibers emanating from grafted tissues. Selected removal of various combinations of the ganglia supplying the iris with nerve fibers permits studies of interaction between defined types of nerves. A further, most valuable feature of the innervation apparatus of the iris is that peripheral iridic nerves are able to invade and, in many instances, functionally innervate grafted brain tissues. This feature is easy to demonstrate by grafting whole embryonic hearts to the eye chamber; they will become innervated by adrenergic and cholinergic nerves from the host iris. Thus, their intraocular beating frequency will be completely controlled by the light input to the eye since the same set of nerve fibers regulates the pupillary diameter.[34]

Third, it is possible to graft more than one tissue piece to the eye chamber. By double simultaneous or, preferably, sequential grafting of two brain areas, isolated living replicas of known CNS pathways can be created in the eye chamber.[36] Sequential grafting can also be used to study whether or not a given brain area is able to functionally innervate another area. Recently, competition for common target areas has been evaluated using the intraocular approach by grafting three pieces to the eye chamber.

INTRAOCULAR GRAFTS OF CENTRAL MONOAMINE NEURON SYSTEMS

All areas of the central nervous system hitherto tested have survived grafting to the eye chamber and have developed more or less organotypically, provided that the right stage is chosen for grafting.[27,28,37] For certain areas, such as the cerebellar cortex, it is critical to take the early developing bud in order to obtain good survival, while for other areas, such as the adrenergic nucleus locus coeruleus, good neuronal survival is obtained from a wider range of developmental stages. Dopamine neurons from the substantia nigra area, noradrenaline neurons from locus coeruleus, and serotonin neurons from the raphe nuclei all survive grafting to the eye chamber and are all able to extend neurites into the peripheral environment of the iris.[32,33,36,44] Interestingly, central adrenergic neurons in locus coeruleus grafts form a halo of fluorescent fibers in surrounding areas of the host iris, irrespective of whether or not the iris has been sympathetically denervated by extirpation of the superior cervical ganglion.[33] Thus, apparently central noradrenergic neurons do not recognize and are unable to react to a peripheral noradrenergic denervation. A series of denervation and transplantation experiments, described in detail elsewhere (see Ref. 33), have instead demonstrated that the sensory innervation of the host iris exerts an inhibitory influence on outgrowing central noradrenergic fibers. Thus if the host iris is denervated with regard to its sensory innervation by "lesioning" of the trigeminal input, a vigorous nerve fiber growth will be reinitiated from a locus coeruleus transplant, resulting in a complete noradrenergic reinnervation of the host iris. It is possible that a similar kind of relation between locus-coeruleus-derived nerve fibers and sensory-type nerve fibers explains the normal course of development of the adrenergic innervation of the cortices, which are adrenergically overinnervated during an early developmental period, after which the proliferation of the noradrenergic terminals is inhibited at about the time of arrival of the sensory input to layer 4 of cortex.

Just as central noradrenergic nerve fibers are able to innervate a peripheral territory, peripheral sympathetic noradrenergic nerves are also able to innervate brain target tissues.[22,38,46] If cortical tissue (for example, hippocampus) is grafted to the eye chamber, it will not receive its normal locus-coeruleus-derived adrenergic innervation. However, peripheral adrenergic (as well as cholinergic) nerves from the host iris will innervate the CNS tissue grafts and substitute for the lacking central input both structurally and functionally. If instead, in a sympathetically denervated eye, a graft of locus coeruleus is combined with a graft of hippocampus, a coeruleo-hippocampal pathway will form. Eventually, however, locus coeruleus will cause an extreme degree of hyperinnervation of its hippocampal target,[38] paralleled by pathologic hyperfunction.[46] Thus, in this case, somewhat surprisingly, those neurons that normally innervate hippocampus will hyperinnervate a graft of that area, while peripheral adrenergic neurons will cause a more normal innervation density. The explanation of these findings is probably that there are basic differences in the mechanisms that regulate peripheral and central adrenergic nerve growth. Thus peripheral neurons, but in all probability not central adrenergic neurons, are sensitive to and dependent upon the presence of nerve growth factor (NGF).[12,29] In addition, it seems as if central,but not peripheral, adrenergic nerve fibers are able to react to the heavily deafferentated state of the grafted hippocampal target by innervating numerous nonadrenergic vacant synaptic sites.

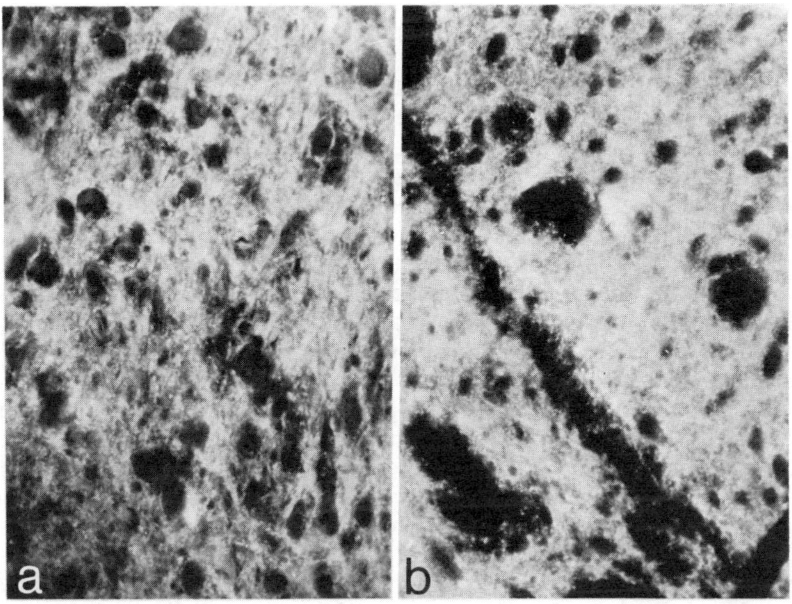

FIGURE 3. Intraocular caudate transplant with densely aggregated fluorescent dopamine nerve terminals originating from a substantia nigra transplant. Note striking similarity in innervation pattern between graft (**a**) and normal caudate tissue (**b**). Falck–Hillarp fluorescence histochemistry of tissue preincubated in alpha-methyl-noradrenaline; original magnification × 330; reduced by 25%. (From Olson *et al.*[36] Reprinted by permission from *Experimental Brain Research.*)

Since the time course of prenatal development of the dopaminergic neuroblasts in mesencephalon is known,[31,43] it is also possible to dissect, with reasonable precision, tissue pieces containing the developing substantia nigra neurons. Stage dependency for optimal cell survival and fiber production from this nucleus was determined by intraocular grafting.[44] Dopamine neuroblasts have to be taken from earlier stages than noradrenaline neuroblasts for optimal survival. It is worth noting in this context that it has never been possible to obtain neuronal survival when one attempts to graft adult mammalian brain tissue. In fact, even the supportive glial cells show a most limited survival when adult tissue transplantation is attempted. Using sequential intraocular grafting, we could demonstrate that substantia nigra grafts were able to innervate adjacent grafts of their normal target area, the striatum. The innervation became organotypic, that is, in most instances a very dense, almost confluent network of fine varicose terminals was seen in the target (FIG. 3). Two conclusions can be drawn from these experiments: nigral neurons are able to reinnervate striatum; and the target tissue determines the morphology of the ingrowing nerve fibers to a large extent since dopamine fibers invading the iris were coarse and with larger varicosites, and thus more similar to peripheral sympathetic nerve fibers, while dopamine terminals in the striatal target, derived from the same grafted neurons, had their typical CNS morphology.

THE CHROMAFFIN CELL HAS A LABILE PHENOTYPE

Chromaffin tissue is derived from the neural crest, as are sympathetic ganglia. In an attempt many years ago to determine whether the scattered ganglion cells seen in the adrenal medulla were adrenergic or cholinergic, adrenal medullary pieces were grafted to sympathetically denervated eyes. An outgrowth of adrenergic nerve fibers from the grafts into the host iris was to be taken as evidence for the presence of adrenergic neurons in the grafts. The somewhat surprising result was that it became difficult to answer the original question since the chromaffin cells themselves transformed towards more neuron-like phenotypes.[24] They migrated on the iris, elongated, and produced nerve fibers that were strongly fluorescent on Falck–Hillarp fluorescence histochemical studies,[10,13] thus being similar to chromaffin tissue, close to their cell body origin, but indistinguishable from peripheral sympathetic nerve fibers at longer distances from the cell bodies (FIG. 4). In the time since the nerve fiber production by adult chromaffin cells was discovered in the rat, much knowledge has been gathered about this transformation. It can occur also in man[30] and in various tumor lines derived from chromaffin tissue. The transformation from a chromaffin towards a neuronal phenotype is driven by the presence of NGF and inhibited by the presence of high local concentrations of glucocortical steroids. Finally, we could also demonstrate in the eye chamber that chromaffin tissue was able to provide a co-grafted CNS target with an adrenergic innervation.[35]

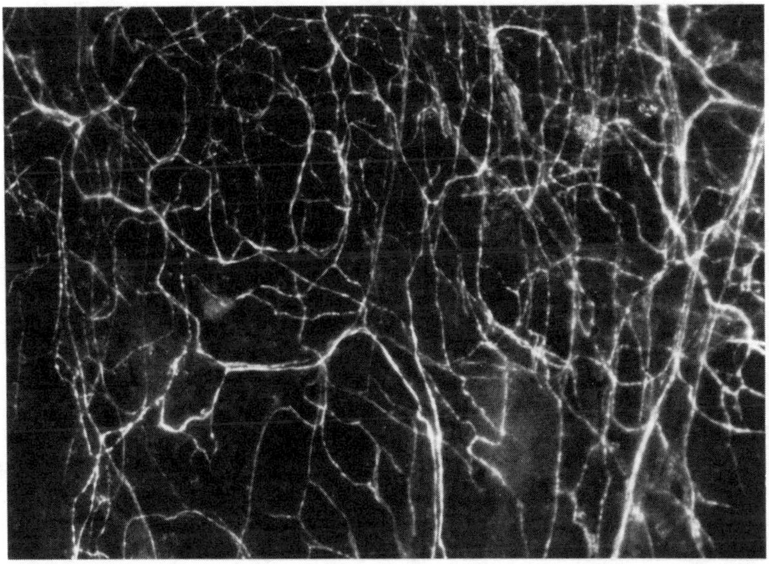

FIGURE 4. Falck–Hillarp fluorescence histochemical micrograph of catecholamine-containing nerve terminals formed in a sympathetically denervated host iris by an intraocular graft of adrenal medullary tissue. Original magnification ×120.

TREATMENT STRATEGIES IN PARKINSON'S DISEASE

Idiopathic parkinsonism is a common so-called extrapyramidal disorder of motor function characterized by slowing and enfeeblement of voluntary and emotional movements, muscular rigidity, and tremor.[4,40] Its neuropathology is highly characteristic. There is a loss of melanin pigment that can be seen with the naked eye in sections through substantia nigra. The depigmentation is due to degeneration of melanin-containing nerve cells, particularly the dopamine neurons in substantia nigra. Degeneration of the nigrostriatal dopamine system leads to decreased levels of dopamine in striatum, which in turn is generally believed to be the major cause of the characteristic symptoms.

Current therapy of Parkinson's disease is aimed at reinstalling proper stimulation of the dopamine receptors in striatum. A dramatic breakthrough was the introduction of L-dopa treatment. L-dopa passes the blood–brain barrier and is converted in the brain to dopamine that becomes available for dopamine receptors in striatum, thereby improving the balance between excitatory and inhibitory influences in this brain region. Several additional types of drug therapy have been continuously introduced. Despite these pharmacologic advances in treatment, however, there remains no cure for parkinsonism. What is worse, after some good years, drug therapy becomes less effective and the patients become more and more troubled by freezing or akinesias on walking and at other times. This hypokinesia can become more severe and the "on-off effects" remain an almost impossible problem of management.[4] Obviously, one major problem with drug therapy is that the drugs employed will reach not only the afflicted area of the brain, but the entire central nervous system as well as the rest of the body, where they can cause various unwanted side effects. Thus, L-dopa therapy seems to be the third best treatment of parkinsonism.

Clearly, the best treatment of Parkinson's disease would be an early diagnosis followed by a way of preventing neuronal death in substantia nigra. The cause of the disease is not known, however, and there is no known way to rescue the degenerating neurons. Perhaps the second best approach would be to replace the missing nerve cells by a transplantation procedure. Transplantation therapy can be suggested in Parkinson's disease because it is caused by disappearance of one defined set of neurons with a known transmitter substance and it is known that L-dopa therapy works. It seems merely necessary to implant a system of cells able to release dopamine or closely related substances within striatum to counteract some of the symptoms. Apparently, restoration of a normal impulse flow in transplanted fiber systems seems unnecessary or L-dopa therapy would not work.

Although there may be a few other central nervous system disease entities where transplantation therapy is at least theoretically an alternative, it is important to emphasize the limitations of this type of replacement therapy. Thus, in the near future brain tissue transplantation seems to offer very little hope in cases of major brain injury, and perhaps only limited hope in spinal cord injury.

ANIMAL MODELS OF PARKINSONISM

Parkinsonism does not occur spontaneously in animals. It is, however, possible to obtain a highly selective degeneration of the nigrostriatal dopamine system in rodents by stereotaxic injections of the neurotoxic drug 6-hydroxydopamine.[47] Bilateral denervations cause a severe syndrome of adipsia, aphagia, and akinesia, and such animals must be fed by intragastric tube to stay alive. If, instead, only one side of the brain is treated with 6-hydroxydopamine, animals will show a unilateral parkinsonism. Such animals have a somewhat asymmetric posture and behavior. When challenged with drugs that interfere with dopaminergic transmission and cause locomotion, unilaterally denervated animals will show a circling behavior which can be precisely quantitated with "rotometers."[48] Dopamine receptors on the denervated side will become supersensitive and react much more strongly to dopamine receptor stimulants, such as apomorphine.[47] Low doses of this drug will cause the animals to rotate towards the normal side. Conversely, if, for instance, amphetamine (a drug that causes release of dopamine from dopamine terminals) is given, animals will rotate towards the denervated side because dopamine can only be released on the intact side. Unilaterally dopamine-denervated animals have become a standard model in which to test various drugs for their use as treatment for parkinsonism. Similarly, such animals have been used to study the effectiveness of transplantations as a way to counteract symptoms of parkinsonism. However, to obtain a complete picture of the behavioral sequelae of transplantation, several other behavioral tests have to be performed to study other aspects of the dopamine deficiency syndrome.

Recently, the meperidine analog, 1-methyl-4-phenyl,1,2,3,6 tetrahydropyridine (MPTP), has been shown to cause severe parkinsonism in man and primates.[9,23] Thus it is now possible to induce Parkinson's disease in monkeys. If MPTP can be used also in rodents,[20] it should constitute a valuable alternative to the 6-hydroxydopamine model.

INTRACRANIAL FETAL SUBSTANTIA NIGRA GRAFTS IN ANIMALS

The first report[41] of a reduction of the motor abnormalities in a unilaterally dopamine-denervated rat by grafted dopamine neurons was published in 1979. Since then, the technique has been improved in several ways and it is now well established that dopamine-neuron-containing grafts can alleviate most, although not all, of the symptoms of experimental parkinsonism.[5–7,11,15,19,25,41,42] Until recently (see the articles in this volume by Price *et. al.* and Björklund and Gage) it has been deemed necessary to graft the dopamine neurons directly into contact with striatum. If grafted back to their normal place in the mesencephalon, axons cannot grow all the way to the denervated target. Structurally and functionally successful grafts have been placed either at the surface of striatum or inside it. Medially one can take advantage of the natural striatal surface facing the lateral ventricle by simply implanting fetal substantia nigra tissue pieces into the lateral ventricle.[19,41] They will attach to the medial surface of striatum and from multiple points of attachment a new dopaminergic innervation will form, innervating dorsomedial aspects of the nucleus. In a technique pioneered by Björklund and his colleagues, striatal surfaces are exposed dorsally or laterally by making cavities through overlying cortex and corpus callosum, and in a second operation transplants are placed in these cavities.[5,7,11] Such experimentation has revealed a functional subdivision of striatum, accumbens, and ventral limbic structures. The rotational behavior is best reversed by grafts reinnervating dorsolateral parts of striatum, while the sensory motor integration is best improved by grafts in more ventral, lateral, and caudal areas of striatum.[11] The locomotion and akinesia symptoms seem to be localized to an area including accumbens and more ventral parts. An experimentally useful alternative to solid tissue grafting is the use of dissociated cell suspensions prepared from fetal substantia nigra. This technique, also pioneered by Björklund and coworkers,[6,42] permits multiple deposits of dopamine neuroblasts at deep brain sites with minimal damage to the host brain.

HOW SUBSTANTIA NIGRA GRAFTS MAY WORK

There is ample evidence that the grafted dopamine neuroblasts are able to provide neighboring areas of host striatum with a rich network of newly formed dopamine nerve terminals. The terminals have been demonstrated by Falck–Hillarp histochemical techniques to reveal their catecholamine content and with tyrosine hydroxylase immunohistochemical methods to show the detailed distribution of dopaminergic, i.e., tyrosine hydroxylase-immunoreactive newly formed nerve terminals. There is a clear correlation between the extent and location of reinnervation and recovery of function. It has also been shown that more inert tissue grafts, such as a piece of sciatic nerve or a piece of frontal cortex, an area that normally innervates striatum but does not provide dopamine, or tectum, an area that is normally physically close to substantia nigra but not projecting to striatum, all are unable to reverse the functional deficits.[15,19] Thus one can conclude that the grafts must contain dopamine neuroblasts and that they must reinnervate striatum for a functional recovery to occur.

It is interesting and important to note that a very low number of surviving dopamine neuroblasts and a very small degree of reinnervation (perhaps 5%) can be of functional benefit. This may relate to the fact that dopamine receptors on the denervated side are supersensitive and/or that striatum is normally supplied with a far greater innervation than is needed for minimal maintenance of function. It is also possible that a low number of neurons and terminals may increase their synthesis and turnover of dopamine to help compensate for the deficit.

Dopamine Levels

Dopamine has been measured biochemically in nigral grafts placed in the lateral ventricle.[19] Within the grafts, dopamine levels are significantly higher than in zona compacta of substantia nigra *in situ*. This is probably due to the large number of dopamine nerve fibers formed within the graft itself. Dopamine levels in adjacent host caudate are high close to the graft and decrease with increasing distance from the graft. Thus, biochemical determinations parallel histochemical observations of reinnervation in host striatum.

Electrical Activity of Nigral Grafts

In zona compacta of substantia nigra the dopaminergic neurons have firing rates between 0.5 and 10.0 Hz.[1] When electrical activity is recorded extracellularly from intraocular as well as intraventricular nigral grafts, cells with similar characteristics are found.[49,50] Thus the grafts are able to maintain spontaneously active nerve cells, despite the isolation and the lack of normal afferent inputs. It has also been shown that transplanted neurons in intraventricular grafts having the zona compacta characteristics respond to dopamine agonists and antagonists in a typical manner. Local application of epinephrine and apomorphine produces dose-dependent inhibition of those neurons. Local application of 6-flupenthixol increases their firing rate. These and other electrophysiological experiments suggest that neurons with many of the characteristics of normal substantia nigra dopamine neurons are present in the graft and spontaneously active. These activities, one must assume, lead to the release of dopamine in host striatum.

Dopamine Receptors in Host Caudate

Dopamine receptors in the caudate can be visualized by *in vitro* light microscopic autoradiography using ^{3}H-labeled spiroperidol.[39] When striatum is denervated, the receptors become supersensitive and there is an increased binding of this dopamine receptor ligand. The distribution of receptor binding is demonstrated by placing treated brain sections in contact with a tritium-sensitive film. The film is then developed and the autoradiograms are analyzed by computerized densitometry and image enhancement using a computerized image analysis system. It was clearly demonstrated that in areas of host striatum that had been reinnervated by nigral grafts, the receptor density returned to normal levels.[17] Thus nigral grafts are able to produce a long-term normalization of dopamine receptors in host brain tissue.

Does the Host Influence the Graft?

As of yet, there are no clear indices of innervation from the host to the graft. Thus, in all likelihood, the host exerts minimal or no influence on graft activity. It is unlikely that an input from the host to the graft, should it occur, could be beneficial since the input would not be derived from the right region of the brain. Clearly, an input from host to graft is not necessary for recovery of function to occur. Although an input from host to graft has not been demonstrated, it is interesting to note that nigral transplants that reinnervate striatum are able to sustain self-stimulation.[14] Experiments with electrodes implanted in nigral grafts showed a functional coupling between graft-related events controlled by the animal through self-stimulation and behavior.

INTRACRANIAL ADRENAL MEDULLARY GRAFTS IN RATS

Fetal dopamine neuroblasts from the substantia nigra region can probably not be used in patients. Stringent ethical, immunologic, and technical constraints suggest that one should look for alternatives to nigral grafts. The ethical issues involved are of a particularly problematic and unresolved

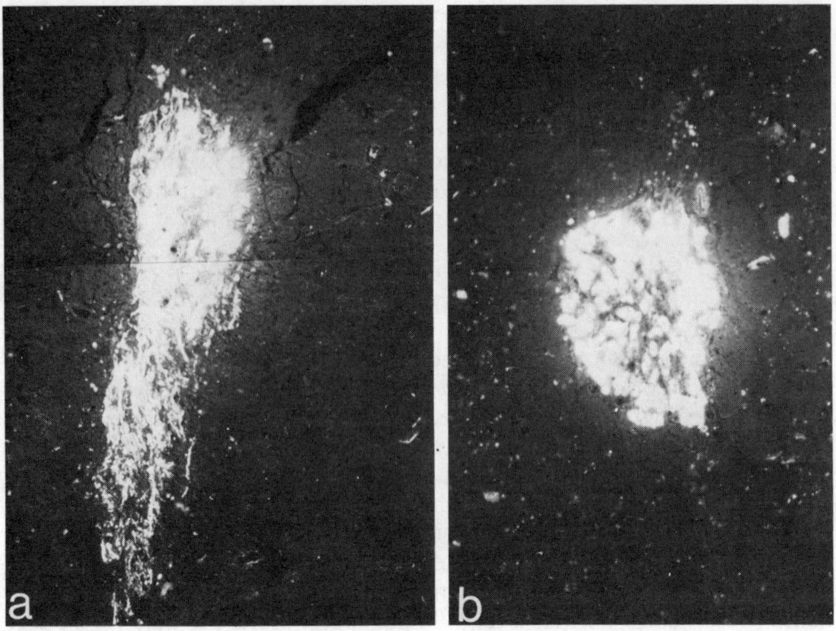

FIGURE 5. Examples of intrastriatal grafts of adrenal medullary tissue. Pieces of adrenal medulla were stereotaxically implanted into the center of the caudate in rats. Nerve growth factor was added at transplantation and 1 and 2 weeks postoperatively. In both (**a**) and (**b**) the strongly catecholamine-fluorescent chromaffin cells have been overexposed (they appear more or less as confluent white areas) in order to illustrate the fluorescent halo of catecholamines spreading in surrounding host brain tissue. (**a**) Graft taken 1 month after implantation. A strongly fluorescent bundle of nerve fibers is seen leaving the graft and entering host brain parenchyma. (**b**) Graft after 15 months. A large number of cells have survived in this graft and a clear fluorescent halo is seen. There are, however, almost no nerve fibers emanating from the graft, suggesting a continuous need for nerve growth factor. The surrounding host striatum is aged and contains numerous autofluorescent lipofuscin pigment granules. Original magnification ×135; reduced by 30%.

nature, but are outside the scope of this review. It has been suggested that the brain is an immunologically privileged site. Thus, rejection processes would be less severe inside the brain. However, when solid pieces of brain tissue are grafted, for example, between mouse and rat brain, most of the grafted mouse brain tissue is rejected.[8] If human fetal brain tissue must not be used, and animal fetal brain tissue cannot be used, other catecholamine-producing cell systems in the human body should be looked for. Clearly, several of the technical and ethical problems, and probably all of the immunologic problems, would be solved if catecholamine-producing cells from the patient's own body could be used. Starting from the observation that adult adrenal medullary chromaffin cells are able to form nerve fibers after grafting to the eye chamber,[24,30,35] we therefore carried out a series of experiments grafting adrenal medullary tissue to the brain of rats with unilateral experimental parkinsonism.

Adrenal medullary tissue was first grafted to the lateral ventricle.[18] It became attached to the medial surface of host striatum, just like fetal substantia nigra grafts. Functionally, such grafts were also able to counteract the apomorphine-induced rotational behavior. The effects were quantitatively similar to those of nigral grafts. When animals with grafts were examined histochemically they were found to have produced very few nerve fibers. This contrasts to the marked fiber production seen to emanate from intraocular chromaffin tissue grafts. The most probable explanation for the lack of fiber formation intracranially is a lack of nerve growth factor.[29] It seemed instead as if the grafted chromaffin cells maintained a more endocrine function. Thus the grafts were always surrounded by a halo of catecholamine fluorescence diffusing through host neuropil after having been released by the grafts. The intraventricular chromaffin grafts were functional for many months. In order to be able to scale up from rat to human brain it was also deemed necessary to explore intrastriatal implantation sites. It was found that intrastriatal grafts were also surrounded by a halo of catecholamines (FIGURES 5, and 6) and that they could also counteract apomorphine-induced rotations.[26]

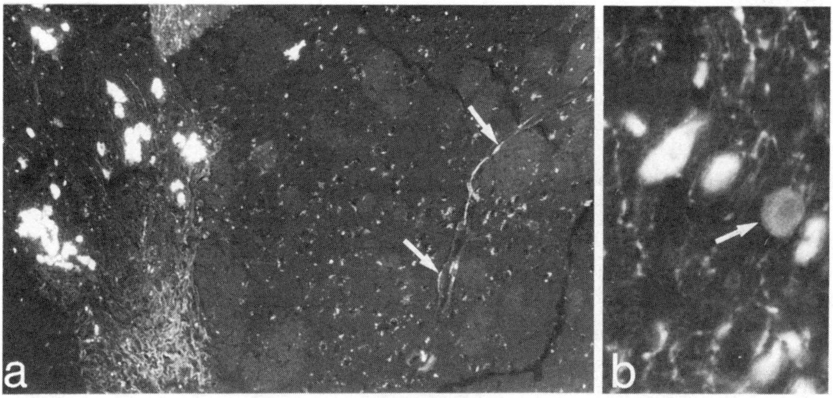

FIGURE 6. Details from intrastriatal grafts of chromaffin tissue as illustrated by Falck–Hillarp fluorescence histochemical techniques. (**a**) Intrastriatal graft with scattered chromaffin cells is shown to the *left*. At a considerable distance from the graft within host striatum, strongly fluorescent adrenergic nerve fibers are seen (*arrow*) associated with blood vessels. These fibers are derived from the graft and illustrate a tendency for the nerve fibers from the chromaffin tissue graft to associate with blood vessels. (**b**) High-power view of part of a chromaffin graft illustrating the presence of a cell with considerably less fluorescence and a larger nucleus than the chromaffin cells, thus having the characteristics of an adrenal ganglion cell. Graft survival, 15 months; original magnification ×120 (**a**) and ×300 (**b**); reduced by 30%.

Acute Effects of Adrenal Medullary Grafts

When chromaffin tissue is implanted into the center of a dopamine-denervated striatum, the rat will begin rotating vigorously towards the contralateral side immediately upon waking. We have shown that the amount of rotation is largely dependent upon the amount of grafted tissue and upon the location of the grafts within striatum.[21] Histochemically, the grafts can be shown to release large amounts of catecholamines that spread 1000–1500 microns in all directions around the graft within minutes. Computerized image analysis of sections processed for Falck–Hillarp fluorescence histochemistry has been used to describe the catecholamine gradient from the grafts in quantitative terms. Considerable amounts of catecholamines were also present around the grafts 100 minutes after grafting, while most of the fluorescent halo had disappeared 400 minutes after grafting.[45] These histochemical results are supported by biochemical measurements using HPLC and electrochemical detection, and the time course of appearance and disappearance of catecholamines in surrounding host striatum[45] correlates well with the time course of rotational behavior.[21] The acutely released catecholamines were mainly adrenaline and noradrenaline, with only trace amounts of dopamine. Nevertheless, dopamine receptor antagonists such as cis-flupenthixol or haloperidol were able to block the rotational behavior in a dose-dependent manner. These experiments suggest that the acutely induced behavior is caused by diffusion of catecholamines (mainly adrenaline and noradrenaline) from the adrenal grafts acting upon supersensitive dopamine receptors.

When catecholamines were measured in chronic grafts it was found that they had ceased to produce adrenaline, a finding that agrees with the known dependency on high local glucocorticoid concentrations for adrenaline synthesis to occur. Perhaps even more interesting is the fact that there was also a shift towards larger amounts of dopamine in the intrastriatal grafts.[16]

We conclude from these experiments that adrenal medullary tissue survives in the lateral ventricle opposed to striatum and in striatum itself, produces few nerve fibers, but considerable amounts of catecholamines, and is able to normalize rotational behavior in denervated animals.

Possible Future Improvements of Adrenal Graft Performance

It would probably be advantageous if chromaffin tissue could be dissociated into viable single cells that could be injected in the form of cell suspensions, thereby achieving a more effective spread of catecholamine-producing cells. Initial experiments indicate, however, that it is considerably more difficult to dissociate adult chromaffin tissue than fetal brain tissue. The use of proper enzymatic and mechanical dissociation procedures should, however, improve the recovery of viable cells enough that this procedure could be used. Obviously, if the procedure is to be useful in a clinical setting also, the recovery must be good enough that one adrenal gland from the patient can supply enough material for grafting.

A second future improvement would be cryopreservation of pieces to be grafted or cell suspensions. This would enable repeated delivery of cells over a longer time period. Thus, the dosage of grafted cells could be better controlled.

Is There a Role for Nerve-Growth-Stimulating Drugs?

The reason for the poor nerve fiber production by intracranial adrenal medullary grafts seems to be the lack of nerve growth factor.[27] Experiments have therefore been initiated where NGF is added to the grafts. Preliminary results indicate survival of a larger number of adrenal medullary cells and a considerably larger amount of nerve fiber formation in the presence of nerve growth factor (FIG. 5). One problem is that grafts may depend continuously upon nerve growth factor. This problem might be solved by implanting miniature osmotic pumps and an intracerebral drug delivery system. Recent results suggest that gangliosides, in particular GM1, are able to stimulate regenerative nerve growth in general.[2] It will be interesting to see what treatment with GM1 ganglioside alone can do experimentally and clinically. It should also be interesting to test whether grafts of substantia nigra or chromaffin tissue could be improved by ganglioside treatment.

FIRST CLINICAL TRIALS WITH ADRENAL MEDULLARY AUTOGRAFTS IN PATIENTS WITH SEVERE PARKINSONISM

Autologous transplantation of adrenal medullary tissue has been tried in two patients suffering from severe parkinsonism, including on-off phenomena, which could not be adequately controlled by drug treatment.[3,26] The first patient was operated on in March 1982 at the Department of Neurosurgery at the Karolinska Hospital. The patients were carefully selected and evaluated clinically; measurements were made of catecholamine metabolites in cerebrospinal fluid; and various self-assessment scales and physiological tests were performed before and after operation. The presence of two adrenal glands was confirmed by CT scan. Two-thirds of one adrenal gland was then removed through a retroperitoneal approach and small pieces of medullary tissue were carefully prepared and freed of cortical tissue using dissection stereomicroscopes. The tissue pieces were trimmed to a size of approximately 1 mm^3 each and loaded into a specially designed implantation cannula. In the cannula they were carried by a stainless steel spiral which was used to deposit the material stereotaxically into the head of the caudate nucleus on one side. Surplus tissue was analyzed by Falck–Hillarp fluorescence histochemistry for the presence of chromaffin tissue and the absence of adrenal cortical tissue. The operations were uneventful. The patients woke up promptly, and in the first patient a skull X-ray film showed the metal marker to be in the desired position in the caudate nucleus. This first patient showed transient and relatively minor signs of improvement during the first couple of weeks after surgery, after which his clinical status has remained essentially unchanged (in contrast to a relatively rapid deterioration during several months prior to surgery). We believe that this first case shows that in a patient with severe parkinsonism, it is feasible to perform an autotransplantation of adrenal chromaffin tissue to the basal ganglia without causing adverse effects.

The second patient, a 45-year-old woman, was given twice as much chromaffin tissue. The tissue pieces were implanted in two places close to each other in the head of the caudate nucleus on one side. This patient developed transient symptoms of paranoia suggestive of an overdosage, and when the dose of L-dopa was lowered, the mental symptoms promptly disappeared. Although it is still too early to draw any definite conclusions, it seems as if rigidity was clearly reduced in the arms of the second patient and that, in addition, there was perhaps an increased amount of voluntary movements and a more normal facial expression.

The experience from the two first cases, we believe, justifies further clinical trials. Several improvements of the technique may be incorporated in the future. It seems as if the putamen is an important part of neostriatum in man and is particularly crucial for motor functions. Dopamine levels are also higher in the putamen than in the caudate nucleus and they are more decreased in putamen than in the caudate nucleus in postmortem cases of Parkinson's disease. The putamen is therefore an interesting target area for adrenal medullary grafts in man.

It is worth mentioning that the stereotaxic neurosurgery involved is of a routine nature and the lesioning effect of the cannula minimal. Much more damage is caused, for instance, by the thalamotomy that is sometimes performed to counteract severe tremor in parkinsonism.

It should also be mentioned that the newly discovered drug MPTP which can induce parkinsonism in primates, promises to aid in the evaluation of the relative importance of the graft to the caudate nucleus and the putamen, respectively.

CONCLUDING REMARKS

Intensive research efforts are presently devoted to the development of transplantation techniques suitable for treatment of neurologic disorders such as Parkinson's disease. Although many problems remain to be solved, it is now proven beyond doubt that grafts of substantia nigra can counteract the symptoms of experimentally induced parkinsonism in rodents. Considerable evidence also exists that suggests that chromaffin tissue from the adrenal medulla can be useful. Results from animal experimentation have recently led to initiation of clinical tests with intrastriatal implantation of adrenal medullary tissue in patients with severe parkinsonism. Several different changes may be incorporated into future clinical trials, such as increasing amount of grafted tissue, varying the target areas, and using dissociated cells.

Although a limited human experimentation has begun, it is important to stress that a transplantation therapy for Parkinson's disease does not exist today. More animal experimentation and further clinical trials are needed before it can be decided whether transplantation is going to be a useful procedure in parkinsonism and before any predictions can be made about the possible role of transplantation therapies in other neurologic diseases. A certain general conservatism concerning new principles for treatment often holds back the initiation of clinical trials. Nevertheless, we have "broken the ice" in trying transplantation therapy in Parkinson's disease.

ACKNOWLEDGMENTS

We thank Lena Hultgren for technical assistance and Ida A. Engqvist for expert typing.

[NOTE ADDED IN PROOF: Since the completion of this manuscript, two more patients with severe Parkinson's disease have been treated with intracranial chromaffin autografts.[51] Chromaffin implants were made into the center of putamen on the right side. Clear-cut improvements of the clinical condition on the contralateral side of the body were seen immediately after transplantation. These improvements included better hand function and less rigidity. In addition, particularly in the younger patient, the percentage time spent in on-periods versus off-periods was significantly increased. The beneficial effects slowly vanished during the first 2–3 months postoperatively. Animal experimentation supports the notion that it is the lack of nerve growth factor in the central nervous system that causes a slow deterioration of the chromaffin grafts. Addition of nerve growth factor for a limited time period after grafting should further improve the clinical results.]

REFERENCES

1. AGHAJANIAN, G. K. & B. S. BUNNEY. 1973. Central dopaminergic neurons: Neurophysiological identification and responses to drugs. *In* Frontiers in Catecholamine Research. E. Usdin, Ed.: 643–648. Pergamon Press. New York, NY.
2. AGNATI, L. F., K. FUXE, L. CALZA, F. BENFENATI, L. CAVICCHIOLI, G. TOFFANO & M. GOLDSTEIN. 1983. Gangliosides increase the survival of lesioned nigral dopamine neurons and favour the recovery of dopaminergic synaptic functions in striatum of rats by collateral sprouting. Acta Physiol. Scand. **119:** 347–363.
3. BACKLUND, E.-O., P. O. GRANDBERG, B. HAMBERGER, E. KNUTSSON, A. MÅRTENSSON, G. SEDVALL, Å. SEIGER & L. OLSON. 1985. Transplantation of adrenal medullary tissue to striatum in parkinsonism: First clinical trials. J. Neurosurg. **62:** 169–173.
4. BANNISTER, R. 1981. Brain's Clinical Neurology, 2nd ed. Oxford University Press. Oxford.
5. BJÖRKLUND, A., S. B. DUNNETT, U. STENEVI, M. E. LEWIS & S. D. IVERSEN. 1980. Reinnervation of the denervated striatum by substantia nigra transplants: Functional consequences as revealed by pharmacological and sensorimotor testing. Brain Res. **199:** 307–333.
6. BJÖRKLUND, A., R. H. SCHMIDT & U. STENEVI. 1980. Functional reinnervation of the neostriatum in the adult rat by use of intraparenchymal grafting of dissociated cell suspensions from the substantia nigra. Cell Tissue Res. **212:** 39–45.
7. BJÖRKLUND, A. & U. STENEVI. 1979. Reconstruction of the nigrostriatal dopamine pathway by intracerebral nigral transplants. Brain Res. **177:** 555–560.

8. BJÖRKLUND, A., U. STENEVI, S. B. DUNNETT & F. H. GAGE. 1982. Cross-species neural grafting in a rat model of Parkinson's disease. Nature **298:** 652–654.
9. BURNS, R. S., C. C. CHIUEH, S. P. MARKEY, M. H. EBERT, D. M. JACOBOWITZ & I. J. KOPIN. 1983. A primate model of parkinsonism: Selective destruction of dopaminergic neurons in the pars compacta of the substantia nigra by N-methyl-4-phenyl-1,2,3,6-tetrahydropyridine. Proc. Natl. Acad. Sci. USA **80:** 4546–4550.
10. CORRODI, H. & G. JONSSON. 1967. The formaldehyde fluorescence method for the histochemical demonstration of biogenic monoamines. A review on the methodology. J. Histochem. Cytochem. **15:** 65–78.
11. DUNNETT, S. B., A. BJÖRKLUND, U. STENEVI & S. D. IVERSEN. 1981. Grafts of embryonic substantia nigra reinnervating the ventrolateral striatum ameliorate sensory motor impairments and akinesia in rats with 6-OHDA lesions of the nigro-striatal pathway. Brain Res. **229:** 209–217.
12. EBENDAL, T., L. OLSON & Å. SEIGER. 1980. Nerve growth factors in the rat iris. Nature **286:** 25–28.
13. FALCK, B., N.-Å. HILLARP, G. THIEME & A. TORP. 1962. Fluorescence of catecholamines and related compounds condensed with formaldehyde. J. Histochem. Cytochem. **10:** 348–354.
14. FRAY, P. J., S. B. DUNNETT, S. D. IVERSEN, A. BJÖRKLUND & U. STENEVI. 1983. Nigral transplants reinnervating the dopamine-depleted neostriatum can sustain intracranial self-stimulation. Science **219:** 416–419.
15. FREED, W. J., B. Hoffer, L. OLSON & R. J. WYATT. 1984. Transplantation of catecholamine-containing tissues to restore the functional capacity of the damaged nigrostriatal system. *In* Neuronal Transplants, Development and Function. J. Sladek & D. Gash, Eds.: 373–406. Plenum Press. New York, NY.
16. FREED, W. J., F. KAROUM, H. E. SPOOR, J. M. MORIHISA L. OLSON & R. J. WYATT 1983. Catecholamine content of intracerebral adrenal medulla grafts. Brain Res. **269:** 184–189.
17. FREED, W. J., G. N. KO, D. L. NEIHOFF, M. KUHAR, B. J. HOFFER, L. OLSON, E. SPOOR, J. M. MORIHISA & R. J. WYATT. 1983. Normalization of spiroperidol binding in the denervated rat striatum by homologous substantia nigra transplants. Science **222:** 937–939.
18. FREED, W. J., J. M. MORIHISA, E. SPOOR, B. HOFFER, L. OLSON, Å. SEIGER & R. J. WYATT. 1981. Transplanted adrenal chromaffin cells in rat brain reduce lesion-induced rotational behaviour. Nature **292:** 351–352.
19. FREED, W. J., M. J. PERLOW, F. KAROUM, Å. SEIGER, L. OLSON, B. J. HOFFER & R. J. WYATT. 1980. Restoration of dopaminergic function by grafting of fetal rat substantia nigra to the caudate nucleus: Long-term behavioural, biochemical, and histochemical studies. Ann. Neurol. **8:** 510–519.
20. HALLMAN, H., L. OLSON & G. JONSSON. 1984. Neurotoxicity of the meperidine analogue 1-methyl-4-phenyl-1,2,5,6-tetrahydropyridine on brain catecholamine neurons in the mouse. Eur. J. Pharmacol. **97:** 133–136.
21. HERRERA-MARSCHITZ, M., I. STRÖMBERG, D. OLSSON, L. OLSON & U. UNGERSTEDT. 1984. Adrenal medullary implants in the dopamine-denervated rat striatum. II. Acute behavior as a function of graft amount and location and its modulation by neuroleptics. Brain Res. **297:** 53–61.
22. HOFFER, B., L. OLSON, Å. SEIGER & F. BLOOM. 1975. Formation of a functional adrenergic input to intraocular cerebellar grafts: Ingrowth of inhibitory sympathetic fibers. J. Neurobiol. **6:** 565–585.
23. LANGSTON, J. W., P. BALLARD, J. W. TETRUD & I. IRWINE. 1983. Chronic parkinsonism in humans due to a product of meperidine-analog synthesis. Science **219:** 979–980.
24. OLSON, L. 1970. Fluorescence histochemical evidence for axonal growth and secretion from transplanted adrenal medullary tissue. Histochemie **22:** 1–7.
25. OLSON, L. 1985. On the use of transplants to counteract the symptoms of Parkinson's disease: Background, experimental models and possible clinical applications. *In* Synaptic Plasticity and Remodelling. C. Cotman, Ed.: 485–505. Guilford Press. New York, NY.
26. OLSON, L., E. O. BACKLUND, G. SEDVALL, M. HERRERA-MARSCHITZ, U. UNGERSTEDT, I. STRÖMBERG, B. HOFFER & Å SEIGER. 1984. Intrastriatal chromaffin grafts in experi-

mental and clinical parkinsonism: First impressions. *In* Catecholamines, Part C. Neuropharmacology and Central Nervous System: Therapeutic Aspects, E. Usdin, A. Carlsson, A. Dahlström & J. Engel, Eds.: 195–201. Alan R. Liss. New York, NY.
27. OLSON, L. H. BJÖRKLUND, R. FREEDMAN, D. GOLDOWITZ, B. J. HOFFER, M. PALMER, Å. SEIGER, D. TAYLOR & D. WOODWARD. 1983. Intrinsic and extrinsic determinants of brain development, as evidenced by grafting of fetal brain tissue. *In* Development and Regenerating Vertebrate Nervous Systems: Proceedings of the Fourth Tarbox Parkinson's Disease Symposium. Lubbock, Texas, Sept. 30–Oct. 2, 1982. P. W. Coates, R. R. Markwald & A. D. KENNY, Eds.: 121–150. Alan R. Liss. New York, NY.
28. OLSON, L., H. BJÖRKLUND & B. HOFFER. 1984. Camera bulbi anterior: New vistas on a classical locus for neural tissue transplantation. *In* Neruronal Transplants, Development and Function. J. Sladek & D. Gash, Eds.: 125–165. Plenum Press. New York, NY.
29. OLSON, L., T. EBENDAL & Å. SEIGER. 1979. NGF and anti-NGF: Evidence against effects on fiber growth in locus coeruleus from cultures of perinatal CNS tissues. Dev. Neurosci. **2:** 160–176.
30. OLSON, L., B. HAMBERGER, B. HOFFER, R. MILLER & Å SEIGER. 1981. Nerve fiber formation by grafted adult adrenal medullary cells. *In* Chemical Neurotransmission: 75 years: Second Nobel Conference. L. Stärne, P. Hedqvist, H. Lagercrantz & Å. Wennmalm, Eds.: 35–48. Academic Press. London
31. OLSON, L. & Å SEIGER. 1972. Early prenatal ontogeny of central monoamine neurons in the rat: Fluorescence histochemical observations. Z. Anat. Entwicklungsgesch. **137:** 301–316.
32. OLSON, L. & Å. SEIGER. 1972. Brain tissue transplanted to the anterior chamber of the eye. I. Fluorescence histochemistry of immature catecholamine and 5-hydroxytryptamine neurons reinnervating the rat iris. Z. Zellforsch. Mikrosk. Anat. **135:** 175–194.
33. OLSON, L. & Å. SEIGER. 1983. Adrenergic nerve growth regulation: Nerve fiber formation by the superior cervical ganglion, the adrenal medulla, and locus coeruleus: Similarities and differences as revealed by grafting. *In* Autonomic Ganglia. L. G. Elfvin, Ed.: 507–522. John Wiley, Ltd. Chichester, England.
34. OLSON, L. & Å. SEIGER. 1976. Beating intraocular hearts: Light-controlled rate by autonomic innervation from host iris. J. Neurobiol. **7:** 193–203.
35. OLSON, L., Å. SEIGER, R. FREEDMAN & B. HOFFER. 1980. Chromaffin cells can innervate brain tissue: Evidence from intraocular double grafts. Exp. Neurol. **70:** 414–426.
36. OLSON, L., Å. SEIGER, B. HOFFER & D. TAYLOR. 1979. Isolated catecholaminergic projections from substantia nigra and locus coeruleus to caudate, hippocampus and cerebral cortex formed by intraocular sequential double brain grafts. Exp. Brain Res. **35:** 47–67.
37. OLSON, L., Å. SEIGER & I. STRÖMBERG. 1983. Intraocular transplantation in rodents: A detailed account of the procedure and examples of its use in neurobiology with special reference to brain tissue grafting. *In* Advances in Cellular Neurobiology, Vol. 4. S. Fedoroff & L. Hertz, Eds.: 407–442. Academic Press. New York, NY.
38. OLSON, L., Å. SEIGER, D. TAYLOR, R. Freedman & B. HOFFER. 1980. Conditions for adrenergic hyperinnervation in hippocampus: I. Histochemical evidence from intraocular double grafts. Exp. Brain Res. **39:** 277–288.
39. PALACIOS, J. M., D. L. NIEHOFF & M. J. KUHAR. 1981. (^{3}H) spiperone binding sites in brain: Autoradiographic localization of multiple receptors. Brain Res. **213:** 277–289.
40. PARKINSON, J. 1917. An Essay on the Shaking Palsy. Sherwood, Neely and Jones. London.
41. PERLOW, M. J., W. J. FREED, B. J. HOFFER, Å. SEIGER, L. OLSON & R. J. WYATT. 1979. Brain grafts reduce motor abnormalities produced by destruction of nigrostriatal dopamine system. Science **204:** 643–647.
42. SCHMIDT, R. H., A. BJÖRKLUND & U. STENEVI. 1981. Intracerebral grafting of dissociated CNS tissue suspensions: A new approach for neuronal transplantation to deep brain sites. Brain Res. **218:** 347–356.
43. SEIGER, Å. & L. OLSON. 1973. Late prenatal ontogeny of central monoamine neurons in the rat: Fluorescence histochemical observations. Z. Anat. Entwicklungsgesch. **140:** 281–318.
44. SEIGER, Å. & L. OLSON. 1977. Quantitation of fiber growth in transplanted central

monoamine neurons. Cell Tissue Res. **179:** 285–316.

45. STRÖMBERG, I., M. HERRERA-MARSCHITZ, L. HULTGREN, U. UNGERSTEDT & L. OLSON, 1984. Adrenal medullary implants to the dopamine-denervated rat striatum. I. Acute catecholamine levels in grafts and host caudate as determined by HPLC-electrochemistry and fluorescence histochemical image analysis. Brain Res. **297:** 41–51.
46. TAYLOR, D., R. FREEDMAN, Å. SEIGER, L. OLSON & B. HOFFER. 1980. Conditions for adrenergic hyperinnervation in hippocampus: II. Electrophysiological evidence from intraocular double grafts. Exp. Brain Res. **39:** 289–299.
47. UNGERSTEDT, U. 1976. 6-Hydroxydopamine-induced degeneration of the nigro-striatal dopamine pathway: The turning syndrome. Pharmacol. Ther. B **2:** 37–40.
48. UNGERSTEDT, U. & G. ARBUTHNOTT. 1970. Quantitative recording of rotational behaviour in rats after 6-hydroxydopamine lesions of the nigro-striatal dopamine system. Brain Res. **24:** 485–493.
49. WUERTHELE, S. M., W. J. FREED, L. OLSON, J. MORIHISA, L. SPOOR, R. J. WYATT & B. HOFFER. 1981. Effect of dopamine agonists and antagonists on the electrical activity of substantia nigra neurons transplanted into the lateral ventricle of the rat. Exp. Brain Res. **44:** 1–10.
50. WUERTHELE, S. M., L. OLSON, W. FREED, R. WYATT & B. HOFFER. 1984. Electrophysiology of substantia nigra transplants. *In* Catecholamines. Part B. Neuropharmacology and Central Nervous System: Theoretical Aspects. E. Usdin, A. Carlsson, A. Dahlström & J. Engel, Eds.: 333–341. Alan R. Liss. New York, NY.
51. OLSON, L., E. O. BACKLUND, G. GERHARDT, B. HOFFER, O. LINDVALL, G. ROSE, Å. SEIGER & I. STRÖMBERG. 1986. Nigral and adrenal grafts in parkinsonism: Recent basic and clinical studies. *In* Proceedings of the VIII International Symposium on Parkinson's Disease. M. D. Yahr, Ed. In press.

Neurogenesis and Plasticity of the Olfactory Sensory Neurons[a]

P. P. C. GRAZIADEI AND G. A. MONTI GRAZIADEI

Department of Biological Science
Florida State University
Tallahassee, Florida 32306

INTRODUCTION

By a phenomenon called primary neural induction, the competent cubic epithelium of the ectoderm becomes the vertebrate nervous system upon contact with the roof of the archenteron.[54,55] The simple cubic epithelium of the ectoderm gives origin subsequently to different populations of neurons which acquire such extreme morphologic and functional complexity that generalization about their behaviors requires great caution. Although some of the basic epithelial characteristics are maintained in the adult nervous system,[52] the capacity to repair cellular losses is greatly impaired.[8,10,34] On the other hand, in a system where specific cell recognition and storage–retrieval of information are of paramount importance, anatomic stability of the cellular elements, after development, has been always considered essential. Consequently, the characterization of the neurons as perennial elements, first put forward by Bizzozero[8] in 1894, has been widely accepted until recently.[10,42] It was also established that in the central nervous system of mammals not only were neurons irreplaceable, but also severed axons could not regrow because of the intrinsic inability of the damaged central perikarya to sustain regeneration of their axons.[53]

The inability of the mammalian CNS to sustain recovery has been recently challenged by a number of new observations. Postnatal development of microneurons from the subependymal regions of the brain has been documented in rodents.[2–4,7,33] Transplantation experiments, resumed after the pioneering work done at the beginning of this century,[5,16,18] have shown that lesioned neuronal populations can be substituted in selected brain regions.[9,15,17,37] The phenomenon of sprouting[40,60] and the capacity of the central neurons to regrow their axons when proper environment is provided [1,17] have challenged the well-established rule proposed by Arnemann[6] since 1787 that regrowth of nerve fibers cannot occur in the postnatal central nervous system. Even if reestablishment of new circuitries with recovery of function has not been so far obtained in mammals, the new observations have great practical and theoretical importance and provide hope for unsuspected capacity of repair of the nervous system. Furthermore, these results

[a] This work was supported by Grant BNS 8006803 from the National Science Foundation and by Grant NS 16421 from the National Institutes of Health.

allow us to examine in a variety of new experimental designs fundamental properties of the system, such as cellular mechanisms of neuronal recognition and plasticity in the postdevelopmental period.

If we consider the neurons, in spite of their morphologic and functional diversity, to be endowed with some basic common properties, the comparative study of different populations of neurons may help us to discover that characteristics that are more obvious in one population may be present in others as well.

In the attempt to pursue this comparative approach we have chosen the olfactory sensory neurons, which seem to have features desirable for the study of repair mechanisms in the central nervous system.[45] So far, the olfactory neurons are the only elements of the adult nervous system known to undergo turnover and to be replaced after experimental degeneration[19–23,44,51] (but see also Bayer[61] and Nottebohm[62]), providing a unique example of anatomic and functional recovery in a sensory pathway. Moreover, the olfactory neurons have the unique experimental advantage of being discretely arranged in an easily accessible neuroepithelium where their stem cells can be selectively identified[43] and their axons can be followed to a specific cortical area in spatially defined glomerular structures.

In the last 10 years we have investigated the olfactory neurons in several vertebrate species and in a number of experimental conditions. While some of the properties of the olfactory neurons seem to be peculiar to this population of elements, the mechanisms subserving these properties may provide insights into more general phenomena of nerve growth and neuronal replacement. We intend to provide here an overview of these observations that illustrate the capacity of morphologic and functional recovery of the system.

TURNOVER AND EXPERIMENTAL AXOTOMY

The olfactory cells, consistently present in all vertebrate classes, are typical Golgi I neurons. They are of early embryologic origin,[12,35] and their relatively long axons, forming a major sensory nerve, are unbranched till they reach the terminal territory in the olfactory bulb glomeruli. These characteristics distinguish them from the short axon cells or Golgi II neurons, which can be defined as those cells of the CNS whose axons never leave the area of the perikaryon to enter major tracts or nerves[39] and are usually of later development.[31] While in the adult animal the olfactory neurons have a peripheral location in the sensory neuroepithelium of the nasal cavity, and during development are commonly believed to originate from a thickening of the cranial ectoderm, embryologic studies have shown that the nasal *anlage* of the olfactory neurons is a portion of the nervous layer of the ectoderm adjacent to the neural plate.[12,35,57]

The continuous replacement of the olfactory neurons (turnover) and their short life-span (in the range of some weeks) are important to our understanding of their behavior and are valuable characteristics for experimentation. By light and electron microscope autoradiography, it has been possible to identify the neurogenetic matrix, which supports the process of neuronal replacement, with the so-called basal cells.[19,20,22,23] The basal cells regulate, by mitotic activity, the maintenance of the neuronal population through the adult life of the animal. Continuous substitution of perikarya implies turnover of their central synapses in the olfactory bulb glomeruli and the persistence of a mechanism of axonal guidance and target recognition, in order to account for the maintenance of a relatively regular pattern of projections from the periphery to the center.[14,38,49,50]

Severance of the olfactory nerves produces total degeneration of the mature neurons whose axons have been cut. The neurogenetic matrix, stimulated by the experimental degeneration of the neurons, responds with an outburst of mitotic activity, which results in the reconstitution of a new population of neurons. The reconstituted neurons send their axons intracranially, where they grow into the bulbar cortex and reestablish synaptic connections, assuring anatomic and functional recovery.[21,27,29,44,46,51] The above experiments thus indicate that in mammals the olfactory pathway is the only sensory pathway where total experimental deafferentiation can be repaired. The anatomic and functional recovery occurs not only during development, but also in adult animals.

BULBECTOMY AND TRANSPLANTATION

Partial removal of the olfactory bulb does not impair the regrowth of the sensory axons. They regrow towards the remaining olfactory bulb, but once they penetrate into their target they not only form glomeruli in the glomerular layer, but also send processes indiscriminately into the external plexiform, mitral, and granule cell layers, thus disrupting the orderly, normal arrangement of the olfactory bulb.[28,45]

When the olfactory bulb is totally removed, the olfactory axons grow into several regions of the spared forebrain, where they establish synaptic contacts with the local neurons in newly formed, ectopic glomerular structures.[11,24,25,30]

Transplantation of cerebellar or occipital cortex from rat embryos (E15) into the olfactory bulb of neonatal rats results in the random invasion by the olfactory axons of the remaining olfactory bulb, the transplanted occipital or cerebellar cortex, and portions of the host's frontal cortex.[26,45]

After the above experiments, which have demonstrated the ability of the olfactory axons not only to regrow from the nasal cavity into several regions of the CNS, but also to alter the morphologic organization of the invaded regions, we are now exploring in our laboratory other aspects of the olfactory matrix in a number of different experimental settings. The rationale for the new experiments derives also from studies in lower vertebrates, where it was observed that damage to the forebrain, involving the olfactory nerves, was often followed by migration of neurons from the sensory epithelium.[13,32,34,36,58,59] The neural elements undergoing migration were claimed to participate in the central regeneration of the removed telencephalic regions. Confirmation of these observations would prove that the olfactory matrix can generate not only sensory, but central neurons as well.

MIGRATION OF OLFACTORY NEUROBLASTS

Olfactory neuroblasts are neuroblasts formed by stem cells from the olfactory epithelium. We report here our preliminary results of migration of olfactory neuroblasts in mammals in two experimental paradigms: (a) migration of the olfactory neuroblasts from the olfactory neuroepithelium *in situ* after brain damage, and (b) migration of olfactory neuroblasts from intracerebrally transplanted olfactory neuroepithelium.

Lesion of the olfactory bulb, both in neonatal and adult rats, induces the migration of neuronal elements from the nasal olfactory neureopithelium.[47] We have identified these neurobalsts in the lamina propria of the olfactory mucosa and intracranially in the plexiform nerve layer of the olfactory bulb both at light and electron microscope levels (FIGS. 1, 2, and 3). Attempts to recognize the migrating neurons by their specific marker, the olfactory marker protein (OMP), with immunohistochemical techniques have been unsuccessful because these migrating cells are either still immature or have lost the capacity to express OMP. Their morphologic recognition in the bulbar parenchyma is consequently quite demanding. The intracranial migration of these neuroblasts leaves open the possibility that in the olfactory neurogenetic matrix, under abnormal conditions, neural elements may originate that have the ability to integrate into the olfactory bulb.

The relationships of the olfactory neurons with the brain parenchyma have been studied by transplanting fragments of olfactory neuroepithelium from neonatal rats into the brain of recipient neonatal and adult animals.[48] Three locations have been chosen for these experiments: the cerebellar cortex, the parietal cortex, and the olfactory bulb. Our observations have been conducted at light and electron microscope levels and with the aid of immunohistochemical techniques for the demonstration of OMP. The postoperative survival periods have extended from 10 days to 8 months. The mature neurons of the transplanted neuroepithelium rapidly degenerate because of the severance of their axons during surgery. The neurogenetic matrix survives well for the entire period of our observations and continuously produces new neurons.

In discrete regions of the transplant the neuroepithelium maintains its normal structure; basal cells, differentiating and mature neurons, and supporting cells can be recognized. From these portions of the neuroepithelium

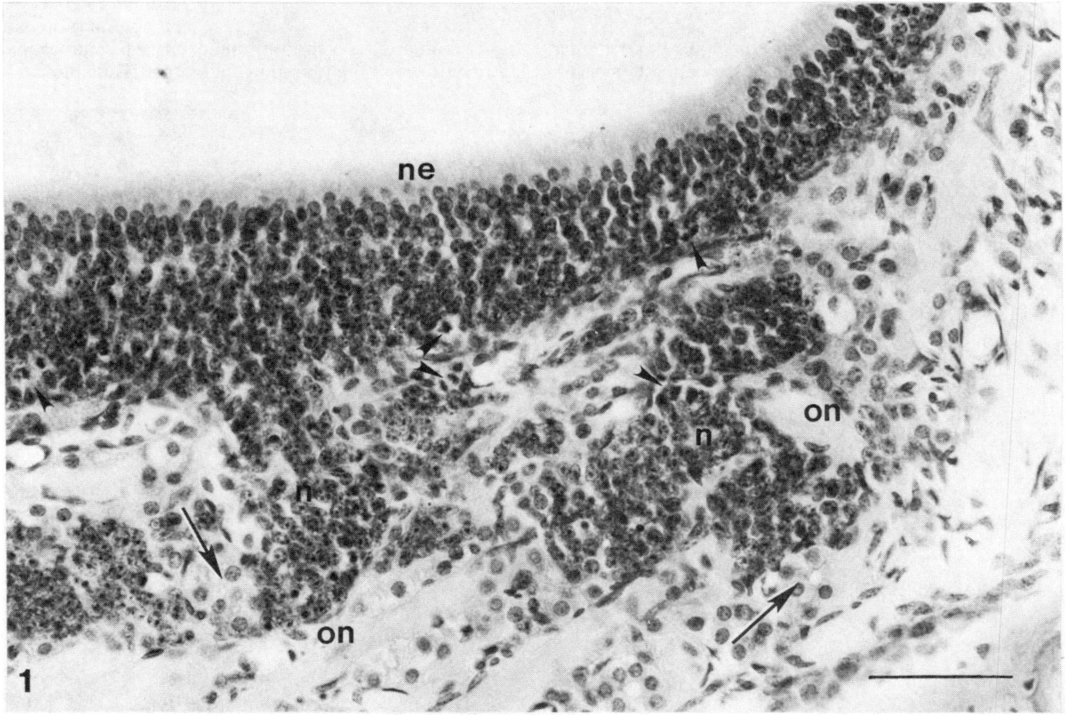

FIGURE 1. Olfactory mucosa of mouse unilaterally, partially bulbectomized; 24-day postoperative survival. From the neuroepithelium (ne) clusters of olfactory neuroblasts (n) migrate into the lamina propria in close proximity to the olfactory nerves (on). Mitotic figures are present at the base of the epithelium and among the migrating neuroblast (*arrowheads*; see also FIGURE 3). Bowman's glands are indicated by *arrows*. Gill's hematoxylin stain. Bar = 50 μm.

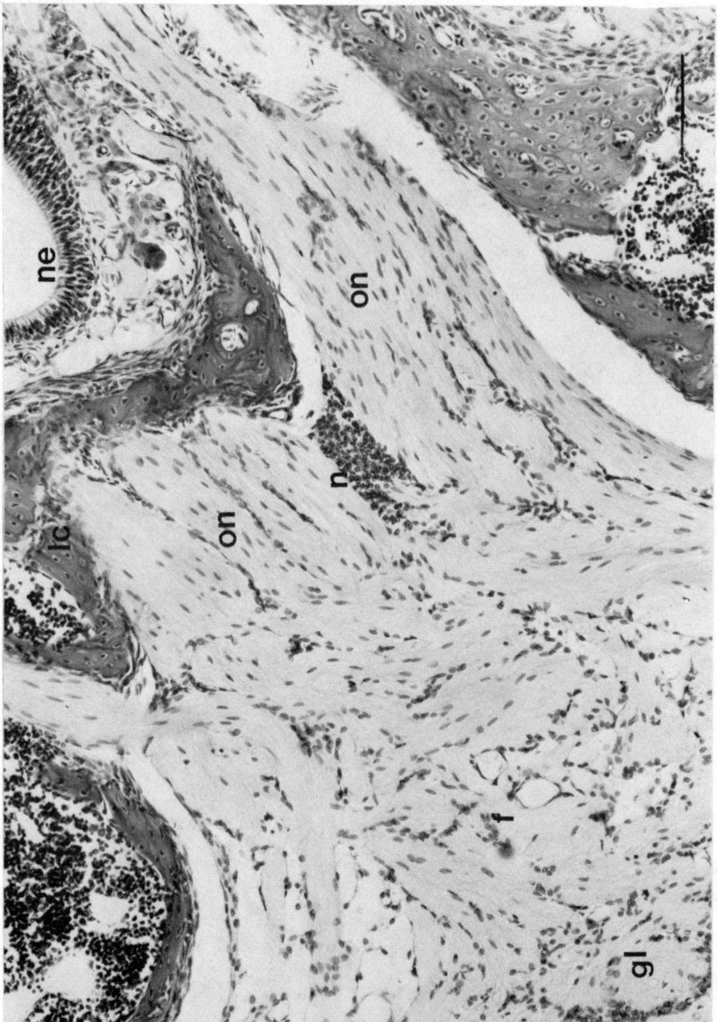

FIGURE 2. From the olfactory neuroepithelium (ne) a cluster of neuroblasts (n) has migrated along the olfactory nerves (on) into the cranial cavity. Rat was partially bulbectomized as a neonate and was sacrificed after 12 days. Lamina cribrosa (lc); fibrous layer of the olfactory bulb (f); glomeruli (gl). Gill's hematoxylin stain. Bar = 50 μm.

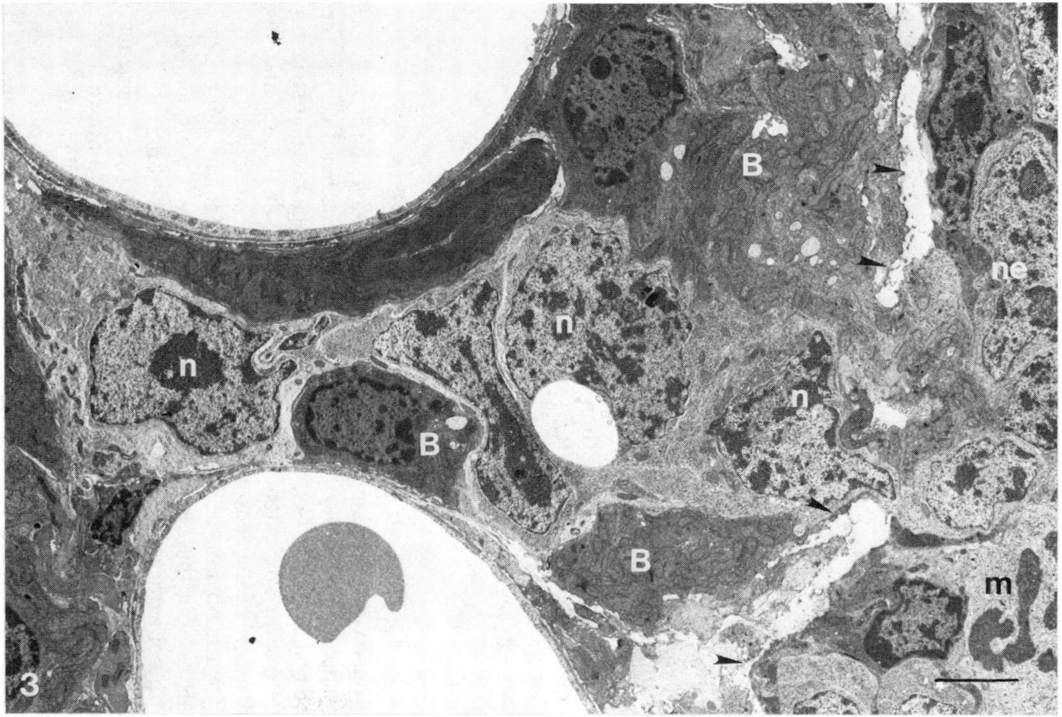

FIGURE 3. Mouse was partially bulbectomized as a neonate and was sacrificed after 12 days. From the neuroepithelium (ne) several neuronal elements (n) migrate into the lamina propria among Bowman's gland cells (**B**). A mitotic figure is observed at the base of the epithelium (m). *Arrowheads* indicate the base of the neuroepithelium. Bar = 2 μm.

bundles of sensory axons deeply penetrate into the brain parenchyma, but consistently fail to form glomeruli. The failure of the olfactory axons to organize in glomeruli is characteristic of these experimental conditions and contrasts with the ability of these axons to glomerulize in several regions of the brain when their perikarya are not removed from the nasal cavity.[24,25] Even when the olfactory neuroepithelium is transplanted into the olfactory bulb, the bundles of olfactory axons do not form glomeruli and do not preferentially orient themselves towards the preexisting glomeruli of the host's bulb.

In other regions of the transplant where the neuroepithelium becomes relatively thin, cubic unicellular cords of neuronal elements deprived of basal lamina migrate directly into the surrounding brain tissue (FIGS. 4 and 5) and several mitotic figures are present among them. In proximity to the transplant, these neuronal elements can be easily recognized. The olfactory cells are often in direct contact with the host's neurons and do not seem to stimulate obvious glial reaction. These elements can be recognized as derived from the transplant by their relatively dense cytoplasm, their relatively small diameter of some 10 microns, and for the presence, in the more mature cells, of lipofuscin granules (FIGS. 6 and 7). We do not know at present whether the transplanted neurons are synaptically connected with the host's neurons. In immunohistochemical preparations only a few transplanted cells appear to be weakly positive to OMP, both in the neuroepithelium and when freely migrating into the brain parenchyma. We have not observed substantial differences in the migratory behavior and in the survival of these neurons in the three brain regions studied so far.

CONCLUSIONS

Several observations in amphibians and mammals have in the past indicated that when the olfactory neurons are located in the nasal cavity, their axons, upon reaching the CNS, induce the formation of glomerular structures and modify to a variable extent the organization and synaptologic and morphologic structure of the neuronal populations with whom they come in contact.[30,41,56] More obvious in amphibians during development, but observed in mammals as well, these phenomena seem to indicate a considerable influence of the olfactory input on other neuronal populations.[30,41,56] This capacity of the olfactory neurons, however, requires that these elements be located in the olfactory organ as a whole. It is interesting to notice that the olfactory *anlage* produces more than a single population of neurons, each with specific function, connections, and biochemical characteristics. In fact, the olfactory neurons, the vomeronasal neurons, and the neurons of the nervus terminalis are all a product of the olfactory *anlage*. However, we do not presently know the limits of the competence of the olfactory matrix.

Phenomena of migration of olfactory neuroblasts in amphibians seem to support the notion that once the neuronal elements have left their epithelial position they can acquire greater plasticity.[34] The preliminary observations

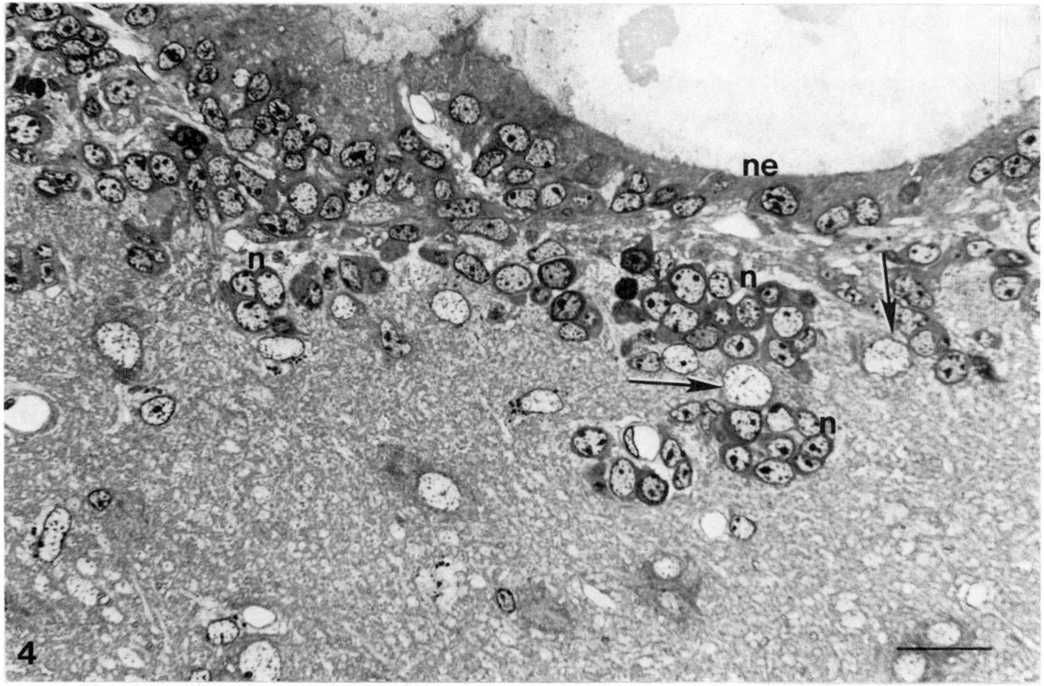

FIGURE 4. Transplant of olfactory neuroepithelium into the parietal cortex of a neonatal rat. The animal survived 30 days. From the olfactory neuroepithelium, which has become cuboidal (ne), several olfactory neuroblasts (n) migrate into the brain parenchyma. Some of them are in intimate contact with the host's neurons at *arrows*. Araldite-embedded material; semi-thin section stained with toluidine blue. Bar = 20 μm.

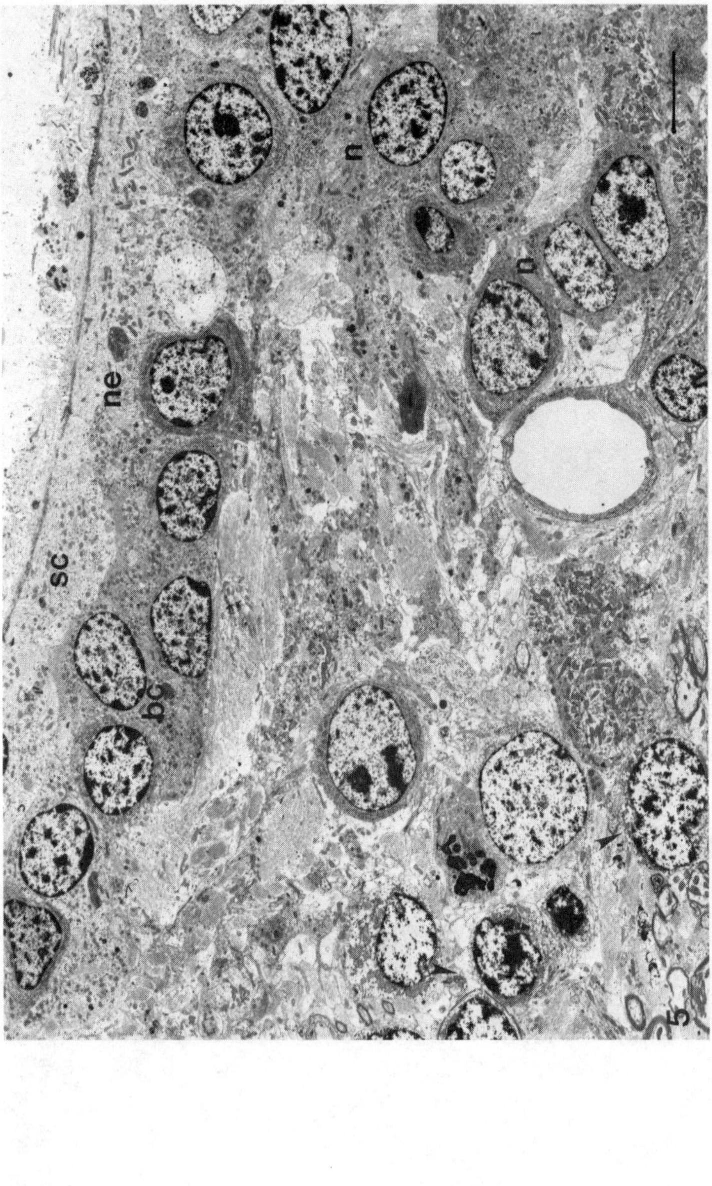

FIGURE 5. Transplant of olfactory neuroepithelium into the cerebellum of an adult rat that survived 60 days. The cubic olfactory neuroepithelium (ne) contains basal (bc) and supporting cells (sc). Some olfactory neuroblasts (n) are seen migrating in extraepithelial position. Cerebellar granule cells are indicated by *arrowheads.* Bar = 5 μm.

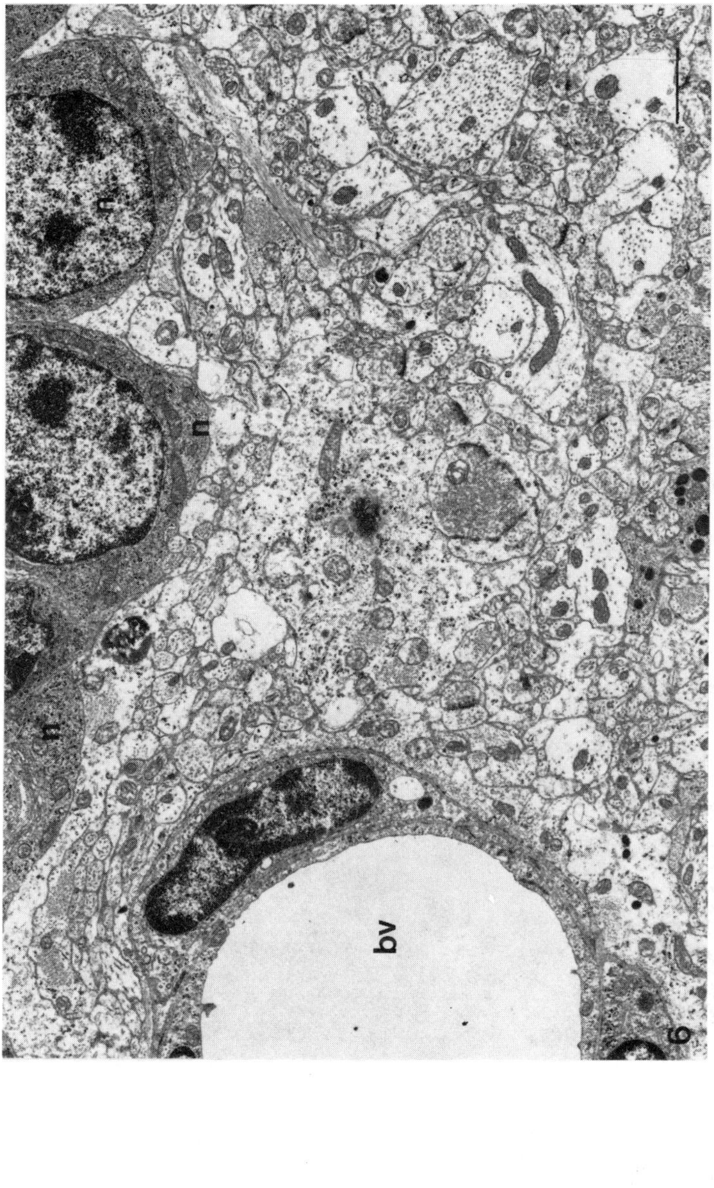

FIGURE 6. Transplant of olfactory neuroepithelium into the parietal cortex of an adult rat that survived 60 days. Olfactory neuroblasts (n) are in intimate contact with the brain parenchyma without intervening basal lamina. Blood vessel (bv). Bar = 1 μm.

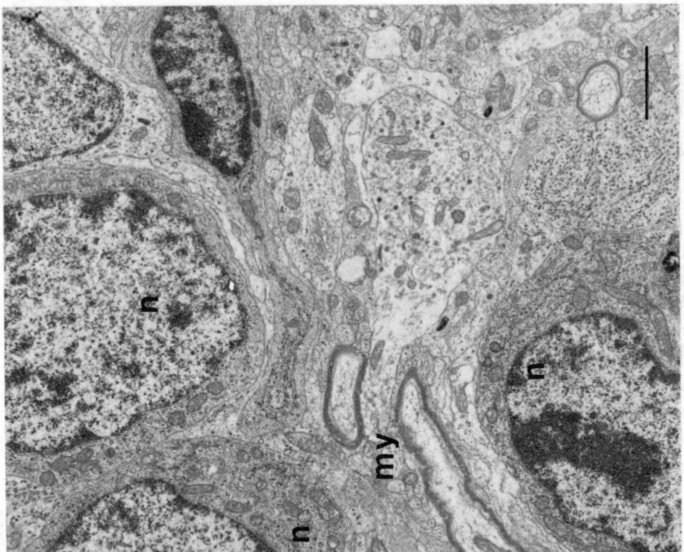

FIGURE 7. Transplant of olfactory neuroepithelium into the olfactory bulb of a neonatal rat that survived 30 days. Olfactory neuroblasts can be identified in close proximity to myelinated axons in the granule layer of the olfactory bulb. Bar = 1 μm.

in our laboratory also demonstrate that after surgical lesions of the olfactory bulb are created, neuronal elements migrate centrally from the olfactory epithelium; however, we do not know the functional significance of this migration. Further studies are required to establish the destiny of these elements and the possibility that they integrate with the host brain.

In any event, we have in the migratory property of these cells a dynamic chracteristic of considerable interest, at least from a theoretical point of view.

It may seem unlikely that olfactory neuroblasts could become convenient "spare" elements for use in brain repair, but from what we know this may not be impossible. We have in the stem cells of the young and adult olfactory epithelium a very robust source of new neurons in all vertebrates studied so far, and the ensuing neuroblasts give rise to axons that grow unhindered into the brain parenchyma of adult mammals. It seems fair to suggest that this system may play an important role in the understanding of regenerative phenomena of the developing and adult brain.

ACKNOWLEDGMENTS

Brain transplantation of olfactory neuroepithelium is carried on in our laboratory in collaboration with Dr. E. E. Morrison.

REFERENCES

1. Aguayo, A. J., P. M., Richardson, S. David & M. Benfey. 1982. Transplantation of neurons and sheath cells. A tool for the study of regeneration. *In* Repair and Regeneration of the Nervous System. J. C. Nicholls. Ed.: 91–105. Springer Verlag. Berlin.
2. Altman, J. 1963. Autoradiographic investigation of cell proliferation in the brain of rats and cats. Anat. Rec. **145:** 573–591.
3. Altman, J. & G. D. Das. 1965. Post-natal origin of microneurons in the rat brain. Nature **207:** 953–956.
4. Altman, J. 1969. Autoradiographic and histological studies of postnatal neurogenesis. III. Dating the time of production and onset of differentiation of cerebellar microneurons in rats. J. Comp. Neurol. **136:** 269–294.
5. Altobelli, R. 1914. Innesti cerebrali. Gazz. Int. Med. Chir. **17:** 25–34.
6. Arnemann, J. 1787. Versuche ueber die Regeneration an lebenden Thieren. I. Bd. Ueber die Regeneration der Nerven. Joh. Christian Dieterich. Goettingen.
7. Bayer, S. A. 1983. ^{3}H-thymidine-radiographic studies of neurogenesis in the rat olfactory bulb. Exp. Brain Res **50:** 329–340.
8. Bizzozero, G. 1894. Accrescimento e rigenerazione nell'organismo. Arch. Sci. Med. **18:** 245–287.
9. Björklund, A. & U. Stenevi. 1979. Regeneration of monoaminergic and cholinergic neurons in the mammalian central nervous system. Physiol. Rev. **59:** 62–100.
10. Brody, H. 1955. Organization of the cerebral cortex. III. A study of aging in the human cerebral cortex. J. Comp. Neurol. **112:** 511–556.
11. Butler, A. B., P. P. C. Graziadei, G. A. Monti Graziadei & B. M. Slotnick. 1984. Neonatally bulbectomized rats with new olfactory-neocortical connections are anosmic. Neurosci. Lett. **48:** 247–254.
12. Carpenter, E. 1937. The head pattern in amblystoma studied by vital staining and transplantation methods. J. Exp. Zool. **75:** 103–129.

13. CLAIRAMBAULT, P. 1976. Development of the prosencephalon. *In* Frog Neurobiology, R. Llinas & W. Precht, Eds. Springer Verlag. Berlin.
14. CLARK LE GROS W. E. 1951. The projection of the olfactory epithelium on the olfactory bulb in the rabbit. J. Neurol. Neurosurg. Psychiat. **14:** 1–10.
15. DAS, G. D. 1983. Neural transplantation in mammalian brain: Some conceptual and technical considerations. *In* Neural Tissue Transplantation Research. R. B. Wallace and G. D. Das, Eds. Springer Verlag. New York.
16. DEL CONTE, G. 1907. Einpflanzungen von embryonalen Gewebe ins Gehirn. Beitr. Pathol. Anat. **42:** 193–201.
17. DUNNET, S. B., A. S. BJÖRKLUND & U. STENEVI. 1983. Transplant induced recovery from brain lesions: A review of the nigrostriatal model. *In* Neural Tissue Transplantation Research. R. B. Wallace & G. D. Das, Eds.: 191–216. Springer Verlag. New York, NY.
18. GLEES, P. 1955. Studies on cortical regeneration with special reference to cerebral inplants. *In* Regeneration in the Central Nervous System. W. F. Windle, Ed: 94–111. Charles C Thomas. Springfield, IL.
19. GRAZIADEI, P. P. C. & J. F. METCALF. 1971. Autoradiographic and ultrastructural observations on the frog's olfactory mucosa. Z. Zellforsch Mikrosk. Anat. **116:** 305–318.
20. GRAZIADEI, P. P. C. 1973. Cell dynamics in the olfactory mucosa. Tissue and Cell **5:** 113–131.
21. GRAZIADEI, P. P. C. & R. S. DEHAN. 1973. Neuronal regeneration in frog olfactory system. J. Cell Biol. **59:** 525–530.
22. GRAZIADEI, P. P. C. & G. A. MONTI GRAZIADEI. 1978. Continuous nerve cell renewal in the olfactory system. *In* Handbook of Sensory Physiology, Vol. IX, M. Jacobson, Ed.: 55–83. Springer Verlag. Berlin.
23. GRAZIADEI, P. P. C. & G. A. MONTI GRAZIADEI. 1978. Neurogenesis and neuron regeneration in the olfactory system of mammals. I. Morphological aspects of differentiation and structural organization of the olfactory sensory neurons. J. Neurocytol. **8:** 1–18.
24. GRAZIADEI, P. P. C., R. R. LEVINE & G. A. MONTI GRAZIADEI. 1978. Regeneration of olfactory axons and synapse formation in the forebrain after bulbectomy in neonatal mouse. Proc. Natl. Acad. Sci. USA **75:** 5230–5234.
25. GRAZIADEI, P. P. C., R. R. LEVINE & G. A. MONTI GRAZIADEI. 1979. Plasticity of connections of the olfactory sensory neurons: Regeneration into the forebrain following bulbectomy in the neonatal mouse. Neuroscience **4:** 712–727.
26. GRAZIADEI, P. P. C. & M. S. KAPLAN. 1980. Regrowth of olfactory sensory axons into transplanted neural tissue. I. Development of connections with the occipital cortex. Brain Res. **201:** 39–44.
27. GRAZIADEI, P. P. C., M. S. KAPLAN, G. A. MONTI GRAZIADEI & J. J. BERNSTEIN. 1980. Neurogenesis of sensory neurons in the primate olfactory system after section of the *fila olfactoria*. Brain Res. **186:** 289–300.
28. GRAZIADEI, P. P. C. & D. W. SAMANEN. 1980. Ectopic glomerular structures in the olfactory bulb of neonatal and adult mice. Brain Res. **187:** 467–472.
29. GRAZIADEI, P. P. C. & G. A. MONTI GRAZIADEI. 1980. Neurogenesis and neuron regeneration in the olfactory system of mammals. III. Deafferentation and reinnervation of the olfactory bulb following section of the *fila olfactoria* in rat. J. Neurocytol. **9:** 145–162.
30. GRAZIADEI, P. P. C. & G. A. MONTI GRAZIADEI. 1985. Neuronal changes in the forebrain of mice following penetration by regenerating olfactory axons. J. Comp. Neurol. Submitted for publication.
31. JACOBSON, M. 1978. Developmental Neurobiology. Plenum Press. New York, NY.
32. JORDAN, M. 1958. Regeneration of the endbrain in post-metamorphic *Xenopus*. Folia Biol. Praha **6:** 103–116.
33. KAPLAN, M. S. & J. W. HINDS. 1977. Neurogenesis in the adult rat: Electron microscopic analysis of light radioautographs. Science **197:** 1092–1094.
34. KIRSCHE, W. 1983. The significance of the matrix zone for brain regeneration and brain transplantation with special consideration of lower vertebrates. *In* Neural Transplantation Research R. B. Wallace & G. D. Das, Eds.: 65–104. Springer Verlag. New York. NY.

35. KLEIN, S. L. & P. P. C. GRAZIADEI. 1983. The differentiation of the olfactory placode in *Xenopus laevis:* A light and electron microscope study. J. Comp. Neurol. **217:** 17–30.
36. KOSCIUSZKO, H. 1958. The influence of the olfactory nerves on the regeneration of the endbrain in *Xenopus laevis* tadpoles. Folia Biol. Praha **6:** 117–130.
37. KROMER, L. F. 1983. Utilization of neural transplants to analyze regeneration in the adult mammalian central nervous system. *In* Neural Tissue Transplantation Research. R. B. Wallace & G. D. Das, Eds.: 135–164. Springer Verlag. New York, NY.
38. LAND, L. J. & G. M. SHEPHERD. 1974. Autoradiographic analysis of olfactory receptor projections in the rabbit. Brain Res. **70:** 506–510.
39. LENHOSSEK, M. V. 1895. Der feinere Bau des Nervensystem. Fisher. Berlin.
40. LIU, C. N. & W. W. CHAMBERS. 1958. Intraspinal sprouting of dorsal root axons. Arch. Neurol. Psychiatr. **79:** 46–61.
41. MAGRASSI, L. & P. P. C. GRAZIADEI. 1985. Olfactory placode transplantation in *Xenopus laevis* embryos. Neuroscience **15:** 903–921.
42. MESSIER, B. & LEBLOND, C. P. 1960. Cell proliferation and migration as revealed by radioautography after injection of thymidine H3 in male rats and mice. Am. J. Anat. **106:** 247–285.
43. MONTI GRAZIADEI, G. A., F. L. MARGOLIS, J. W. HARDING & P. P. C. GRAZIADEI. 1977. Immunocytochemistry of the olfactory marker protein. J. Histochem. Cytochem. **25:** 1311–1316.
44. MONTI GRAZIADEI, G. A. & P. P. C. GRAZIADEI. 1979. Neurogenesis and neuron regeneration in the olfactory system of mammals. II. Degeneration and reconstitution of the olfactory sensory neurons after axotomy. J. Neurocytol. **8:** 197–213.
45. MONTI GRAZIADEI, G. A. & P. P. C. GRAZIADEI. 1979. Studies on neuronal plasticity and regeneration in the olfactory system: Morphologic and functional characteristics of the olfactory sensory neurons. *In* Neuronal Growth and Differentiation, E. Meisami and M. A. B. Brazier, Eds.: 373–396. Raven Press. New York, NY.
46. MONTI GRAZIADEI, G. A., M. S. KAPLAN, J. J. BERSTEIN & P. P. C. GRAZIADEI. 1980. Reinnervation of the olfactory bulb after section of the olfactory nerve in monkey (*Saimiri sciureus*). Brain Res. **189:** 343–354.
47. MONTI GRAZIADEI, G. A. & P. P. C. GRAZIADEI. 1983. Experimentally induced extra-epithelial migration of olfactory neurons in neonatal and adult rodents. Soc. Neurosci. Abstr.: 1019 (295.3).
48. MORRISON, E. E. & P. P. C. GRAZIADEI. 1983. Transplant of olfactory mucosa in the rat brain. I. A light microscopic study of transplant organization. Brain Res. **279:** 241–245.
49. MOULTON, D. G. 1976. Spatial patterning of response to odors in the peripheral olfactory system. Physiol. Rev. **56:** 578–593.
50. MOZELL, M. M. 1966. The spatiotemporal analysis of odorants at the level of the olfactory sheet. J. Gen. Physiol. **56:** 46–63.
51. OLEY, N., R. S. DEHAN, D. TUCKER, J. C. SMITH & P. P. C. GRAZIADEI. 1975. Recovery of structure and function following transection of the primary olfactory nerves in pigeons. J. Comp. Physiol. Psychol. **88:** 477–495.
52. PALAY, S. L. 1967. Principles of cellular organization in the nervous system. *In* The Neurosciences. G. C. Quarton, T. Melnechuk and F. O. Schmitt, Eds.: 24–30. Rockefeller Universitv Press. New York, NY.
53. RAMON Y CAJAL, S. 1928. Degeneration and Regeneration of the Nervous System (R. M. May, trans.). Hafner. New York, NY (1959).
54. SPEMANN, H. & H. MANGOLD. 1924. Ueber Induktion von Embryonalanlagen durch Implantation artfremder Organisatoren. Arch. Mikroskop. Anat. Entwicklungsmech. **100:** 599–638.
55. SPEMANN, H. 1936. Experimentelle Beitrage zu einer Theorie der Entwicklung. Springer Verlag. Berlin.
56. STOUT, R. P. & P. P. C. GRAZIADEI. 1980. Influence of the olfactory placode on the development of the brain in *Xenopus laevis* (Daudin). Neuroscience **5:** 2175–2186.
57. VAN OOSTROM, C. G. & C. D. A. VERWOERS. 1972. The origin of the olfactory placode. Acta Morphol. Neerl. Scand. **9:** 160.

58. WEISSFEILER, J. 1924. Regeneration des lobes olfactifs et des hemispheres cerebraux. C. R. Soc. Biol. **91:** 543–544.
59. WEISSFEILER, J. 1925. Regeneration du cerveau et du nerf olfactif chez lex Batraciens urodeles. Rev. Suisse Zool. **32:** 1–43.
60. COTMAN, C. W. & M. NIETO-SAMPEDRO. 1985. Progress in facilitating the recovery of function after central nervous system trauma. Ann. N.Y. Acad. Sci. **457:** 83–104 (this volume).
61. BAYER, S. A. 1985. Neuron production in the hippocampus and olfactory bulb of the adult rat brain: Addition or replacement? Ann. N.Y. Acad. Sci. **457:** 163–172 (this volume).
62. NOTTEBOHM, F. 1985. Neuronal replacement in adulthood. Ann. N.Y. Acad. Sci. **457:** 143–161 (this volume).

Neuronal Replacement in Adulthood

FERNANDO NOTTEBOHM

The Rockefeller University
New York, New York 10021

My colleagues and I are interested in brain events that control learning. Our work, using canaries, has shown that brain cells can be replaced in adulthood. We suspect that neuronal replacement in adulthood is related to some kinds of learning; it is also a form of brain repair, though it happens in the absence of an external lesion. I will present the background to this work and our most recent findings.

SONG AS A LEARNED BEHAVIOR

Neuronal replacement in adulthood is probably widespread among birds. I will use its occurrence in the song control system of canaries to describe it and speculate about its significance.

Male canaries develop their first adult song repertoire during the period between hatching and sexual maturity.[32] The duration of this period can vary from 6 to 10 months, depending on whether a canary hatched late or early in the breeding season. However, unlike many other songbirds which learn their song once, during a "critical period" before reaching sexual maturity, canaries continue to modify their song in adulthood. They do this by altering existent syllable types as well as by eliminating some syllables and adding many new ones.[32] Because of this ability, canaries are called "open-ended" learners.[24–26]

Song-learning requires that vocal output be modified to match an auditory expectation, for example, a remembered model.[16] A young male canary kept in the same cage with its father will develop a song very similar to that of the latter. If, instead, the same young canary is tutored with recorded song played over a speaker, it will imitate the latter array of sounds. By contrast, a young canary deafened before the onset of singing will develop an overly simple repertoire of sounds.[20,43] Even after the song is learned, maintenance of the learned pattern requires access to hearing. If an adult canary is deafened after it has mastered stable adult song, these learned patterns will be forgotten over a period of months; eventually the song of such a bird becomes no different from that of a male deafened before the onset of singing.[34] We may conclude from this that song-learning requires two steps: (1) the model to be imitated must be acquired as a perceptual memory; and (2) then the vocal output must be modified so that the auditory feedback it creates matches the model. Apparently, the maintenance of learned song in adult canaries requires that there be a sustained opportunity to match feedback and model.

For most canaries in our breeding colony, breeding ends in late June, when the birds are approximately 14 months old. During the months of July through October, when these birds are 15–18 months old, song becomes unstable, so that it resembles the "plastic song" of a 3–4 month old male canary. During this summer and early fall period of unstable song, many new syllables are added and others are modified. After this period of unstable song ends, song becomes once again stereotyped. With a few further changes, this will be the song used during the following breeding season. In this manner the song of adult male canaries continues to be modified in future years.[32,33]

BRAIN PATHWAYS FOR SONG CONTROL

Brain pathways for song control in canaries have been described. A large forebrain nucleus, hyperstriatum ventralis, pars caudalis (HVc), projects to the robust nucleus of the archistriatum (RA). RA projects to the caudal half of the hypoglossal nucleus of the medulla, which houses the motor neurons that innervate the vocal control organ (syrinx).[15,31,34] This pathway is shown in FIGURE 1.

Neurons in nucleus HVc respond to sound, including that of conspecific song.[14,19,21] HVc neurons also start firing before and during song produc-

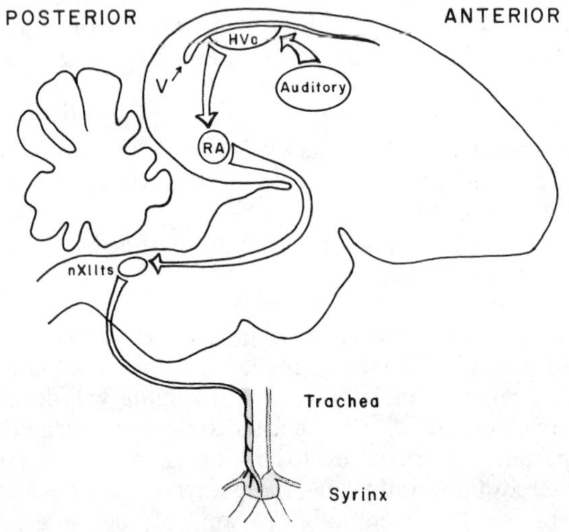

FIGURE 1. Schematic representation of the motor song control pathway in sagittal section of the brain of an adult canary. Notice that nucleus HVc receives auditory input, and that the axons of the motor neurons in nXIIts innervate the muscles of the trachea and syrinx.[34] The distance from the anterior to the posterior end of the brain is 1.2 cm. HVc, hyperstriatum ventralis, pars caudalis; RA, robust nucleus of the archistriatum; nXIIts, part of the hypoglossal nucleus which innervates the muscles of trachea and syrinx; V, lateral ventricle of forebrain. (From Nottebohm.[24] Reproduced by permission from *Condor*.)

tion.[21] Removal of HVc results in aberrant song.[34] Thus HVc may partake in a perceptual and motor involvement in song control.

SONG AS A HORMONE-DEPENDENT BEHAVIOR

It has been known for many years that birdsong is a hormone-dependent behavior.[6,42] Female canaries treated with testosterone develop male-like song.[2,13,18,40] Twenty days after onset of treatment with physiological levels of testosterone the song of an adult intact or ovariectomized female canary becomes stable (unpublished observations). This effect of testosterone apparently requires that two of testosterone's metabolites—estradiol and 5-α-dihydrotestosterone (DHT)—be present. Treatment of adult ovariectomized females with DHT by itself does not induce song.[8] However, DHT will induce song in adult females with intact ovaries (unpublished observation). The song developed by adult female canaries treated with testosterone is male-like in structure, but has only one-third or less as many different syllable types as the song of adult males.

The summer and early fall period of song instability in adult male canaries corresponds to a time of lowered plasma testosterone levels. Testosterone levels rise once more in early fall, as song gradually regains the stereotyped delivery typical of adult canaries in breeding condition.[33] Castrated male canaries fail to develop stable adult song.[22]

SPACE FOR SONG-LEARNING

Sexual Dimorphism and Its Sensitivity to Adult Testosterone Levels

Nucleus HVc is four times larger in adult male than in adult female canaries; RA is three times larger in males than in females.[27,30] This makes sense, since male canaries sing and female canaries normally do not. That is, the amount of brain space related to a learned skill is larger in the sex that develops that skill, or that develops it more. Part of this difference in brain space for song control can be reduced by treating adult females with physiological levels of testosterone, which, as we have seen, induces such birds to sing in a male-like manner. Adult females sacrificed 30 days after onset of testosterone treatment have a neuclus HVc that is 1.9 times larger than that of cholesterol-treated controls, whereas RA is 1.5 times larger than in controls.[22]

Ontogeny of Brain Space for Song-Learning in Males

Nucleus HVc can be first recognized in male canaries 30 days after hatching. It triples in size during the subsequent 30 days, which correspond to the subsong stage of song development. HVc continues to grow while the young bird is in the period of plastic song. Growth stops at 7–8 months, which is also the time when the birds first achieve stable adult song and come into full reproductive condition. (As mentioned earlier, the exact age when this happens depends on whether the bird has hatched early or late in the preceding breeding season.) After then, the size of HVc remains stable for the duration of the breeding season, which stretches roughly from early March to late June (FIG. 2). A similar developmental growth, although somewhat attenuated, also occurs in nucleus RA. The size of both nuclei increases as the behavior is acquired and perfected.

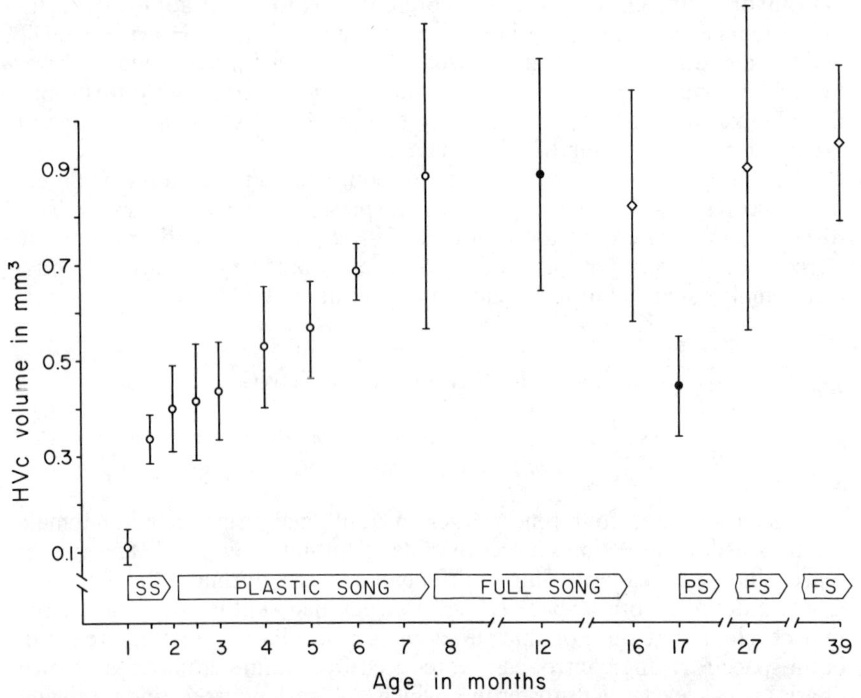

FIGURE 2. Relation between age, HVc volume, and stage in song development in male canaries. Song development, as it normally occurs in male canaries kept under the photoperiod conditions of New York State, is shown as a horizontal progression from subsong (SS) to plastic song (PS) to full song (FS), which is the stable song adult canaries sing during the breeding season. Plastic song recurs again at the end of the breeding season. The vertical axis shows the volume of nucleus HVc, with one standard deviation. *Open circles* (○) correspond to samples of 4 birds each, sacrificed at the age shown in the horizontal axis. *Solid circles* (●) correspond to samples of 9 and 12 birds sacrificed, respectively, at 12 and 17 months of age. *Open diamonds* (◇) correspond to samples of 10, 9 and 8 birds sacrificed, respectively, at the end of their first, second, and third breeding season. Notice that HVc volume grows during the time song is first acquired. This volume shrinks to that of a 3–4-month-old canary in late summer after the breeding season is over and song once more becomes plastic.

Relation between Brain Space for Learning and Amount Learned

Adult male canaries vary in the size of their learned song repertoire. There is a three-fold range between the smallest and largest syllable repertoires recorded from members of our close-bred Wasserschlager colony (15–47 syllables). There is also a three-fold range between the smallest and largest HVc found in those birds. There is a significant correlation between these two variables. Birds with large song repertoires tend to have large HVcs, whereas birds with small HVcs tend to have small repertoires.[30] This correlation, which also applies to nucleus, RA, has also been observed in zebra finches (Nottebohm and Crane, unpublished observation) and in wild populations of marsh wrens.[5] These correlations seem to argue that learned information requires space, much as books in a library require space. Presumably, this "space" has to do with the number, size, and complexity of forebrain circuits controlling song.

SEASONAL CHANGES IN SPACE FOR LEARNING

Twenty-one male canaries born in the month of April were divided in two groups. Twelve males were sacrificed in the following April, when 12 months old and in the middle of the breeding season, when song is stable (*Spring* group). The other nine males bred and were sacrificed in mid-September, when they were finishing the molt of their feathers (*Fall* group). Birds in the Fall group were 5 months older when sacrificed than those in the Spring group. HVc was 1.9 times larger in the Spring group than in the Fall group; RA was 1.6 times larger in the Spring group than in the Fall group.[23] Since we know that HVc and RA size is the same in birds 1, 2, and 3 years old,[30] the inevitable conclusion is that the size of these two nuclei fluctuates seasonally. It is smallest in late summer, at a time when male canaries are silent or producing very unstable song (FIG. 2). The seasonal decrease in the size of HVc and RA is of the same magnitude but inverse sign as that found in adult females treated with testosterone. Quite likely, the reduction in volume is causally related to the decrease in testosterone levels which occurs in males at the end of the breeding season.[33] The late summer size of HVc and RA observed in 17-month-old male canaries is comparable to that of a 3–4-month-old male canary (FIG. 2). It seems possible that this process of circuit rejuvenation is important for the remodeling of song that takes place during the summer months.[33]

TESTOSTERONE INDUCES DENDRITIC GROWTH AND SYNAPTOGENESIS

Type 4 neurons in nucleus RA have a stellate soma and thick spiny dendrites. These dendrites are significantly longer in males than in females.[7] However, after testosterone administration in adulthood, the dendrites of females grow by 49%,[8] and this growth is accompanied by a 51% increase in the number of synapses found in RA.[9] The growth of RA in the testosterone-treated females occurs in the absence of new neurons.[10] It seems likely that the end-of-summer reduction in size of the male RA results from a retraction of the testosterone-sensitive dendrites and synapses. This hormone-dependent plasticity is quite remarkable for an adult brain. Since forebrain pathways for song control exit the forebrain via RA, we may infer that the addition and (presumed) subtraction of dendrites and synapses are related importantly to the motor control of this learned behavior.

NEUROGENESIS IN FEMALES

In view of the marked changes in size of HVc and RA that occurred with changing hormone levels in males and females, it seemed natural to wonder whether such marked changes involved the birth and loss of neurons.[22] As a first experiment aimed at testing this possibility, adult female canaries were treated systemically for 2 days with three daily injections of 50 μCi of [^{3}H]thymidine (2.5 μCi per g body weight).[10] [^{3}H]thymidine is a marker of DNA synthesis and, by extrapolation, of cell birth.[17] Half of the females had been pretreated with cholesterol, the other half with testosterone. This treatment, in the form of a Silastic implant, continued during [^{3}H]thymidine administration. Our expectation was that if neuronal labeling indicative of neurogenesis occurred at all, it would occur in the testosterone-treated group, since only females in that group underwent the doubling in size of HVc.

A High Labeling Index

The results of this experiment were clear and surprising. A mean of 1.5% of all neurons in HVc became labeled per day of [^{3}H]thymidine treatment in both the testosterone- and cholesterol-treated females. Label was concentrated over nuclei (FIG. 3), suggesting that its presence originated from the incorporation of the labeled thymidine into DNA. Thus neurogenesis in these females required neither the presence of exogenous hormone, nor that the females produce male-like song.

A Ventricular Zone Origin

Females that were treated as above, but sacrificed 1 or 2 days after the last [^{3}H]thymidine injection, had no labeled neurons. These birds, however, had many labeled cells in the ventricular zone overlying HVc. From this we inferred that new neurons were born in the ventricular zone and from there migrated into HVc, where they found a place to settle and differentiate. Had neuronal labeling resulted from amitotic DNA replication in existing neurons, leading to polyploidy, or had it resulted from DNA repair, then it would have been expected to occur *in situ*, and labeled neurons would have been found in the birds sacrificed soon after the [^{3}H]thymidine treatment.

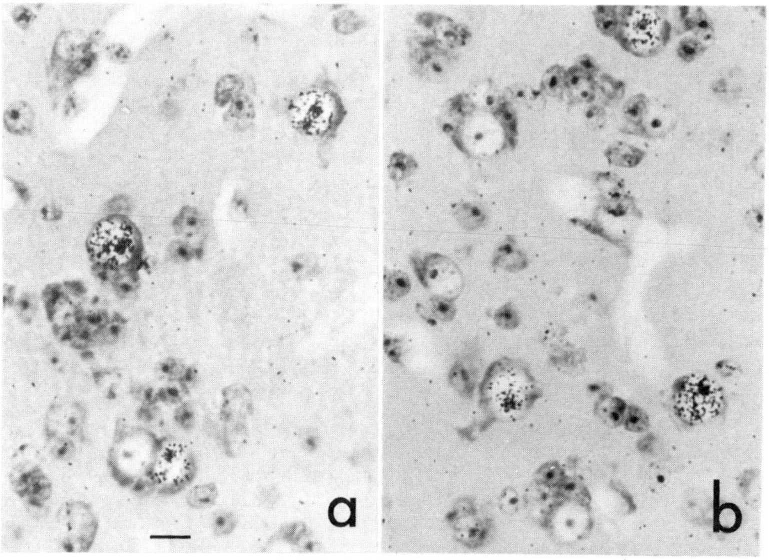

FIGURE 3. Examples of labeled neurons in left (**a**) and right (**b**) neostriatum caudalis (N in FIGURES 5 and 6). Three labeled neurons are shown on each side. The sections, which are representative of labeling in adult canary forebrain, were obtained from the same adult female canary as shown in FIGURE 6. The bird was sacrificed 26 days after the last of 28 intramuscular injections of [^{3}H]thymidine given at 12-hr intervals over a 14-day period. Sections were exposed for autoradiography for 4 weeks, then counterstained with cresyl violet. See Goldman and Nottebohm[10] for other details on histologic and autoradiography methods. Notice the concentration of exposed silver grains over the nuclei of neurons recognized by their clear karyoplasm; notice also the single dark staining nucleoli. One of the labeled neurons in **a** is in close opposition to an unlabeled neuron. Calibration bar in **a** represents 10 μm.

Labeling as Evidence of Birth

There are other ways of testing for the origin of the neuronal labeling observed. The occurrence of gliogenesis and birth of endothelial cells in the adult brain is widely accepted.[2] Therefore, we argued, if the numbers of exposed silver grains in birds that received [^{3}H]thymidine and whose brains were treated for autoradiography were to be similar over the nuclei of labeled neurons, glia and endothelial cells, then in all cases the presence of label could be explained by the same mechanism, the incorporation of [^{3}H]thymidine into DNA during the S-phase that precedes mitosis.[29] We tested this possibility in an adult female canary that received 50 μCi of [^{3}H]thymidine intramuscularly at 12-hr intervals for 14 days. The purpose of giving that many injections was to increase the time period during which new cell birth would be recorded. [^{3}H]thymidine is metabolized promptly after one injection, so that virtually all of the unincorporated nucleoside is cleared from the blood in about 30 minutes.[1,39] Since the S-phase in most cases of

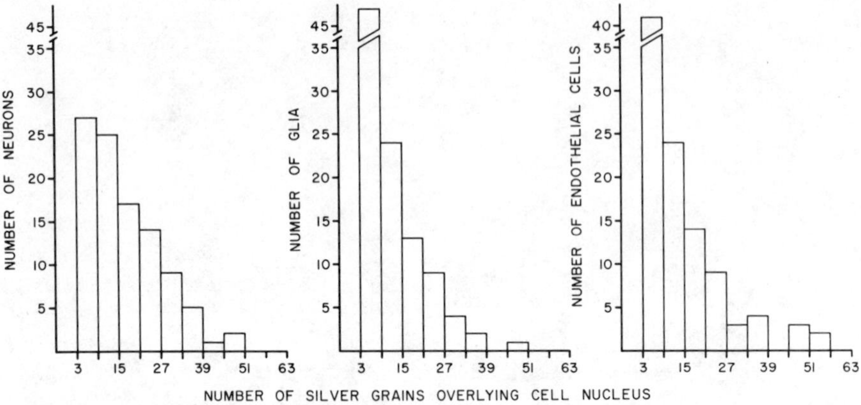

FIGURE 4. Histograms showing the relative frequency with which various numbers of exposed silver grains occurred over the nuclei of 100 labeled neurons (*left*), 100 labeled glia (*middle*), and 100 labeled endothelial cells (*right*). The sample of labeled cells was obtained from HVc and adjacent neostriatum. This material came from the same adult female canary that generated the sections shown in FIGURE 3; however, exposure time was only 10 days. Criterion for labeling was 3 exposed silver grains per nucleus, which corresponds here to 10 × background. The short exposure time was chosen to reduce the instances in which the number of exposed silver grains over the nucleus was too high to allow for the indentification of the underlying cell.

postnatal neurogenesis studied lasts 8–12 hr, it seemed very unlikely that the S-phase of any one cell would be exposed to more than one pulse of label. Brain sections from this bird were cut at 6 μm and exposed to autoradiography for 10 days. After such a brief exposure it is possible to count all exposed silver grains even over the heaviest of labeled nuclei. Criterion for accepting a cell as labeled was set at ten times background, which in this case corresponded to 3 grains per nucleus. Our sample consisted of 100 labeled neurons, 100 labeled glia, and 100 labeled endothelial cells from HVc and its immediate surrounds. The mean number of silver grains per nucleus of labeled cell was well above criterion and comparable for neurons (16.4 grains), glia (11.8 grains) and endothelial cells (14.3 grains) (FIG. 4). It seems most parsimonious to conclude that the new neurons were generated in the ventricular zone as the result of mitosis of ventricular zone cells.[29]

Neuronal Identity Ascertained

We tried to confirm the neuronal identity of the labeled putative neurons in several ways. Initial identification was based on light and electron microscopic criteria. A neuron in a 6-μm-thick paraffin-embedded section stained with cresyl violet was a cell with a clear nucleus, one or two darkly stained nucleoli, and no heterochromatin. A better look at such cells was then obtained by using 1-μm-thick plastic-embedded sections which were then processed for transmission electron microscopy. These revealed a well-developed Golgi apparatus and one instance of an embedded cilium.[10] Soon thereafter it was possible to demonstrate synapses on [^{3}H]thymidine-labeled HVc neurons,[4] but even this did not constitute final proof of neuronal identity. There are precedents of synapse formation on glia.[12,35,44] We wanted to show that a ^{3}H-labeled cell that looked like a neuron also acted like a neuron.

Final neuronal identification was obtained as follows: Adult canaries received two intramuscular injections of [^{3}H]thymidine for 14 days. We hoped that this would label some 10% of the neurons in HVc. These birds were allowed to survive 30 days after the last [^{3}H]thymidine injection and were then anesthetized. Glass electrodes filled with HRP were used to impale HVc cells. Changes in their membrane potential could be used to judge the neuronal identity of these cells. In addition, white-noise clicks were played over a speaker. Many of the HVc cells impaled responded to sound stimulation with typical neuronal action potentials. At this point the intracellular electrode used for physiological recording filled the cells iontophoretically with HRP. The birds were then sacrificed and their brains prepared for histologic examination. A total of 74 HRP-filled cells with neuronal physiological profiles were recovered. Of these, 7 had radioactively labeled nuclei; four of these seven cells had produced synaptic potentials in response to sound.[36] This work showed beyond reasonable doubt that neurons born in adulthood are recruited into existing circuits.

New Neurons are Local Interneurons

This same experiment yielded other valuable information. The axons of the seven HRP and [^{3}H]thymidine double-labeled neurons branched repeatedly within HVc without ever leaving this nucleus. This suggests that the HVc neurons born in adulthood assume the function of local interneurons.

Other work since then has pointed to the same conclusion.[37] In this case adult male and female canaries received the same 14-day treatment with [^{3}H]thymidine as described for the previous experiment. Thirty or sixty days after the last injection of [^{3}H]thymidine, HRP was injected into either of two parts of the brain known to receive a heavy projection from HVc—nucleus RA and area X of lobus parolfactorius. As expected, HRP was carried retrogradely into HVc neurons projecting to either of these two nuclei. As a result, many HVc neurons were now filled with HRP. Many neurons in HVc were also labeled with [^{3}H]thymidine. However, only a handful of the many thousands of HVc neurons examined was labeled by both HRP and [^{3}H]thymidine. The conclusion, as before, is that in the great majority of cases axons of HVc neurons born in adulthood do not leave HVc.

Survivorship of New Neurons

Survival of neurons born in adulthood must be quantified if one is to understand the significance of neurogenesis in adulthood. Preliminary results indicate that only half of the labeled HVc neurons present 26 days after a

14-day series of [^{3}H]thymidine injections survive yet another 26 days. After this initial loss, virtually all of the survivors persist for at least another 26 days. Exceedingly few labeled neurons are seen 1 year after [^{3}H]thymidine treatment (unpublished observations). It is possible that the initial mortality results from an overproduction of neurons, as has been described in embryos,[11] so that this initial mortality does not reflect the half-life of new neurons successfully incorporated into functioning circuits. Clearly, though, the great majority of labeled neurons does not live past the 12-month mark. However, we must still show that the doses of [^{3}H]thymidine used do not affect the survival of labeled neurons.

NEUROGENESIS IN MALE CANARIES

Soon after neurogenesis was established for nucleus HVc of adult female canaries, the observation was extended to HVc of males.[28] Quantitative analysis of neurogenesis in adults of both sexes for every month of the year is now in progress. In males, as in females, the new HVc neurons are interneurons,[36,37] and few, if any, seem to survive in excess of 12 months.

NEURONAL REPLACEMENT IN ADULTHOOD

Our initial finding that 1.5% of the HVc neurons of adult female canaries were labeled per day of [^{3}H]thymidine treatment was perplexing. At this rate, if a compound-interest formula is applied, the number of HVc neurons would double in 49 days. Yet other data[30] indicated that nucleus HVc in adult female canaries 15 and 27 months old was remarkably similar in size. Counts of HVc neurons in females of these two age groups ($n = 10$ and $n = 9$, respectively) has revealed that in both cases females have a mean of approximately 15,000 neurons per left HVc (Nottebohm and O'Loughlin, in preparation). The inescapable conclusion is that there must be neuronal death in nucleus HVc of adult female canaries, and that its extent must offset the numbers of new neurons added.

We have also counted neurons in the left HVc of males sacrificed in the spring ($n = 9$) at 12 months of age or in the fall ($n = 12$) at 17 months of age. These are the same birds for which we had obtained gross measurements on size of nucleus HVc.[23] Males in the Spring group had a mean of 41,000 neurons per left HVc; those in the Fall group, 25,000. The numbers within each group clustered sufficiently around the mean, with little overlap between groups, so that the difference was significant (t test; $p < 0.001$). Thus, a large number of the HVc neurons present in the spring, when males are producing stable adult song, has been dismissed by late summer, when song is in the process of undergoing significant change and relearning. This observation suggests that the demise of HVc neurons may be narrowed in time, so that most of it occurs over a period of 1 or 2 months. The neurogenesis observed during the ensuing 12-month period may make up for this loss. The rates of neurogenesis observed in adult males, corrected for the possible loss of one-half of the new neurons due to overproduction, would yield a daily recruitment rate of approximately 0.20. At that rate the number of HVc neurons observed in the fall would be approximately doubled over the ensuing 12-month period (Nottebohm, Kasparian and O'Loughlin, in preparation).

We do not know whether the numbers of HVc neurons of female canaries undergo similar seasonal oscillation. This would be predicted if the process of death and replacement were similar in the two sexes.

The observation that a population of 16,000 neurons, possibly all interneurons, undergoes relatively sudden demise, almost halving the population of neurons in a part of the forebrain concerned with a learned behavior, has no precedent. Neither is there a precedent for such a loss then being made up by the production of new neurons. Not surprisingly, then, we have as yet no philosophy of brain function that can easily accommodate these facts. Some testable hypotheses are now offered.

SIGNIFICANCE OF NEURONAL REPLACEMENT IN THE SONG CONTROL SYSTEM

Neurogenesis and neuronal replacement occur in nucleus HVc of adult male and female canaries, although males sing and females normally do not. Neurogenesis in adult nucleus HVc also occurs in male zebra finches after the end of the critical period for song-learning.[24] Thus, it seems unlikely that adult neurogenesis and neuronal replacement in HVc are exclusively related to the learning of song as a motor skill.

It was mentioned earlier that HVc receives auditory input and may partake in a perceptual function. This perceptual function could consist of laying down perceptual memories of songs heard. Males would use such perceptual memories for song learning, as well as for identification of neighbors. Females would use such perceptual memories for recognizing the song of their mate and that of their neighbors. The relevance of memories used in such social interactions would possibly fade after the end of the breeding season, as the pair bond is discontinued and the birds forage singly or in flocks. The replacement of HVc interneurons seen in adulthood may be related to the updating of perceptual memories in a system that has limited space for learning. More specifically, anatomic and functional properties of HVc interneurons may be irreversibly modified by learning. Replacement of such interneurons would result in a loss of the memories they held, as well as in a restoration of the plasticity needed for learning new perceptual memories. I will call this speculation Hypothesis #1; a more expanded version of it has been published elsewhere.[24] This hypothesis predicts that song perceptual memories would have a half-life comparable to that of the interneurons replaced. It also predicts that interference with neurogenesis in nucleus HVc would preclude the formation of new perceptual memories of song.

There is another way of looking at perceptual phenomena and replaceable neurons, which I will call Hypothesis #2. HVc interneurons and the circuits they form may offer a finite and rather stochastic array for encoding a diversity of sounds. Those circuits that match sounds that are actually perceived and remembered may have their connectivity confirmed, and persist. Other circuits not matched by experiential inputs may be less stable, and the HVc interneurons linked to them may undergo turnover. As the latter interneurons are replaced, the new interneurons that replace them may form a new array of stochastic connections, some of which will be novel, thus generating new perceptual possibilities which may or may not correspond to new environmental inputs. In this manner, replacement of interneurons could generate new learning opportunities without encroaching on circuits already holding memories. As this process continued, the memory space of the HVc would eventually be fully occupied, so that neuronal replacement would slow down and come to a halt. Hypothesis #2 predicts that once song perceptual memories are learned, they persist. In this model, too, interference with neurogenesis would hinder learning.

A caveat is pertinent here. Although we know that neurogenesis in adulthood gives rise to new HVc interneurons, we do not as yet know that the cells they replace are interneurons too. Furthermore, there is still no evidence that neurogenesis and neuronal replacement in adulthood have anything to do with learning, although these are testable propositions.

WIDESPREAD NEUROGENESIS IN FOREBRAIN

Neurogenesis is not restricted to the ventricular zone overlying HVc. Four 1-year-old canaries (2 males, 2 females) received injections of [^{3}H]thymidine (2.5 μCi per g body weight) at 12-hr intervals for 14 days. These birds were sacrificed 1 day after the last injection (short-term survival birds). Another six 1-year-old canaries (3 males, 3 females) were similarly treated with [^{3}H]thymidine and sacrificed 26 to 78 days after the last injection (long-term survival birds). Labeling criterion was set at 5 times background; this required that for a neuron to be counted as labeled it had to have at least 5 exposed silver grains overlying its nucleus. Representative sections of all 10 birds, including at least one per bird with nucleus HVc in it, were thoroughly surveyed. Labeled cells were found in the ventricular zone lining the lateral ventricles abutting with many parts of forebrain, and they were found in all birds. The short-term and long-term survival birds differed in that labeled neurons were only found in the brains of the latter group. The distribution of such labeled neurons was carefully mapped in 13 sections from one of the long-term survival birds, a female sacrificed 26 days after the last injection. We mapped the position of each of the 2026 labeled neurons identified in this birds. Of these, 2020 were in forebrain; the other six were in cerebellum, midbrain, and medulla. There were no labeled neurons in hypothalamus and septum. From the number of labeled neurons observed in this bird, it was estimated that 20,000 new neurons were added to the forebrain per day of [^{3}H]thymidine treatment.[29] It is worth noting that whereas very few labeled neurons were found outside of forebrain, numerous labeled glia and endothelial cells were found in nonforebrain areas (FIG. 5). We may infer, from this, that [^{3}H]thymidine label was available throughout the

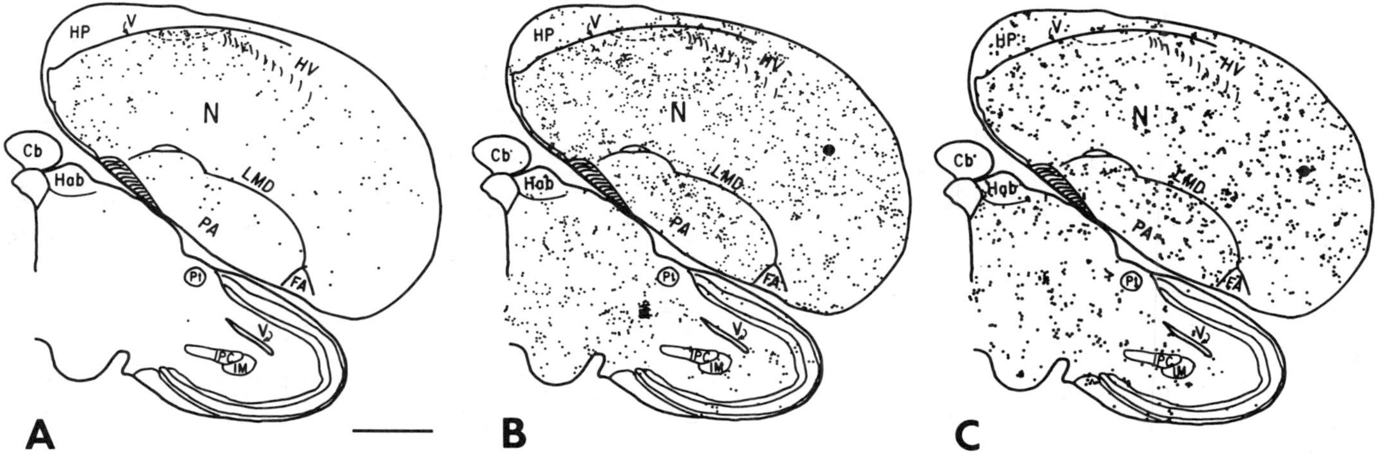

FIGURE 5. Distribution of labeled neurons (**A**), glia (**B**), and endothelial cells (**C**) in a cross section of the right half of the brain of a 1-year-old female canary studied by autoradiography as described in FIGURE 3. The section was taken at the level of nucleus HVc, which is demarcated by a broken line curving under the lateral ventricle of the forebrain (V); the plane of section is close to that of our canary atlas[41]; each point corresponds to a labeled cell. [^{3}H]thymidine was given during the month of April and the bird survived 26 days after the last [^{3}H]thymidine injection. The *solid circle* and the *solid square* in **B** correspond, respectively, to clusters of 13 and 34 labeled glia; the *solid circle* in **C** corresponds to 38 labeled endothelial cells. Notice that whereas labeled glia and endothelial cells can be found throughout the brain, labeled neurons are almost completely restricted to the forebrain. The calibration bar corresponds to 1 mm. Cb, cerebellum; FA, tractus fronto-archistriatalis; Hab, habenula; HV, hyperstriatum ventralis; HP, hippocampus; IM, nucleus isthmi, pars magnocellularis; IPC, nucleus isthmi, pars parvocellularis; LMD, lamina medullaris dorsalis; N, neostriatum; PA, paleostriatum augmentatum; Pt, nucleus pretectalis.

brain, and that the incidence of labeled neurons in the forebrain of the long-term survival birds and their virtual absence elsewhere were not artifactual.

The 5× background criterion for accepting a cell as labeled may be a bit lenient. However, it seemed the most open-minded way to conduct an initial survey of presence of labeled neurons. Conceivably, [^{3}H]thymidine-labeled neuron-producing stem cells in different parts of the brain may divide one or more times before giving rise to a neuroblast that then would migrate and differentiate into a neuron. Depending on the temporal relation between such multiple division and the [^{3}H]thymidine injections, the label of the new neuron could be concentrated or diluted when compared with the label of a cell produced after a single labeled mitotic event. In order to estimate the extent to which the number of labeled cells and their distribution depended on this lenient criterion, we mapped the position of all labeled neurons in a brain section of another female canary, first using a criterion of 5× background (4 exposed silver grains per nucleus). This yielded a total of 598 labeled neurons for this section, of which 17 were outside of forebrain. Then we mapped once more the position of all labeled neurons using a criterion of 10× background (8 exposed silver grains per nucleus). This second count yielded only 405 labeled neurons, 68% of the previous count, and none of these were outside the forebrain (FIG. 6.) We may conclude from this that in 1-year-old canaries neurogenesis is predominantly a forebrain affair.

It should be noted that all the above counts were biased towards neuronal recognition of cells with relatively large clear nuclei (mean nuclear diameters: 9 μm) with single or double nucleoli. The smallest labeled neurons we recognized had a diameter of 5 μm. Our counts may have underestimated or overlooked the presence of labeled microneurons, which can be quite difficult to distinguish from glia. Thus, the suggestion that neurogenesis in adult canaries is a forebrain phenomenon may have to be revised as microneurons are more easily identified. Labeled neurons have also been found in the forebrain of budgerigars (*Melopsittacus undulatus*) and ring doves (*Streptopelia risoria*) (unpublished observation). Neurogenesis in adulthood seems to be widespread among birds.

Even if the caveat regarding the possible occurrence of labeled microneurons is taken into account, the overrepresentation of neuronal labeling in forebrain, and its underrepresentation elsewhere is impressive. The forebrain of vertebrates is credited with the control of complex learned behaviors. Forebrain neurogenesis may be related to learning.

The brain of a 1-month-old canary weighs the same as that of an 8-month-old adult in reproductive condition (unpublished observations). Brain weight of adult males sampled at 15 months of age was similar to that at 27 and 39 months.[30] From this it would seem that, as in the case of HVc, the new forebrain neurons may replace old forebrain neurons. If the analogy with HVc is extended, then the new neurons in the rest of forebrain may be components of local circuits, possibly interneurons in charge of processing and storing perceptual inputs. A diversity of forebrain perceptual systems

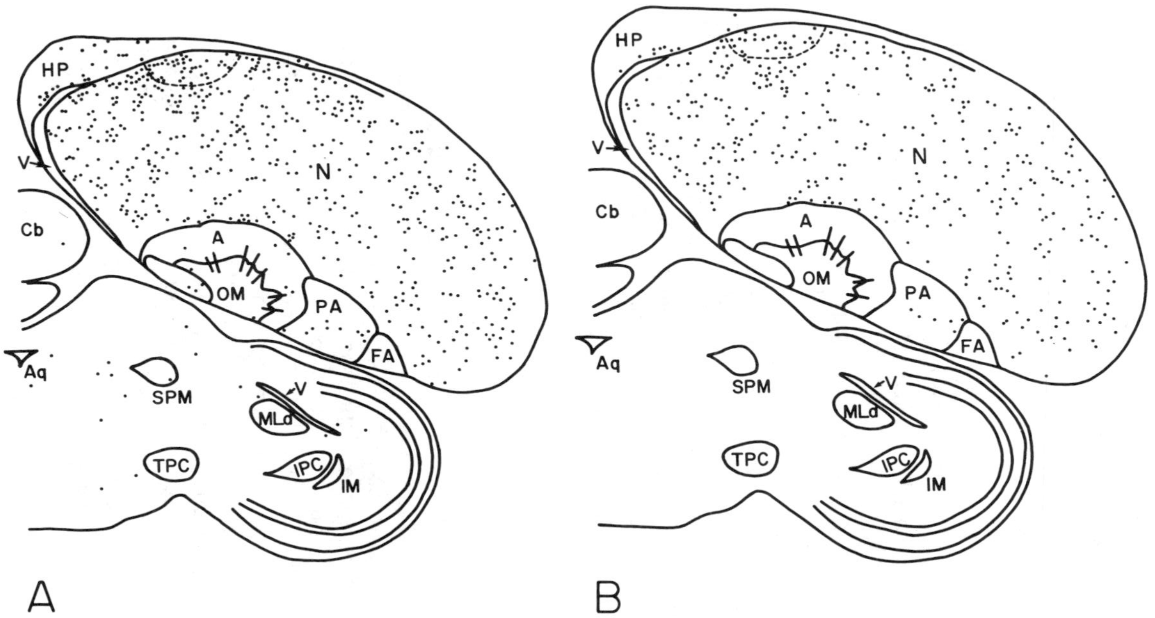

FIGURE 6. Cross section of the right half of the brain of a 1-year-old adult female canary treated with [^{3}H]thymidine as described in the text and in FIGURE 3. The level and plane at which this cross section was obtained is comparable to that shown in FIGURE 5, though not identical. Each *dot* corresponds to a labeled neuron. Labeled neurons were mapped in the same section using first a criterion of 5 × background (**A**), then a criterion of 10 × background (**B**). Notice that when the more stringent criterion is used, no labeled neurons are found in archistriatum, cerebellum, and midbrain. HVc, shown as the region bound by a *broken line* curving under the lateral ventricle (V), has many labeled neurons. This bird, which survived 52 days after the last injection of [^{3}H]thymidine, had more labeled neurons in lateral neostriatum (N) than did the bird shown in FIGURE 5A, which was sacrificed 26 days after the last injection of [^{3}H]thymidine. Presumably the longer survival time allowed more neuroblasts to migrate from their place of origin in the ventricular zone of the forebrain. Calibration bar represents 1 mm. Abbreviations are as in FIGURE 5 and: Aq, aqueduct; MLd, nucleus mesencephalicus lateralis, pars dorsalis; OM, tractus occipitomesencephalicus; SPM, nucleus spiriformis demialis; TPC, nucleus tegmenti pedunculo pontinus, pars compacta.

may rely on replacement of old interneurons by new interneurons to rejuvenate periodically their learning potential. It may not be accidental (or artifactual) that the brain of adult male canaries is 15% lighter in late summer than in the previous spring.[23] Many forebrain circuits, in addition to those in HVc, may go through an acute episode of interneuron death, with vacancies filled during the next 12-month period.

RELEVANCE TO NEUROLOGY

The brain of birds may offer a poor model for studying the human brain. Most birds achieve reproductive age towards the end of their first year. Their life after then goes through marked seasonality, as reproductive and nonreproductive periods alternate. This sets the stage for sex hormones or other hormones sensitive to day length to play a major role in regulating brain performance.[23,26,33] However, reproductive seasonality is by no means restricted to birds. The great majority of mammals, including many primates, are seasonal breeders. Even in nonseasonal mammals, such as most populations of humans, there is a marked change in plasma levels of sex hormones during development and particularly at puberty. It is believed by many that early brain damage is followed by better prognosis for recovery than is late brain damage. The reasons for this are not fully understood. Blood hormone levels typical of those of infancy may be conducive to functional recovery after occurrence of a lesion. Neurologists may find that inducing prepuberal hormone levels in postpuberal individuals encourages processes of brain repair and functional recovery. This is an area where insights from research on other animals might be well worth testing in primates, and eventually humans.

On the narrower issue of neurogenesis and neuronal replacement in adulthood, we do not know if it occurs in humans. Neurogenesis is reported to be absent in postpuberal macaques.[38,45] However, if neurogenesis were not to occur normally in postpuberal humans, this need not close the door to addition of new cells as a tool for brain repair, as demonstrated by the papers in this volume by Björklund and Gage[46], Cotman and Nieto-Sampedro,[47] and Olson *et al.*[48] Furthermore, it may be possible to induce neurogenesis in ventricular zone cell populations that are no longer dividing, or that are only giving rise to ependymal cells or glia. The key to success in such an endeavor will be to discover the chemicals or other physical signals that normally control neurogenesis. However, even if this effort were to succeed, functional success would require that neurogenesis be followed by migration of the resulting neuroblasts and their differentation and incorporation into the correct circuits. The effective stimuli to achieve this may be common to adult lampreys,[49] adult birds, adult rats,[50] and human embryos.

Whatever the outcome of these potential applications, it seems fair to say that the work on animal systems in which neurogenesis has been shown in adulthood has brought about a change in perspective. The dogma that neurogenesis and neuronal replacement does not occur and is not possible in adulthood is dead. From now on, those who fail to find neurogenesis in the adult brain cannot hold their findings as confirmatory of a law of nature. Instead, they must ask "why not?" or "how could it be brought about?" Birth and functional replacement of neurons in an adult, warm-blooded vertebrate brain is now a well-established fact.

ACKNOWLEDGMENTS

Special credit for the work on neurogenesis reported here goes to Gail D. Burd, Steven A. Goldman, Robert Morrison and John A. Paton, as well as to research assistants Susan Kasparian and Barbara O'Loughlin. The skills and enthusiasm of these individuals opened up new possibilities and got the work done.

REFERENCES

1. Altman, J. 1969. DNA Metabolism and cell proliferation. *In* Structural Neurochemistry. A. Lajtha, Ed. Plenum Press. New York, NY.
2. Alberts S., D. Bray, J. Lewis, M. Raff, K. Roberts & J. D. Watson. 1983. Molecular biology of the cell. Garland Publishing. New York, NY.
3. Baldwin, F. M., Goldin, H. S. & Metfessel. M. 1940. Effects of testosterone propionate on female Roller canaries under complete song isolation. Proc. Soc. Exp. Biol. **44:** 373–375.
4. Burd, G. D. & F. Nottebohm. 1985. Ultrastructural characterization of synaptic terminals formed on newly-generated neurons in a song control nucleus of the adult canary forebrain. J. Comp. Neurol. **240:** 143–152.
5. Canady, R. A., D. E. Kroodsma & F. Nottebohm. 1984. Population differences in complexity of a learned skill are correlated with brain space involved. Proc. Natl. Acad. Sci. USA **81:** 6232–6234.
6. Collard, J. & L. Grevendal. 1946. Etudes sur les caractères sexuels des Pinsons, *Fringilla coelebs* et *F. montifringilla.* Gerfaut **2:** 89–107.
7. DeVoogd, T. J. & F. Nottebohm. 1981. Sex differences in dendritic morphology of a song control nucleus in the canary. A quantitative Golgi study. J. Comp. Neurol. **196:** 309–316.
8. DeVoogd, T. J. & F. Nottebohm. 1981. Gonadal hormones induce dendritic growth in the adult brain. Science **214:** 202–204.
9. DeVoogd, T. J., B. Nixdorf & F. Nottebohm. 1985. Synaptogenesis and changes in synaptic morphology related to acquisition of a new behavior. Brain Res. **329:** 304–308.
10. Goldman, S. A. & F. Nottebohm. 1983. Neuronal production, migration and differentiation in a vocal control nucleus of the adult female canary brain. Proc. Natl. Acad. Sci. USA **80:** 2390–2394.
11. Hamburger, V. & R. Levi-Montalcini. 1949. Proliferation, differentiation and degeneration in the spinal ganglia of the chick embryo under normal and experimental conditions. J. Exp. Zool. **111:** 457–502.
12. Henrikson, C. K. & J. E. Vaughn. 1974. Fine structural relationship between neurites and radial glial processes in developing mouse spinal cord. J. Neurocytol. **3:** 659–675.
13. Herrick, E. H. & J. O. Harris. 1957. Singing female canaries. Science **125:** 1299–1300.
14. Katz, L. C. & M. E. Gurney. 1981. Auditory responses in the zebra finch's motor system for song. Brain Res. **221:** 192–197.
15. Kelley, D. B. & F. Nottebohm. 1979. Projections of a telencephalic auditory nucleus—field L—in the canary. J. Comp. Neurol. **183:** 455–470.

16. KONISHI, M. 1965. The role of auditory feedback in the control of vocalization in the white-crowned sparrow. Z. Tierpsychol. **22:** 770–783.
17. KORR, H. 1980. Proliferation of different cell types in the brain. Adv. Anat. Embryol. Cell. Biol. **61** (monograph).
18. LEONARD, S. L. 1939. Induction of singing in female canaries by injections of male hormone. Proc. Soc. Exp. Biol. **41:** 229–230.
19. MARGOLIASH, D. 1983. Acoustic parameters underlying the responses of song-specific neurons in the white-crowned sparrow. J. Neurosci. **3:** 1039–1057.
20. MARLER, P. & M. S. WASER. 1977. The role of auditory feedback in canary song development. J. Comp. Physiol. Psychol. **91:** 8–16.
21. MCCASLAND, J. S. & M. KONISHI. 1981. Interaction between auditory and motor activities in an avian song control nucleus. Proc. Natl. Acad. Sci. USA **78:** 7815–7819.
22. NOTTEBOHM, F. 1980. Testosterone triggers growth of brain vocal control nuclei in adult female canaries. Brain Res. **189:** 429–436.
23. NOTTEBOHM, F. 1981. A brain for all seasons: Cyclical anatomical changes in song control nuclei of the canary brain. Science **214:** 1368–1370.
24. NOTTEBOHM, F. 1984. Birdsong as a model in which to study brain processes related to learning. Condor **86:** 227–236.
25. NOTTEBOHM, F. 1984. Learning, forgetting and brain repair. *In* Cerebral Dominance. Norman Geschwind & Albert M. Galaburda, Eds.: 93–113. Harvard University Press. Cambridge, MA.
26. NOTTEBOHM, F. Plasticity in the adult central nervous system: A possible relation between hormones, learning and brain repair. *In* Handbook of Physiology, Section 1: Higher Functions of the Nervous System. Fred Plum, Ed. The American Physiological Society. Bethesda, MD. In press.
27. NOTTEBOHM, F. & A. P. ARNOLD. 1976. Sexual dimorphism in vocal control areas of the songbird brain. Science **194:** 211–213.
28. NOTTEBOHM, F. & S. A. GOLDMAN, 1982. Connectivity and kinetics of neurons born in adulthood. Soc. Neurosci. Abstr. **8:** 140.
29. NOTTEBOHM, F. & S. KASPARIAN. 1983. Widespread labeling of avian forebrain neurons after systemic injections of ^{3}H-thymidine in adulthood. Soc. Neurosci. Abstr. **9:** 380.
30. NOTTEBOHM, F., KASPARIAN, S. & PANDAZIS, C. 1981. Brain space for a learned task. Brain Res. **213:** 99–109.
31. NOTTEBOHM, F., KELLEY, D. B. & J. A. PATON. 1982. Connections of vocal control nuclei in the canary telencephalon. J. Comp. Neurol. **207:** 344–357.
32. NOTTEBOHM, F. & M. E. NOTTEBOHM. 1978. Relationship between song repertoire and age in the canary, *Serinus canarius*. Z. Tierpsychol. **46:** 298–305.
33. NOTTEBOHM, F., M. E. NOTTEBOHM, L. A. CRANE & J. C. WINGFIELD. Seasonal changes in adult canary song learning and their possible relation to gonadal hormone levels. Behav. Neural Biol. In press.
34. NOTTEBOHM, F., T. M. STOKES & C. M. LEONARD. 1976. Central control of song in the canary, *Serinus canarius*. J. Comp. Neurol. **165:** 457–486.
35. OPPENHEIM, R. W., I. W. CHU-WANG & J. L. MADERDRUT. 1978. Cell death of motoneurons in the chick embryo spinal cord. III. The differentiation of motoneurons prior to their induced degeneration following limb-bud removal. J. Comp. Neurol. **177:** 87–112.
36. PATON, J. A. & F. NOTTEBOHM. 1984. Neurons born in adult brain are recruited into functional circuits. Science **225:** 1046–1048.
37. PATON, J. A., B. E. O'LOUGHLIN & F. NOTTEBOHM. Cells born in adult canary forebrain are local interneurons. J. Neurosci. **5:** in press.
38. RAKIC, P. 1985. Limits of neurogenesis in primates. Science **227:** 1054–1056.
39. RUBINI, J. R., E. P. CRONKITE, V. P. BOND T. M. & FLIEDNER. 1960. The metabolic fate of tritiated thymidine in man. J. Clin. Invest. **39:** 909–919.
40. SHOEMAKER, H. H. 1939. Effect of testosterone propionate on the behavior of the female canary. Proc. Soc. Exp. Biol. **41:** 229–302.
41. STOKES, T. M., C. M. LEONARD & F. NOTTEBOHM. 1974. The telencephalon, diencephalon, and mesencephalon of the canary, *Serinus canarius*, in the stereotaxic coordinates. J. Comp. Neurol. **156:** 337–374.

42. Thorpe, W. H. 1958. The learning of song patterns by birds, with special reference to the song of the chaffinch, *Fringilla coelebs*. Ibis **100:** 535–570.
43. Waser, M. S. & P. Marler. 1977. Song learning in canaries. J. Comp. Physiol. Psychol. **91:** 1–7.
44. Wolff, J. R., M. Rickmann & B. M. Chronwall. 1979. Axo-glial synapses and GABA—accumulating glial cells in the embryonic neocortex of the rat. Cell Tissue Res. **201:** 239–248.
45. Rakic, P. 1985. DNA synthesis and cell division in the adult primate brain. Ann. N.Y. Acad. Sci. **457:** 193–212 (this volume).
46. Björklund, A. & F. H. Gage. 1985. Neural grafting in animal models of neurodegenerative diseases. Ann. N.Y. Acad. Sci. **457:** 53–82 (this volume).
47. Cotman, C. W. & M. Nieto-Sampedro. 1985. Progress in facilitating the recovery of function after central nervous system trauma. Ann. N.Y. Acad. Sci. **457:** 83–104 (this volume).
48. Olson, L., E.-O. Backlund, W. Freed, M. Herrera-Marschitz, B. Hoffer, Å. Seiger & I. Stromberg. 1985. Transplantation of monoamine producing cell systems *in oculo* and intracranically: Experiments in search of a treatment for Parkinson's disease. Ann. N.Y. Acad. Sci. **457:** 105–126 (this volume).
49. Anderson, M. J. & S. G. Waxman. 1985. Neurogenesis in adult vertebrate spinal cord *in situ* and *in vitro*: A new model system. Ann. N.Y. Acad. Sci. **457:** 213–233 (this volume).
50. Bayer, S. A. 1985. Neuron production in the hippocampus and olfactory bulb of the adult rat brain: Addition or replacement? Ann. N.Y. Acad. Sci. **457:** 163–172 (this volume).

Neuron Production in the Hippocampus and Olfactory Bulb of the Adult Rat Brain: Addition or Replacement?[a]

SHIRLEY A. BAYER

Department of Biology
Indiana-Purdue University
Indianapolis, Indiana 46223

INTRODUCTION

In 1962, Altman[1] proposed that neurogenesis takes place in the cerebral cortex of adult rats. Between 1963 and 1969, Altman and coworkers found adult and juvenile neurogenesis to be especially prominent in the granule cell populations of both the hippocampus and olfactory bulb.[2–6] Kaplan and Hinds[20] subsequently showed that these newly formed cells had the ultrastructural characteristics of neurons. In the meantime, Bayer and Altman[10] obtained circumstantial evidence that the number of granule cells in the hippocampus was increasing in the adult period, while Roselli-Austin and Altman[29] found the number of granule cells in the olfactory bulb to remain constant during adult life. This paper summarizes recent studies[7,8,12] comparing the patterns of adult neurogenesis in these two populations of the rat brain.

METHODS AND RESULTS

Volumetric Analysis of Hippocampal Granule Cells

The total number of granule cells was estimated in the hippocampus of 17 male Purdue-Wistar rats, four animals each at 30, 120, and 200 days, and five at 365 days. After a transcardial perfusion with 10% neutral formalin and Bouin's fixative, the brains were stored in 10% neutral formalin until the block containing the entire right hippocampus was embedded in methacrylate. Serial 3-μm slices were cut in the horizontal plane with a JB-4 microtome (Sorvall) and stained with cresyl violet. A running count was made of all slices containing the granular layer; care was taken to assure that slices were of uniform thickness.

Two previous volumetric estimates of granule cell numbers in rats used modified Abercrombie correction factors to count neuronal nucleoli.[16,30] This method was unworkable in our preparations since the Purdue-Wistar

[a] This work was supported by Grant BNS 79-21303 from the National Science Foundation.

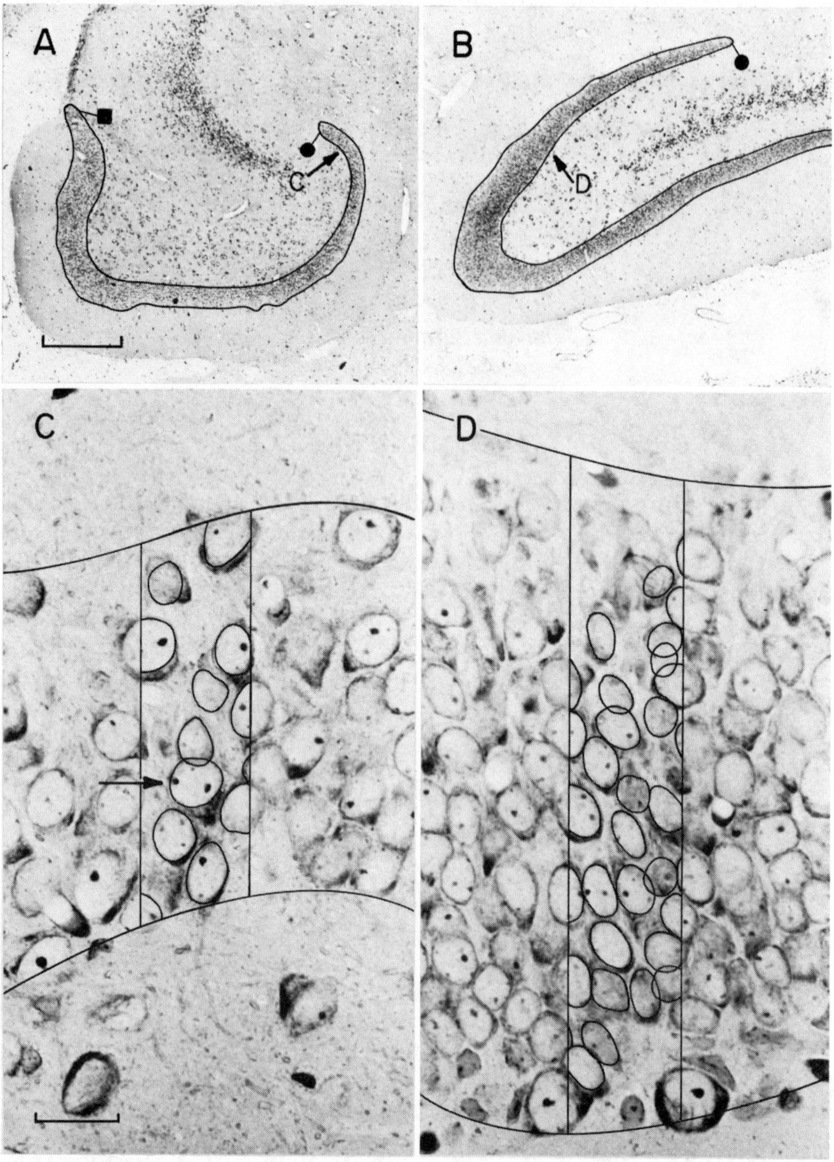

FIGURE 1. (**A** and **B**) Low-magnification (bar = 0.4 mm) views of ventral (**A**) and dorsal (**B**) horizontal sections of the dentate granular layer in a P30 rat; only the posterior part of the granular layer is shown in **B**. The length at the base of the layer was measured starting with the point indicated by the *solid circle*, and ending at the point indicated by the *solid square* to determine the total number of available samples in each section to be quantified. (**C** and **D**) High-magnification views (bar = 20 μm) of samples randomly drawn from either **A** or **B** (the location of **C** is indicated by *arrow* in **A**, while that of **D** is indicated by *arrow* in **B**). The areas of the outlined features in each photograph were measured and formed the data base needed to determine both V_t and V_a. *Arrow* in **C** indicates a granule cell with two nucleolus-like bodies. Notice that the ventral granule cell nuclear profiles (**C**) tend to be larger than the nuclear profiles in the dorsal section (**D**). (3-μm methacrylate sections stained with cresyl violet.) (From Bayer.[7] Reprinted by permission from *Experimental Brain Research.*)

strain consistently shows two or more nucleolus-like bodies in many granule cell nuclei (arrows in FIGURE 1). Consequently, the nucleus was quantified. The method was based on the equation:

$$N = V_t/V_a$$

where N is the total number of cells, V_t the total volume of cell nuclei, and V_a the average nuclear volume. V_t was experimentally determined from low-magnification photomicrographs of dorsal (FIG. 1A) and ventral (FIG. 1B) granular layer slices at regularly spaced intervals. The granular layer was divided into 25-μm wide strips running perpendicular to the length; each strip was a possible sample. Two hundred strips from the total sample pool in all selected slices were randomly chosen for examination at high magnification (FIG. 1C and D). The sampling technique was adjusted so that the experimental error was sensitive to a 10% change in cell number. For each slice examined, the areas of all complete and partial granule cell nuclear profiles (outlined in FIGURE 1C and D) within the samples were measured with a digitizer (Summagraphics) connected to a Wang 2200 computer (accuracy within 0.75%). These measurements provided the basis for the final estimation of V_t (for more details of the method, see Ref. 7).

To estimate V_a in the ventral part of the granular layer, for example, the nuclear profiles completely contained in all ventral samples (between 700 to 1000 in each animal) were used to form empirical distributions of observed ventral granule cell nuclear sizes. Complete profiles contained in all dorsal samples (usually 2000 or more observations for each animal) were similarly processed. In both parts, V_a was estimated by applying a modification[28] of the method of Hendry[18] to the empirical distributions.

Final cell numbers ranged from means of 890,146 at 30 days to 1,276,734 at 365 days (FIG. 2A).[b] Between 1 month and 1 year there is a 43% gain in cell number which the analysis of variance showed to be primarily due to age differences ($F = 34.16$, $p < 0.0001$). There is a high positive correlation with age and cell number (Pearson $r = 0.86$, $p < 0.0001$), which regression analysis shows to be linear (solid line, FIG. 2A; $F = 38.93$, $p < 0.0001$), and cells are added at the approximate rate of 1149 per day between 30 and 365 days. Assuming that the left hippocampus has similar gains, nearly 770,000 granule cells originate between 1 month and 1 year. During this time, the granular layer increased 35% in total volume (FIG. 2B) in an age-related linear pattern (regression analysis: $F = 25.68$, $p < 0.0001$: Pearson $r = 0.80$). There was also an 18% decrease in V_a in the ventral granular layer (FIG. 2C) with a negative correlation between age and cell volume (Pearson $r = -0.64$), and ventral nuclear packing density increased by approximately 50,000 cells

[b] One of the animals (#161) at P365 had an abnormal total cell count 4.74 standard deviations below the mean of the other four animals in this age group. When #161 is included, the mean at P365 is 1,206,209, and the increase between P30 and P365 is 35% (dashed line in FIG. 2A: analysis of variance, $F = 14.66$, $p < 0.0021$; Pearson $r = 0.72$, $p < 0.001$; regression analysis, $F = 16.22$, $p < 0.001$). Since #161 is not representative of the age group at one year, it was eliminated from the data shown in FIG. 2B and C.

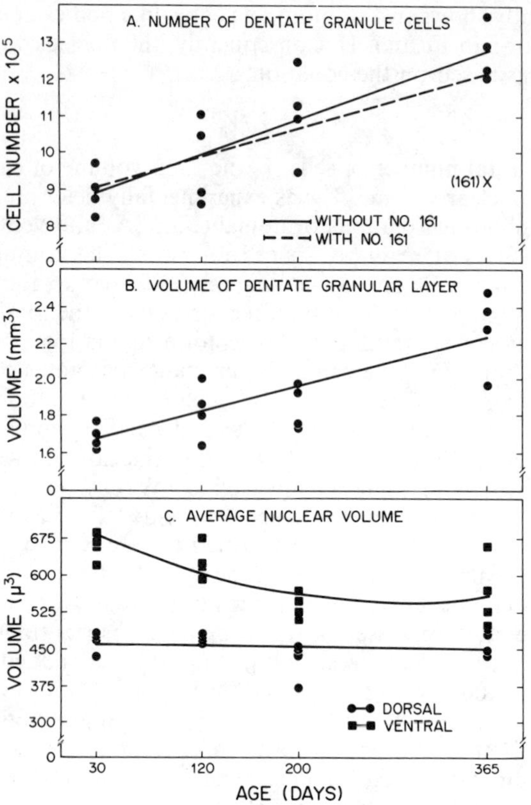

FIGURE 2. Scattergrams with regression lines of best fit showing total number of dentate granule cells (**A**), total volume of the dentate granular layer (**B**), average nuclear volume in dorsal and ventral parts of the granular layer (**C**) in the right hippocampus in rats between 1 month and 1 year of age. (From Bayer.[7] Reprinted by permission from *Experimental Brain Research.*)

per cubic millimeter between 1 month and 1 year. In the dorsal part, V_a was considerably smaller (approximately 465 μm^3) at all ages and remained constant.

Adult Hippocampal Granule Cell Neurogenesis

The proportion of labeled mature granule cells and precursor cells to total cells was determined in groups of Purdue-Wistar male rats after four consecutive daily subcutaneous injections of [^{3}H]thymidine (5 μCi/g body weight) according to the following schedules: postnatal (P) days P30–P33 ($n = 9$), P60–P63 ($n = 5$), P120–P123 ($n = 6$), and P180–P183 ($n = 4$). Three animals from the P30–P33 group were killed on P60; all remaining animals were killed on P200. All animals underwent transcardial perfusion with 10%

neutral formalin. The brains were placed in Bouin's fixative for 24 hr and were then stored in 10% neutral formalin until they were embedded in paraffin. Serial 6-μm sections were cut in the sagittal plane (every 15th section was saved); slides were dipped in Kodak NTB-3 emulsion, exposed for 3 months, developed in Kodak D19, and sections were poststained with hematoxylin and eosin. Anatomically matched sections were selected for cell counts 1.0 and 3.6 mm lateral to the midline. The number of labeled and unlabeled mature granule cells was determined (obvious glial and endothelial cells were eliminated) and the proportion of labeled cells was calculated. A labeled cell had reduced silver grains above background levels in the emulsion layer overlying the nucleus (see FIGURE 5 for examples). Small cells either immediately below the granular layer or embedded into the base were also classed as either labeled or unlabeled, and the proportion of labeled cells was calculated. The analysis of variance was applied to the data to test for age-related changes.

Mature dentate granule cells were routinely labeled after injections of ^{3}H-thymidine in juvenile and adult rats (arrows, FIG. 3B) as were small cells lying beneath the granular layer (asterisk, FIG. 3B). There is evidence that some of these small cells, which cannot be distinguished from glia in paraffin sections, are granule cell precursors,[6,9,30] and mitotic figures have been occasionally observed in this zone in adult animals. FIGURE 3A shows that the

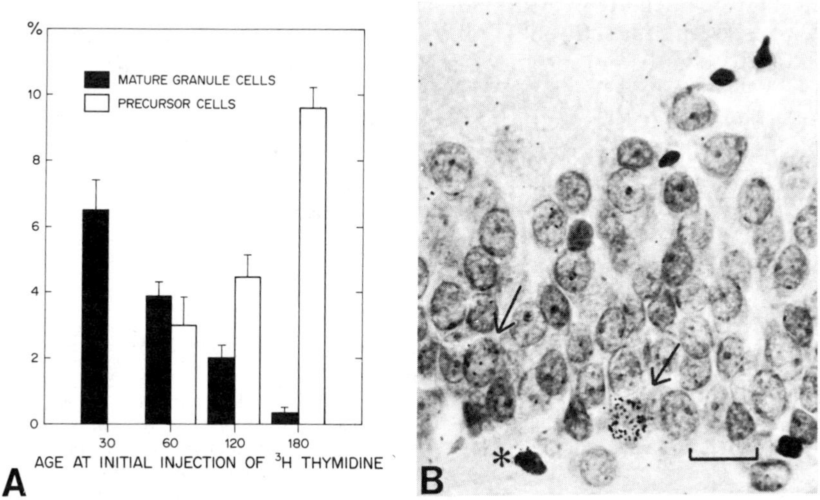

FIGURE 3. (**A**) Means (with standard deviation) of the proportion of labeled mature granule cells (*solid bars*) and labeled precursor cells (*open bars*) in animals injected with [^{3}H]thymidine on four consecutive days beginning with the day indicated. All animals survived to 200 days of age. With a shorter survival after injection (180-day group) there are many precursors and few mature granule cells labeled. Increasing the survival time allows more precursors to mature into granule cells. (**B**) Labeled mature granule cells (*arrows*) and a labeled presumptive granule cell precursor (*asterisk*) in the granular layer of a rat given four injections of [^{3}H]thymidine at 120–123 days of age and killed at 200 days of age. (6-μm paraffin sections; hematoxylin and eosin stain; bar = 20 μm.) (Modified from Bayer.[7]).

proportion of labeled mature granule cells decreases linearly with age (analysis of variance, F = 61.54, $p < 0.0001$) while, at the same time, the proportion of labeled precursor cells increases linearly (analysis of variance, F = 167.55, $p < 0.00001$). The proportion of labeled precursor cells was not quantified in animals injected with [^{3}H]thymidine on 30–33 days because some glial generation is still taking place at this time.[9] Increasing the survival time in the P30–P33 group from P60 to P200 results in a slight increase (2–3%) in the proportion of mature granule cells; these data are not illustrated in FIGURE 3A.

Adult Olfactory Bulb Granule Cell Neurogenesis

The same groups of Purdue-Wistar male rats used in the preceding experiment were also used to study adult olfactory bulb neurogenesis. The proportion of labeled neurons in the granule cell population in the olfactory bulb was determined in serveral randomly selected unit areas (0.04 mm^2), and the effects of both a change in survival time (P30–P33 group) and in injection time were assessed either with the analysis of variance (serveral groups) or the *t* test (two groups). While care was taken to eliminate glial cells from the counts, it should also be noted that small granule cell nuclei are difficult to distinguish from those of astrocytes in paraffin sections. Only nuclei appearing to be definitely "neuronal" were counted. Thus, the data reported are conservative measures of adult neurogenesis. FIGURE 4 shows that there is a decrease in the proportion of labeled cells in injection schedules beyond the P30–P33 group (analysis of variance, F = 10.87, $p < 0.0003$). There is also a significant decrease in the proportion of labeled cells if the survival time in the P30–P33 group is extended from P60 to P200 ($t = 8.72$, $p < 0.0001$, two-tailed probability). FIGURE 5 illustrates the decrease in the proportion of labeled cells with a lengthening of the survival time.

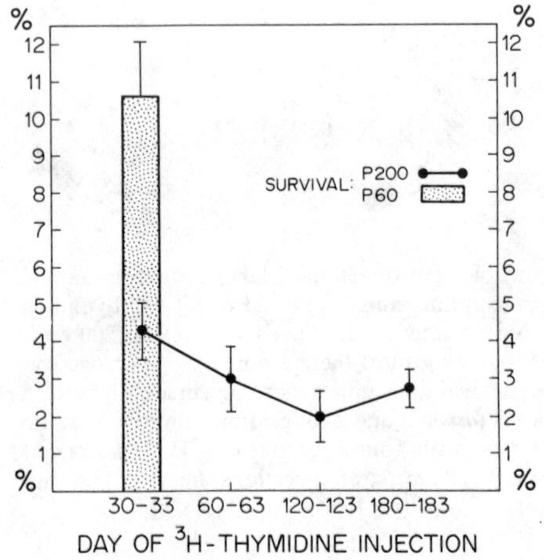

FIGURE 4. The proportion of granule cells in the main olfactory bulb labeled with four consecutive injections of [^{3}H]-thymidine on the days indicated. All *points* are means with standard deviations. *Line graph* is the proportion determined at a P200 survival date; *bar graph* shows that a higher proportion of labeled cells is attained in the P30–P33 group if survival time is decreased to P60. (From Bayer.[8] Reprinted by permission from *Experimental Brain Research.*)

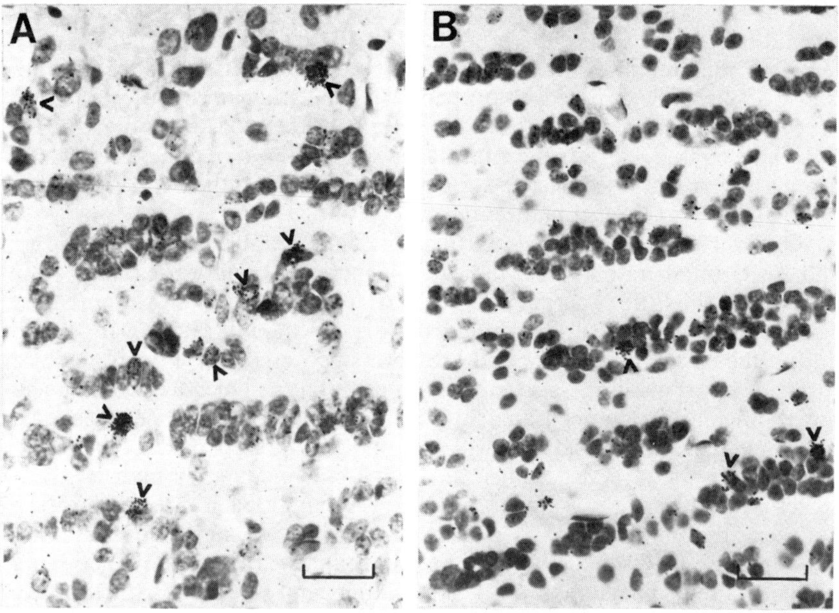

FIGURE 5. Photomicrographs of the main olfactory bulb granule cells in the P30–P33 group with survival times to P60 (**A**) and P200 (**B**). There is a higher proportion of labeled cells (*arrowheads*) in the P60 survival group. (6 μm paraffin sections; hematoxylin and eosin stain; bar = 20 μm.)

DISCUSSION

Hippocampal Granule Cells

It was originally found that approximately 85% of the granule cells in the dentate gyrus originate after birth when rats survive to P60.[9] This must now be considered a conservative estimate since the postnatal part of the granule cell population is continually enlarging. The 43% increase between P30 and P365 (FIG. 2A) is considerable. During this time, two aspects of granular layer morphology are changing, which together reflect the numerical increase. First, new neurons add to total granular layer volume (FIG. 2B); and second, ventral granule cell nuclear volume becomes smaller in older animals (FIG. 2C). So older rats not only have a larger granular layer, but they also tend to have more and smaller cells. Even though morphologic evidence of hippocampal granule cell death, such as pyknotic fragments in the granular layer, is almost never observed, dentate granule cells may also be dying in adult rats. If so, the data of this study indicate that the rate of cell production exceeds the rate of cell death to bring about a net gain.

The volumetric analysis shows that granule cells are added at a constant rate (FIG. 2A), while the autoradiographic analysis shows a sharp decline (FIG. 3B) in the ratio of labeled cells to total cells. However, the proportion of labeled precursor cells increases with age. This is to be expected since

[^{3}H]thymidine will only be incorporated by multiplying precursor cells, not by mature granule cells. Some of the progeny of the precursor cells may remain undifferentiated, while some others may differentiate into granule cells over an undetermined time period. In the earlier injection groups the progeny of the labeled precursors have more time to become mature granule cells, and consequently there is a higher proportion of labeled cells. Confirming this hypothesis, decreasing the survival time in the P30–P33 group resulted in fewer labeled mature granule cells.

One might speculate that the capacity of the granule cell population to add to its numbers may also indicate an increased ability for repair after injury. But the little experimental evidence available does not support this. The losses in granule cells resulting from the exposure of rat pups to X rays during the early postnatal period are never recovered.[10,11] Possibly milder forms of injury with a less severe loss in cell number (such as slight undernutrition) may be compensated for by an increase in adult neurogenesis. To date, there are no data available on this topic. Conceivably, adult neurogenesis may serve another function than repair after injury. Ultrastructural studies of the granular layer show a characteristic direct apposition between adjacent granule cell plasma membranes without any intervening glial processes.[22] This contact may be important for the normal functioning of the granule cell population. As the hippocampus grows with age, the growth pressure will tend to pull adjacent granule cells farther apart. Perhaps adult neurogenesis occurs simply to "fill the gaps" created by increased growth.

Assigning a specific function to the hippocampus is still controversial. Many experiments show it to be involved in short-term memory[19,21,31] especially spatial memory.[26,27] Other studies implicate hippocampal activity in response to inhibition,[13,15,24] which develops in synchrony with the maturation of the dentate gyrus.[14] The growing body of evidence for morphologic and physiological plasticity of the dentate granule cells in both immature and mature animals[23] suggests that the dentate gyrus may be active during the brain's response to changes in the environment. Whatever the function may be, dentate granule cells must play a pivotal role, since their elimination by early postnatal X-irradiation in rats gives behavioral deficits similar to those seen after bilateral hippocampal lesions.[11,17] The continued increase of dentate granule cells in the adult suggests that their influence on total hippocampal function grows with age.

Olfactory Bulb Granule Cells

The level of adult neurogenesis in the granule cells of the olfactory bulb is very prominent, sometimes reaching higher proportions than those found in the dentate granule cell population. If the granule cell populations in both the olfactory bulb and hippocampus are similar, one would predict an even more dramatic increase in the olfactory bulb granule cell population. There are two sets of data that indicate that this is not the case. First, a volumetric determination of total granule cell number in the olfactory bulb showed no significant increase between the ages of 1 month and 1 year.[29] Second, the data of FIGURE 4 and earlier studies by Altman and coworkers[3,29] show that increasing the survival time in the P30–P33 injection group from P60 to P200 results in a *decrease* in the proportion of labeled neurons, possibly due to death of the new neurons. Since neurons are added for several weeks after the injections in the P30–P33 group, the precursors may eventually dilute their supply of [^{3}H]thymidine by repeated cell divisions to undetectable levels and may generate unlabeled new neurons, thus bringing down the proportion of labeled cells. In contrast, the proportion of labeled dentate granule cells slightly *increases* with a longer survival time. The overall implication of these data is that the rate of granule cell production in the main olfactory bulb during adult life is balanced by an equal rate of granule cell death. There is some histologic evidence for cell death since pyknotic fragments are often observed in the granular layer (Bayer, unpublished observations). Cell turnover and regeneration are shown by neurons in the olfactory epithelium,[25] and this phenomenon may also be found in the granule cell population. Thus, prolonged neurogenesis in the olfactory bulb may be more indicative of cell turnover in a numerically stable population rather than cell accumulation in a growing population.

ACKNOWLEDGMENTS

Excellent statistical consultation was provided by P. S. Puri and J. W. Yackel, Department of Statistics, Purdue University. I also wish to thank Joseph Altman for advice and encouragement. Technical assistance was provided by Janis Malone and Ann Hostetler. Connie Flexman typed the manuscript.

REFERENCES

1. ALTMAN, J. 1962. Are new neurons formed in the brains of adult mammals? Science **135:** 1127–1129.
2. ALTMAN. J. 1963. Autoradiographic study of cell proliferation in the brains of rats and cats. Anat. Rec. **145:** 573—592.
3. ALTMAN, J. 1969. Autoradiographic and histological studies of postnatal neurogenesis IV. Cell proliferation and migration in the anterior forebrain, with special reference to persisting neurogenesis in the olfactory bulb. J. Comp. Neurol. **137:** 433–458.
4. ALTMAN, J. & G. D. DAS. 1965. Postnatal origin of microneurons in the rat brain. Nature **207:** 953–956.
5. ALTMAN, J. & G. D. DAS. 1965. Autoradiographic and histological evidence of postnatal hippocampal neurogenesis in rats. J. Comp. Neurol. **124:** 319–336.
6. ALTMAN, J. & G. D. DAS. 1966. Autoradiographic and histological studies of postnatal neurogenesis. I. A longitudinal investigation of the kinetics, migration and transformation of cells incorporating tritiated thymidine in neonate rats, with special reference to postnatal neurogenesis in some brain regions. J. Comp. Neurol. **126:** 337–390.
7. BAYER, S. A. 1982. Changes in the total number of dentate granule cells in juvenile and adult rats: A correlated volumetric and ^{3}H-thymidine autoradiographic study. Exp. Brain Res. **46:** 315–323.
8. BAYER, S. A. 1983. ^{3}H-thymidine-radiographic studies of neurogenesis in the rat olfactory bulb. Exp. Brain Res. **50:** 329–340.

9. Bayer, S. A. & J. Altman. 1974. Hippocampal development in the rat: Cytogenesis and morphogenesis examined with autoradiography and low-level X-irradiation. J. Comp. Neurol. **158:** 55–80.
10. Bayer, S. A. & J. Altman. 1975. Radiation-induced interference with postnatal hippocampal cytogenesis in rats and its long-term effects on the acquisition of neurons and glia. J. Comp. Neurol. **163:** 1–20.
11. Bayer, S. A., R. L. Brunner, R. Hine & J. Altman. 1973. Behavioural effects of interference with the postnatal acquisition of hippocampal granule cells, Nature **242:** 222–224.
12. Bayer, S. A., J. W. Yackel & P. S. Puri. 1982. Neurons in the rat dentate gyrus granular layer substantially increase during juvenile and adult life. Science **216:** 890–892.
13. Douglas, R. J. 1967. The hippocampus and behavior. Psychol. Bull. **67:** 416–422.
14. Douglas, R. J. 1975. The development of hippocampal function: Implications for theory and therapy. *In* The Hippocampus. Vol. 2 Neurophysiology and Behavior. R. L. Isaacson & K. H. Pribram, Eds.: 327–361. Plenum. New York, NY.
15. Douglas, R. J. & K. H. Pribram. 1966. Learning and limbic lesions. Neurophychologia **4:** 197–220.
16. Gaarskjaer, F. B. 1978. Organization of the mossy fiber system of the rat studied in extended hippocampi. I. Terminal area related to number of granule and pyramidal cells. J. Comp. Neurol. **178:** 49–72.
17. Gazzara, R. A. & J. Altman. 1981. Early postnatal X-irradiation of the hippocampus and discrimination learning in adult rats. J. Comp. Phys. Psychol. **95:** 484–495.
18. Hendry, I. A. 1976. A method to correct adequately for the change in neuronal size when estimating neuronal numbers after nerve growth factor treatment. J. Neurocytol. **5:** 337–349.
19. Hirsch, R. 1974. The hippocampus and contextual retrieval of information from memory. Behavioral Biol. **12:** 421–444.
20. Kaplan, M. S. & J. W. Hinds. 1977. Neurogenesis in the adult rat: Electron microscopic analysis of light radioautographs. Science **197:** 1092–1094.
21. Kapp, B. S., M. Gallagher, B. K. Holmquist & C. L. Theall. 1978. Retrograde ammnesia and hippocampal stimulation: Dependence upon the nature of associations formed during conditioning. Behav. Biol. **24:** 1–23.
22. Laatsch, R. H. & W. M. Cowan 1966. Electron microscopic studies of the dentate gyrus of the rat. I. Normal structure with special reference to synaptic organization. J. Comp. Neurol. **128:** 359–375.
23. Lynch, G., B. Stanfield & C. W. Cotman. 1973. Developmental differences in post-lesion axonal growth in the hippocampus. Brain Res. **59:** 155–168.
24. McCleary, R. A. 1966. Response-modulation functions of the limbic system: Initiation and suppression. *In* Progress in Physiological Psychology. E. Stellar & J. N. Sprague, Eds.: 209–272. Academic Press. New York, NY.
25. Monti-Graziadei, G. A. & P. P. C. Graziadei. 1979. Neurogenesis and neuron regeneration in the olfactory system of mammals. II. Degeneration and reconstitution of the olfactory sensory neurons after axotomy. J. Neurocytol. **8:** 197–213.
26. O'Keefe, J. & L. Nadel. 1978. The Hippocampus as a Cognitive Map. Clarendon Press. Oxford, England.
27. Olton, D. S. 1978. The function of septo-hippocampal connections in spatially organized behavior. *In* Functions of the Septo-Hippocampal System. Ciba Foundation Symposium no. 58.: 327–342. Elsevier. Amsterdam.
28. Puri, P. S. & J. W. Yackel. 1983. On a problem of non-identifiability arising in simple stochastic models for stereological counts. Technical Report no. 83-25. Department of Statistics, Purdue University, West Lafayette, IN.
29. Roselli-Austin, L., & J. Altman. 1979. The postnatal development of the main olfactory bulb of the rat. J. Dev. Physiol. **1:** 295–313.
30. Schlessinger, A. R., W. M. Cowan & D. I. Gottlieb. 1975. An autoradiographic study of the time of origin and the pattern of granule cell migration in the dentate gyrus of the rat. J. Comp. Neurol. **159:** 149–176.
31. Scoville, W. & B. Milner. 1957. Loss of recent memory after bilateral hippocampal lesions. J. Neurol. Neurosurg. Psych. **20:** 11–21.

Formation and Turnover of Neurons in Young and Senescent Animals: An Electronmicroscopic and Morphometric Analysis

MICHAEL S. KAPLAN

University of Miami School of Medicine
Miami, Florida 33101

TECHNICAL CONSIDERATIONS

Even though numerous light microscopic studies have been made of neurogenesis and gliogenesis, the identity of the proliferating cells and their eventual fates in normal adult grey matter is still controversial. To determine accurately the types of cells that are formed, the advantages gained by use of [^{3}H]thymidine autoradiography with light microscopy need to be combined with the resolution of electron microscopy. Electron microscopic autoradiography used by itself so limits the sampling that a population of labeled cells is nearly impossible to detect in adult animals. In a large number of earlier studies on neurogenesis and gliogenesis it has been impossible to classify cells with any degree of certainty in sections more than 1 μm thick,[76] and, as a result, it has been difficult to distinguish cells in the light microscope.[23,25,61,82,98] In addition, division of glial cells into the traditional categories (astrocytes, oligodendrocytes, and microglia) often ends up with a large number of indeterminate cells, even when the electron microscope is used. [60,105] Most light microscopic studies using autoradiography of the cerebral cortex of normal adult mammals do not specifically subdivide labeled cells into glial types.[2,35,47,64,82,86,87,112] Likewise, the few microneurons reported to be formed in the newborn[2,10,12,20,41,97,103,106,111] or adult rodent[2,5–9,82–84,87] may be identified inaccurately in light microscopic analysis of thick paraffin sections.[4,41,76] It is generally believed that neurogenesis does not occur in the neocortex of mammals after birth.[51,89,94,116] There are two main technical reasons why reports of neurogenesis in experimental and normal animals[1,3,10,20,82–84,87,97,111] may have been ignored: (1) labeled cells appear to be small neurons, which cannot be distinguished with certainty in light micrographs from neuroglial cells[2,57]; (2) thick paraffin sections were used, which allows the possibility that grazed labeled neuroglial cells could have caused an underlying neuron to appear labeled.[2,57]

The incorporation of [^{3}H]thymidine into newly synthesized DNA should result in a labeled subpopulation of cells. The quantification of this labeled subpopulation could be the basis for the calculations of such parameters as new cell formation or length of the cell cycle. The calculations often assume that if a dividing cell is exposed to [^{3}H]thymidine during the final period of DNA synthesis, the parent cell will become labeled and the number of silver grains per daughter nucleus will be halved with each subsequent division. Conversely, if [^{3}H]thymidine were injected after final division, cells should remain unlabeled. Therefore, the labeling intensities are typically used as a valid index of the proliferating activity of cells. For a given species, increases in the amount of the radiochemical administered increases the number of labeled cells and the intensity of labeling.[24] Curiously, this does not always hold true between species. Although intraperitoneal (i.p.) injections of 5μCi/gram of body weight label glia cells in the rodent,[58] i.p. injections of 10 μCi of [^{3}H]thymidine/gram body weight do not reach the kitten brain.[24] An initial interpretation might be that after i.p. injections in the kitten, the failure for many glial cells to become labeled or for mitotically active cells to be observed is due to lesser cell proliferation. In fact, Das and Altman[24] have contradicted this concept by labeling a very large number of cells in the cat brain after administering [^{3}H]thymidine intracisternally; these injections did not damage the brain itself so that it seems unlikely that the labeled cells were phagocytes.

The best evidence supporting differential uptake of [^{3}H]thymidine is the ultrastructural identification of labeled and mitotic cells of the same cell type; light labeling, which otherwise might be rejected, can then be used as evidence for the birth of new cells. In adult rodents. labeled hippocampal granule neurons and stellate neurons of the visual cortex are obviously more lightly labeled than are adjacent glial cells.[52,54,57,58] In the adult primate, mitotic and lightly labeled subependymal cells indicate that some cells incorporate minute amounts of radioactivity[53] which are near background levels. These low levels of labeling in primates have led to conflicting reports. The subependymal layer in the adult primate may[75] or may not contain proliferative stem cells.[89,92] Previous light microscopic examination suggests the presence of mitotic cells,[75] yet autoradiographic examination after i.p. injections of [^{3}H]thymidine had failed to reveal any mitotic cells or labeled subependymal cells.[89,92]

I have reported the first autoradiographic and ultrastructural evidence that subependymal cells proliferate in the adult primate.[53] To overcome the unreliable identification of cell types at the light microscopic level, we have developed a new procedure. This method allows serial thin sectioning and subsequent electron microscopic examination of 0.5- to 1.5-μm plastic-embedded sections previously prepared for light microscopic autoradiography.[52,55]

Three conclusions result from our studies using these technical procedures: (1) the subependymal layer in the adult rhesus monkey contains mitotic cells; (2) labeled subependymal cells observed after i.p. injection of [^{3}H]thymidine incorporate only minute amounts of radioactivity; and (3) a small percentage of the intraperitoneally injected radioactive DNA precursor is available to the brain. In fact, after i.p. injections of [^{3}H]thymidine, the labeling of subependymal cells is sufficiently light that in standard autoradiographic techniques using single sections our finding might have been dismissed as representing random clustering of silver grains (labeling) over the nucleus.

NEUROGENESIS IN ADULT ANIMALS

Mature neurons may be labeled in adult rodents 30 days after injection of [^{3}H]thymidine. These cells are labeled significantly above background [52,55,56,57] and show clusters of silver grains over the nucleus in several adjacent plastic sections.[52,55,56] Therefore, it is reasonable to conclude that incorporation of label into DNA occurred and that labeling was not a result of random clustering of silver grains. Cells labeled in light microscopic autoradiography were shown in re-embedded thin sections to receive synapses.[57] Our findings represent the first ultrastructural evidence that new neurons are formed in the neocortex, olfactory bulb, and hippocampus of an adult rodent. Nevertheless, it remains necessary to demonstrate that the labeling of the neurons was a result of DNA synthesis and not a result of polyploidy or DNA repair.

Earlier cytophotometric and microspectrophotometric reports have published claims of large deviations of the DNA content of Purkinje cells in various species. These large cells have been measured and found to exceed the normal diploid DNA content and have tetraploid or even octoploid levels of DNA. The species examined were: rat,[15,71,72,90,100] cat,[39,40] rabbit,[65] and human.[66,67] More recently, however, using a variety of methods, investigators have been unable to find evidence of polyploidy in Purkinje cells or labeling of these cells during the period in which the DNA content was believed to increase.[3,5,68,79,81]

Therefore, it seems that these earlier polyploid measurements of DNA content using microspectrophotometric methods might have been inaccurate. Technical improvements of appropriate compensation for light scattered by reflection, diffraction, and refraction in the protoplasmic structures of the tissue[28–30,77,78,88] have since helped to confirm the biochemical and autoradiographic results. In the more recent microspectrophotometric studies, which utilized a variety of species, a thorough consideration of nonspecific light loss was made, and all species showed diploid amounts of DNA in the cells studied, including small granule cells.[28,29,77,78] Only studies that have not controlled for nonspecific factors report a polyploid DNA content of large neurons. Furthermore, even in the earlier microspectrophotometric studies there never was any suggestion that small granule cells may have greater than normal diploid amounts of DNA.[39,40,67,71,95]

Careful autoradiographic studies have not disclosed any evidence for repair or turnover of DNA in mouse Purkinje cells. Mares *et al.*[84] prelabeled pyramidal cells and Purkinje cells prenatally and found that during the first 90 days after birth there was no dilution of labeling, which would have been the result if any DNA repair or turnover had occurred. Also, in the mouse there is no noticeable dilution of labeling in neurons for more than 700 days after injection of [^{3}H]thymidine.[108] These results may be explained by two possibilities: (1) the rate of DNA repair is too low to be detectable; or (2) some nerve cells may have an inability to repair damage to DNA, and this may result in the death of the neuron.[11] Although there appears to be no significant turnover of nuclear DNA in neurons, if only a small portion of DNA was repaired, labeling would be limited to very small segments of the DNA chain, and one would then expect either labeling below background or no labeling at all in the affected neurons. Furthermore, it is difficult to explain why nonspecific repair would be limited specifically to neurons of only one layer in the visual cortex,[52] olfactory bulb,[57] or hippocampus.[55–57] Several divisions of the stem cells may have occurred during the 30 days after injection of [^{3}H]thymidine, thus contributing to the relatively lighter labeling of the neurons. The concentration of DNA within the nuclei does not account for this labeling variability since small neuronal precursors with high concentrations of DNA often are labeled more weakly than cells with larger nuclei.[108]

DO NEUROBLASTS DIVIDE?

The controversy over whether fully formed neuroglia and nerve cells are incapable of multiplication[101,102] or whether they may divide[36,37] began almost 100 years ago. Light microscopic studies of labeled granular neurons support the concept that hippocampal neurons may be formed in mammals just after birth.[12,97,103,114] Serial surivals of animals injected with [^{3}H]-thymidine have demonstrated that shortly after injection, mitotic and labeled cells are present in the base of the granule cell layer. With longer surivals, after [^{3}H]thymidine injection, fewer of the basal cells are labeled and more granular neurons are labeled within the stratum granulosum.[7,8,12,22,34,103] Accordingly, the labeled neurons in the stratum granulosum have a lower mean number of silver grains over the nucleus than the precursor basal stem cells.[34] Although these light microscopic studies have suggested that basal cells of the granule cell layer are neuronal precursors, there has only been one electron microscopic study, in the 2-month-old rabbit,[34] to characterize the labeled stem cells during division. The concept of neurogenesis in the adult as documented by [^{3}H]thymidine incorporation would be much less speculative if mitotic neuroblasts, which incorporated [^{3}H]thymidine shortly before sacrifice, could be demonstrated by electron microscopy[16,42,51,69] and [^{3}H]thymidine autoradiography. Recently we have observed,[56] using electron microscopy and [^{3}H]thymidine autoradiography, that the granule neuron precursors in the postnatal dentate gyrus are indeed mitotic neuroblasts in prophase and telophase with synapses on their cell bodies and axonal-like processes.

Our contention that mitotic neuroblasts may be identified after birth is supported by electron micrographs of synapses on apparently immature axons. Identification of these immature axons rested on the following characteristics: (1) The caliber was fairly uniform throughout their length[43,49,95,113,117]; unlike immature axons, most other processes begin as large cytoplasmic extensions of the perikarya[21,107] and contain more organelles.[21] (2) Neither fascicles of microtubules nor a dense undercoating of the axolemma were present on the proximal parts of immature axons.[43,107] (3) Axonal ribosomes predominate near the nucleus and then become relatively indistinct in the distalmost part of immature axons.[43,107] (4) Filopodial-like processes, "microspikes," are present on developing axons.[43,117] (5) Synapses were observed on processes (FIGS. 1 and 2). Migrating postmitotic neurons have features similar to the neuroblasts described in our study.[91] The nucleus is ovoid in shape, occasionally lobulated, and the cell has an electron-dense karyoplasm (FIGS. 1 and 2). Our observations support the findings of Nowakowski and Rakic[91] that neurons in more advanced maturation stages decrease in electron opacity. It should be emphasized that no suitable cytochemical markers are thought to exist for immature neurons which are still undergoing migration and/or cell division.[38,80,104] Furthermore, neuronal precursors of the hippocampal dentate gyrus do not stain positively for glial fibrillary acidic protein.[73,74] Our observations in mice agree with the work of Levitt *et al.*[74] on the coexistence of neuronal and glial precursor cells in the fetal monkey.

ADDITION OR REPLACEMENT OF NEURONS?

With advancing age there are progressive declines in various areas of physical and mental functioning which have been attributed to morphologic changes in the brain. In conditions such as senile dementia, the functional deficits and correlated morphologic changes in the central nervous system increase significantly with age.[85] Surveys[110,115] demonstrate that 10.9% of those over 65 years of age display mild to moderate cerebral dysfunction, and that 4.4% of those in that age group are seriously demented. Few attempts have been made to compare the morphologic changes of the central nervous system in "normal" elderly people with those in persons with varying degrees of senile dementia. The difficulties in obtaining statistically validated quantitative information on aging humans result from heterogeneity of the genetic and environmental background of people, as well as technical problems such as adequate fixation for microscopy. In contrast, these variables can be controlled in rodent models. Thus, the natural history of lesions in the aged and their possible pathogenetic significance may be better analyzed in animal models.

The possibility that, in certain brain regions, new neuron formation may persist during adult life raises a number of interesting questions. What is the time course of new neuron formation with age? Are the newly formed neurons associated with turnover of existing neurons or do the newly formed neurons add to a population of stable neurons? What is the fate of newly formed cells—do they persist for a month or two and then degenerate or do they live longer? In the last few years, some partial answers to the above

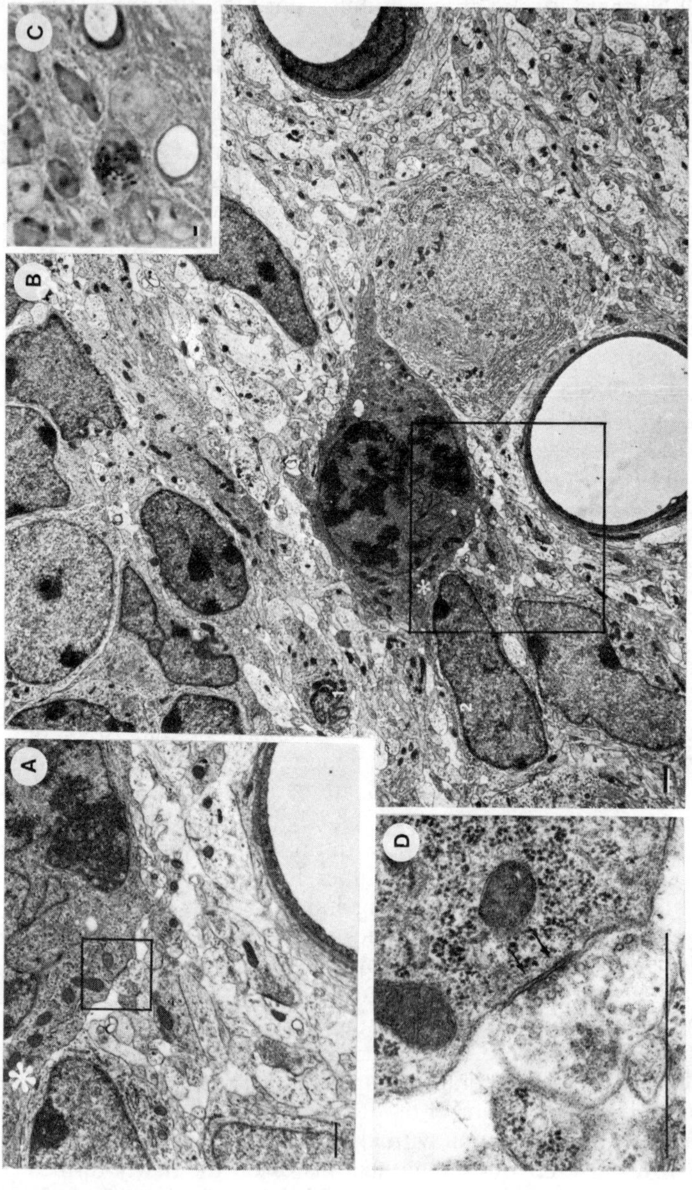

FIGURE 1. Mitotic cell in subgranular zone of the hippocampus in a 9-day-old mouse. The *asterisk* (*) identifies this cell in FIGURES 1 and 2. **(A)** Electron micrograph of a serial thin section through the *boxed region* shown in **(B)**. The labeled cell (*) has a small axon terminal synapsing onto the cell body (in the *box*), which is shown at higher magnification in **(D)**. **(B)** Electron micrograph of the re-embedded labeled cell shown in the light microscopic radioautograph **(C)**; the mitotic cell is labeled several hours after a single tritiated thymidine injection. For orientation between the light microscopic radioautograph **(C)** and the electron micrograph **(B)** of the re-embedded radioautographic section, note the two capillaries and adjacent undifferentiated cells in the same position. **(D)** Higher magnification electron micrograph of axosomatic synapse (*arrows*) on the perikaryon of the labeled mitotic cell (*). Scale bars = 1 μm. (From Kaplan and Bell.[56] Reprinted by permission from the *Journal of Neuroscience*.)

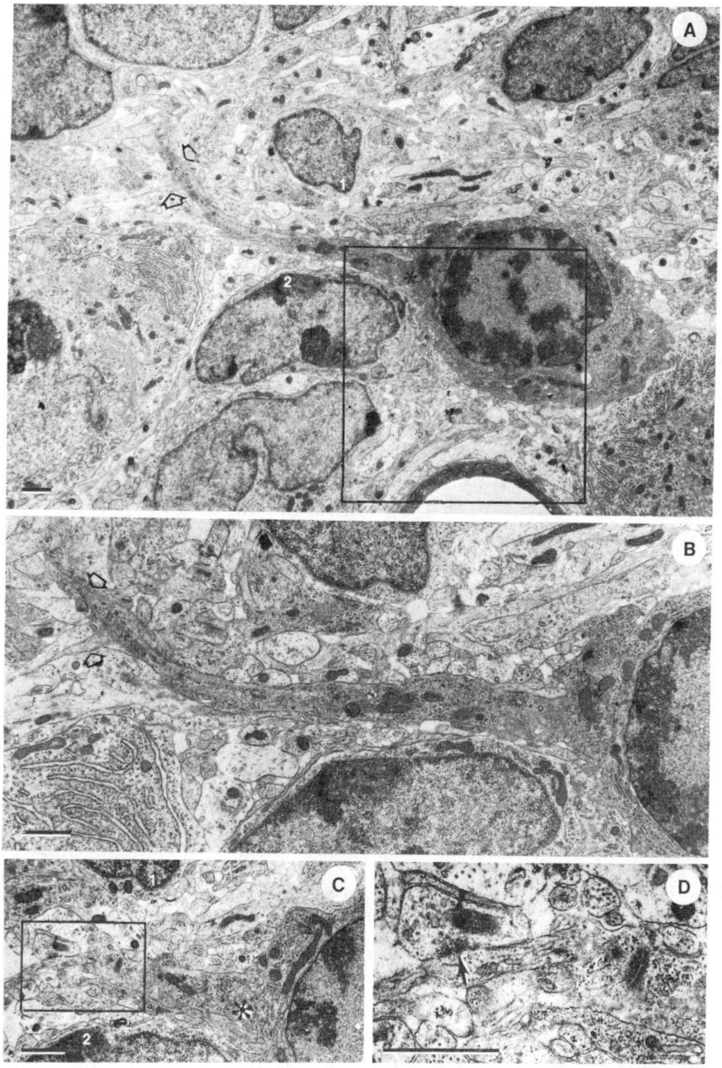

FIGURE 2. Electron micrograph of a serial thin section through the labeled mitotic cell shown in FIGURE 1. The *asterisk* (*) identifies the labeled cell of the previous plate. (**A**) Note the long immature axon (see the text) which courses between two undifferentiated cells numbered 1 and 2. For orientation, these same cells are numbered in both plates. The *boxed region* in FIGURE 1B and the *boxed region* in FIGURE 2A are similar. (**B**) Higher power electron micrograph of the process demonstrated in (**A**); note the thin microspike processes (*open arrowheads*). (**C**) Adjacent serial thin section of immature axon. The labeled cell (*) process is located between previously identified undifferentiated cells (numbered 1 and 2). The region containing a synapse (in the *box*) onto the immature axon is shown at higher magnification in (**D**). (**D**) Electron micrograph of apparent symmetrical synapse (*arrow*) on the immature process. Scale bars = 1 μm. (From Kaplan and Bell.[56] Reprinted by permission from the *Journal of Neuroscience*.)

questions have emerged. For example, Bayer *et al.*[13] have shown increases in numbers of rat dentate gyrus cells by direct enumeration and Kaplan[55] has shown that new neuron formation in the dentate gyrus can persist at least until 11 months of age. Hinds and McNelly[44,45] have demonstrated large increases in the volume of the granule cell layer during adult life, but they have not determined directly whether granule cells themselves are increasing in number with age.

In the rodent some investigators report decreases in the density of cortical neurons,[19,27,93] while others have not been able to demonstrate neuron population reductions.[62] The only demonstration of absolute cell loss in the rodent brain was found for mitral cells of the olfactory bulb in Sprague-Dawley rats.[44] The evidence for nerve cell reductions with age is often conflicting and far from convincing.[31,44,48,63] In a recent study[59] we have attempted to carry out such a comprehensive study for one of the regions—the olfactory bulb—in which new neuron formation exists in the adult. Morphometric studies on the olfactory bulb are interpretable since the internal granule cells in it are contained in a discrete and relatively small layer which lends itself to quantification. Furthermore, the labeling index of granule cells is relatively high after injections into fully adult animals,[57] thus facilitating the accumulation of statistically validated data on numbers of labeled cells. Degeneration can be shown more unequivocally and can be quantified more easily by evaluating labeling index changes after long survivals in autoradiographic studies, utilizing 1-μm plastic sections, than by counting dark "pyknotic" nuclei in paraffin sections.[59]

Most investigations regard neuronal cell death as an abortive process of prenatally formed cells and do not consider the contribution of postnatally formed cells to the population dynamics. Moreover, light microscopic autoradiographic studies have suggested that new neurons may be formed till 1 year after birth.[2,4,6–8,13] Whether these very late-formed neurons serve to replace other granule cells that are formed prenatally or whether they die prematurely without contributing to the cell population may be an important consideration. Only one investigator has evaluated the neuronal changes with regard to tissue volume in the hippocampal dentate gyrus of animals of up to 1 year.[13,14] Bayer[14] reported that there is only circumstantial evidence for turnover of main bulb granule cells during adult life. Although the conclusions of Bayer[14] are similar to those of our studies,[59] her interpretations are based on "circumstantial evidence." For example, Bayer reported that there is a significant decrease in the proportion of labeled cells if the survival time in animals labeled at P30–P33 is extended from P60 to P200. Although Bayer did not report any evidence of actual grain distribution (nuclear labeling) changes after longer survivals, she suggested that these results could result from a dilution of the [^{3}H]thymidine incorporated by neuronal precursors so that after repeated cell divisions it reached undetectable levels. Our results on grain distributions do not substantiate this interpretation (FIG. 3). Bayer[14] also speculated that if new neurons are continuously produced up to 180 days[14] and if the total number of main olfactory bulb granule cells does not significantly change between 1 month and 1 year

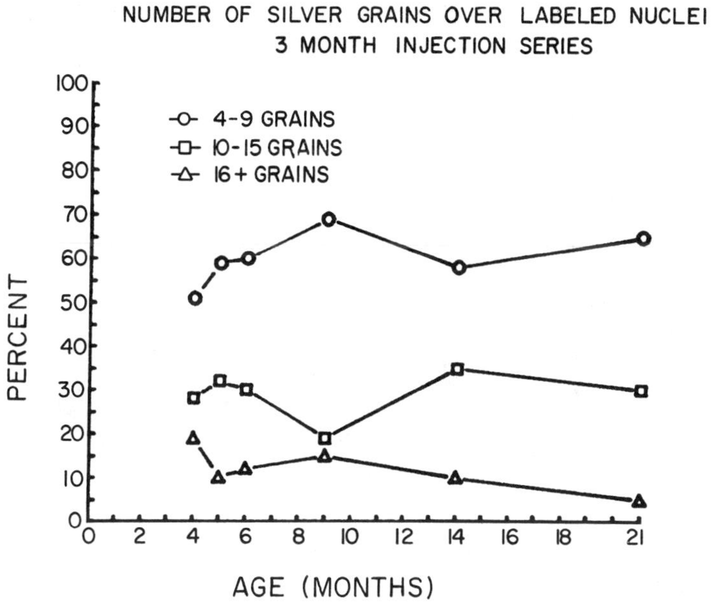

FIGURE 3. Percentage of olfactory granule neurons with 4–9, 10–15 and 16 or more silver grains over nuclei at various survival times after injection of tritiated thymidine at 3 months. χ^2 test was performed to check whether the distribution of grains was the same at different survival times. The χ^2 was not significant ($\chi^2_{10} = 17.6$); there was no dilution of the label in animals that survived 1, 2, 3, 6, 11, or 18 months after injection of tritiated thymidine.

of age,[99] cell death must balance postnatal neurogenesis.[14] Bayer's argument on this point relied heavily on a study done by Roselli-Austin and Altman.[99]

Several important similarities must be considered when comparing our results[59] with those of Roselli-Austin and Altman.[99] Both groups have evaluated volumetric changes, acquisition of granule neurons, packing density, and cell size changes in internal granule cell layer of the rodent olfactory bulb. The important differences in experimental design are: (1) we have evaluated these features in animals up to 32 months after birth, whereas others have examined animals aged up to 12 months; (2) our data were derived from microscopic evaluation of semithin (1 μm or less) plastic embedded sections, while other investigators have used 10-μm paraplast sections; (3) our criteria to distinguish granule neurons from neuroglial cells were based on high-resolution light and electron microscopic studies,[57,76,95] but Bayer's evaluations on paraplast sections used less stringent criteria[112] because of poor resolution[76]; and (4) we used strains of rats different from those used by Roselli-Austin and Altman.[99] Strain differences and resolution features could explain some of the contrasting results.

In contrast to our study, Roselli-Austin and Altman[99] reported that: (1) there was no increase in the total number of internal granular cells from P90 to P360; (2) an analysis of variance performed on the total number of labeled

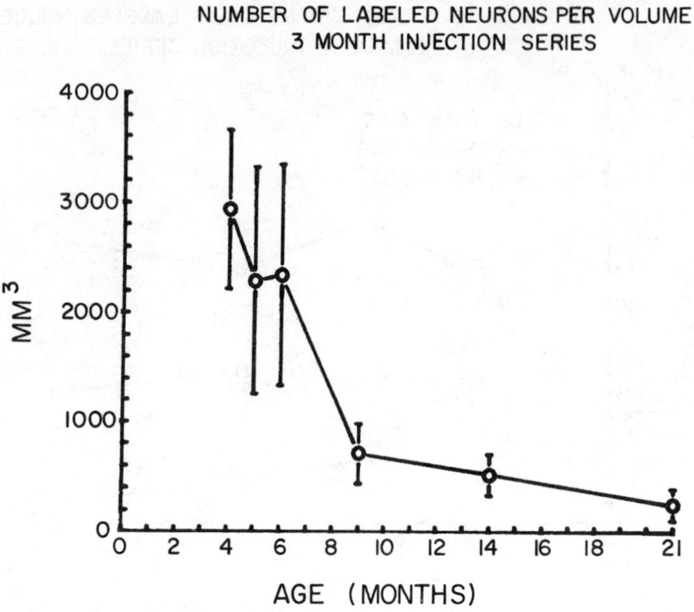

FIGURE 4. Number of labeled granule neurons per volume of granule cell layer at various intervals after injection of tritiated thymidine at 3 months of age. The number of labeled cells per volume of granule cell layer decreased from about 22,800 cells at 1 month survival to about 3000 at 18 months' survival after injection of [^{3}H]thymidine at 3 months; mean and SEM shown. Analysis of variance: $F(5,6) = 5.82$, $p < 0.05$. Newman-Keuls *a posteriori* test; $p < 0.05$, 4/21 and 5/21 months.

granule cells as a function of survival time was not significantly different; and (3) the volume of the internal granular layer did not increase beyond P30. Contrary to Rosselli-Austin and Altman,[99] Kaplan *et al.*[59] documented a significant decrease in the number of postnatally formed neurons within 18 months of the cell birthdate. Cell death was evaluated in animals that were injected with tritiated thymidine at 3 months, then allowed to survive 1–18 months afterward (FIG. 4). The number of labeled granule neurons per unit area significantly decreases, by cell death, with longer survivals (FIG. 4). Nevertheless, the total number of granule neurons increases linearly with age, indicating that many of the postnatally formed neurons survive.

Perhaps the discrepancies between our observations on population dynamics and those of Rosselli-Austin and Altman[99] result from the chronic rhinitis that affected the receptors in the olfactory mucosa of the Rosselli-Austin and Altman study more than it did in our rats. Our rats were kept in a laminar flow enclosure, breathing only highly filtered air at all times to minimize rhinitis. Thus, a difference in the degree of rhinitis is a reasonable possibility. Hinds and McNelly[45] have published evidence suggesting that a decrease in the number of receptor cells leads to decreases in mitral cell size in the olfactory bulb, and that a constant relationship exists between the olfactory receptor cell number and mitral cell perikaryal size from 1 to 12 months of age.[45] Thus a failure of the mitral cells to increase in size in the Rosselli-Austin and Altman[99] study might suggest an explanation for the failure of their olfactory bulb granule cell population to increase. Perhaps, as indicated by Bayer's[14] autoradiographic evidence, granule cells continue to form during adult life but, because mitral cells are not increasing in size, there is no new synaptic surface being added, the new granule cells are unable to form any permanent synapses, and consequently many of them die. In our rats, mitral cells may continue to grow; other workers have shown that mitral cell size increases until 27 months of age.[44,45] Thus, some of the olfactory bulb newly formed granule cells in our rats could form synapses and survive permanently. Our results are consistent with the notion that, once established, a granule cell population may not undergo any automatic turnover; approximately the same number of labeled cells were found after a 6-month survival as after 18 months.[46] The neurons that survive apparently contribute to an overall growth of the olfactory bulb internal granule cell layer. New neurons are being formed throughout adult life, even in senescent animals (FIGS. 4 and 7). The rate of neurogenesis decreases from a high rate in young adults[90] to a lower value in animals aged over 1 year.[59] Indeed, the overall rate of neurogenesis must exceed the rate of cell death; the total number and the areal density of granule cells (labeled and unlabeled) significantly increases in aging animals (FIG. 5).

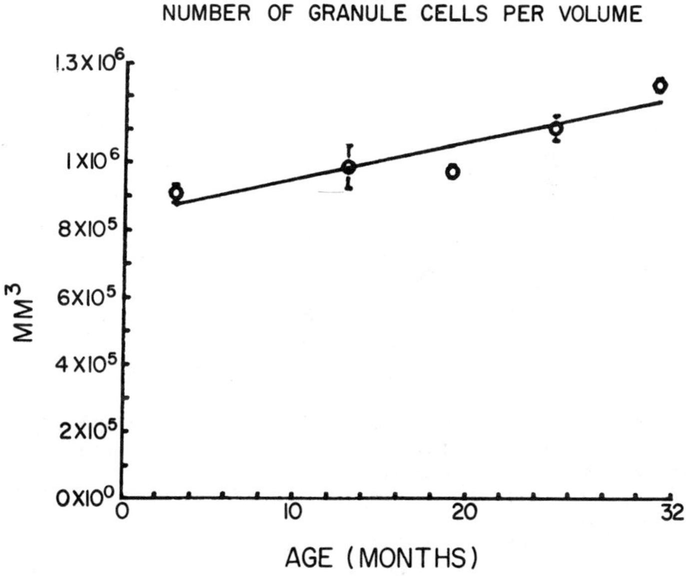

FIGURE 5. The number of granule cells per volume of granule cell layer (mean and SEM at each age studied). Analysis of variance for the linear regression line; $F(1,13) = 30.48, p < 0.0001$. Newman-Keuls *a posteriori* test; $p < 0.01$, 3/31, 13/31, and 19/31 months, $p < 0.05$, 3/13, 3/25, 19/25, and 25/31 months.

Our model of granule cell formation thus resembles that proposed by Hinds *et al.*[46] for receptor cells of the olfactory epithelium; new cells form continuously throughout life and, if postsynaptic space is available, a fraction will survive. Once synaptically established, there may be no significant tendency towards renewal and turnover. Thus, Hinds *et al.*[46] suggest that the demonstration of a turnover of olfactory receptor cells does not necessarily imply a turnover of all cells, as suggested by Graziadei and his associates,[32,33] a distinction that has often not been appreciated in the previous literature. However, Hinds *et al.*[46] report that the time course for labeled cells to disappear is 3 to 6 months (FIG. 6); therefore, it is unlikely that the rapid disappearance of receptors reported by Graziadei and Monti Graziadei[33] to occur 1 month after injection of [^{3}H]thymidine can be explained simply by the turnover of cells failing to form synapses in the olfactory bulb. Instead, one might speculate that Graziadei observed a genuine

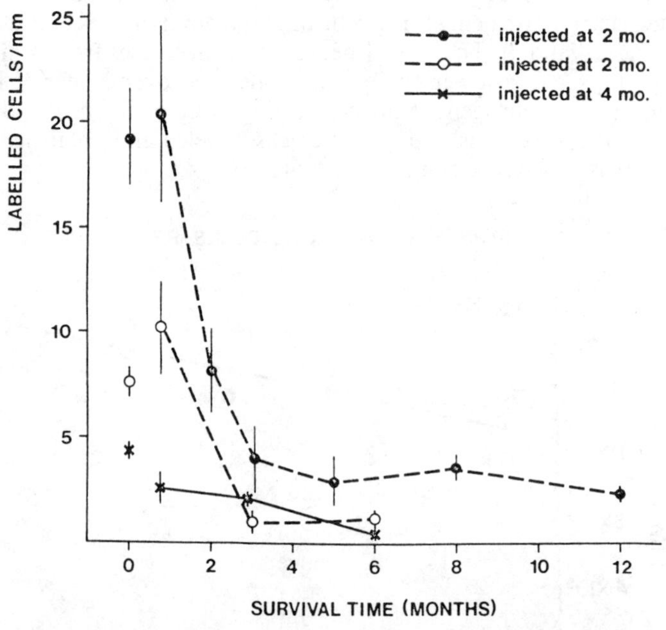

FIGURE 6. The number of labeled basal cells (1-hour survival) or receptor cells (3-week to 12-month survival) per millimeter of septal olfactory epithelium at varying survival times; *solid circles* represent series II animals, *open circles*, series III animals, and *asterisks*, series IV animals. The approximate number of *unlabeled* nuclear profiles of receptor cells per millimeter of septal olfactory epithelium is estimated at 800. Series II analysis of variance: $F(5,23) = 8.16$, $p = 0.000015$; Tukey B *a posteriori* test: $p < 0.001$, 3 wk/3 mo, 3 wk/5 mo, 3 wk/8 mo, 3 wk/12 mo; $p < 0.005$, 3 wk/2 mo. Series III analysis of variance: $F(2,15) = 17.46$, $p = 0.00012$; Tukey B: $p < 0.001$, 3 wk/3 mo, 3 wk/6 mo. Series IV analysis of variance: $F(2,13) = 5.17$, $p = 0.022$; Tukey B: $p < 0.05$, 3 wk/6 mo, 3 mo/6 mo. (From Hinds *et al.*[46] Reproduced by permission from *Anatomical Record.*)

turnover of all receptor cells, but one caused by rhinitic destruction of receptors that in turn led to their replacement by regeneration of new receptors from undifferentiated precursors.

A prediction of the model offered here is that if the olfactory epithelium is destroyed or damaged and prevented from regenerating, newly formed granule cells would continue to be produced, but few of them would become synaptically established and survive. When the olfactory mucosa is allowed to regenerate, however, some of the granule cells produced should survive, synapsing with the mitral cells, which should increase in size in concert with the increase in the number of olfactory nerve receptor cells. Consequently, environment and disease may have an important influence on postnatal cell proliferation and cell death in superficial olfactory receptors and more distant neurons along the transsynaptic chain.

NEUROGENESIS IN ADULT PRIMATE BRAIN: AN UNSETTLED ISSUE

Our studies with [^{125}I]iododeoxyuridine (IUDR), a marker of DNA synthesis (just as [^{3}H]thymidine is), indicate that ^{125}IUDR injected into the ventricles of rats traverses the blood–brain barrier with a half-time of approximately 30 minutes.[53] Once in the blood, because of hepatic breakdown (dehalogenation), ^{125}IUDR in rodents has a half-life of about 3 minutes.[50] After systemic injections, [^{3}H]thymidine disappears from the blood stream of mice in about 7 minutes.[70] Thus, intraperitoneally injected DNA precursors are largely destroyed before they have a chance to cross the blood–brain barrier. The extent of this destruction is demonstrated by the fact that after i.p. injection of ^{125}IUDR into rats, only about 0.002% of the injected radioactivity is incorporated into proliferating cells within the brain. By comparison, 0.18% of the activity is incorporated into the brain after intraventricular adminsitration of ^{125}IUDR. These values represent about a 90-fold increase in the amount of incorporated activity using intraventricular injections as compared to i.p. injections. Not surprisingly, then, i.p. injection of DNA precursors may be an inefficient method of labeling brain cells in primates, and much higher rates of incorporation may be achieved by intraventricular administration. These are important considerations when studying neuronal labeling in search of evidence for neurogenesis, since injected [^{3}H]thymidine competes with endogenous cold thymidine during DNA synthesis.[70] To illustrate the action of the primate blood–brain barrier, one can compare the poor labeling efficiency of subependymal cells to the choroid plexus epithelial cells,[53] located outside the blood–brain barrier.[17,18] These choroid epithelial cells were labeled with 10–28 grains over the nucleus, while subependymal cells were only labeled with 4–8 grains per nucleus.[53]

To date, Rakic and his associates have been the only investigators to evaluate possible neurogenesis in adult primates. Unfortunately, interpretation of their results is complicated by two important procedural inadequacies. First, their use of intravenous injections of low-specific-activity

[^{3}H]thymidine[96] make it difficult to use an autoradiographic labeling index to accurately evaluate neurogenesis (see discussion above). Clearly, their recognition of labeled cells was impaired since they reported that the granule cells generated after E85 must originate exclusively in the hilus of the dentate gyrus, which they report remains as the only proliferative zone in the second half of gestation and after birth in this species.[96] In contrast, we have demonstrated labeled and mitotic subependymal stem cells in an adult rhesus monkey.[53] Second, no clear morphologic criteria can distinguish hippocampal granule neurons from glial cells using thick sections[93,97] with light microscopy.[52,76] Indeed, Rakic and Nowakowski[96] state that they have not explored this issue with electron microscope autoradiography to unequivocally identify labeled cell types.

Nevetheless, Rakic and Nowakowski[96] have reported with light microscopic autoradiography that the genesis of granule neurons in the fascia dentata continues in the rhesus monkey for at least 3 months postnatally. In older animals, the 3- or 8-year-old rhesus, Rakic and Nowakowski[96] observed a few labeled cells, which did not have typical neuronal morphologic structure, situated in proximity to blood vessels. Without better resolution, it remains possible that these few labeled cells near blood vessels may be neurons or neuronal precursors. Indeed, our electron microscopic observations indicate that mitotic cells, with synapses on their cell bodies and processes, are preferentially located near blood vessels, as are many labeled mature neurons.[56]

Nowakowski and Rakic[92] state that although the exact postnatal day when granule cell generation in the rhesus monkey ceases was not precisely identified, their available material suggested that only a small number of granule cells was generated after the second postnatal month. Unlike Rakic and Nowakowski,[96] we believe that small numbers of labeled cells, after a single injection of [^{3}H]thymidine, might indicate a larger increase over time. Indeed, after a single injection of [^{3}H]thymidine, very few cells are labeled in the adult central nervous system. Since [^{3}H]thymidine is available for incorporation during a small fraction of the DNA synthetic phase,[108,109] an injection of [^{3}H]thymidine would be available for just one DNA synthetic cycle. If we assume a synchronous population of dividing cells, then administering [^{3}H]thymidine during the next phase of DNA synthesis would label another equally large population of cells. The percentage increase in the number of newly formed labeled cells could significantly increase the total population of cells during an animal's life.[57] For example, in adult rodents, approximately 0.044% of the hippocampal granule neurons are heavily labeled 30 days after [^{3}H]thymidine injection, 12 labeled neurons per 27,097 unlabeled ones.[55–57] If neuron production continues at this rate from 3 months to 24 months, the total number of heavily labeled cells seen would be (640 days ÷ 11 hr, the probable length of the S-phase) 1396 times the number of heavily labeled cells actually observed after the single injection at 3 months, a 60% increase. Indeed, it appears that the number of newly formed granule neurons is appreciable during adulthood.[55–57] These extrapolated increases of the number of newly formed hippocampal granule neurons are very similar to the volume increases with age shown by the dentate gyrus of the rodent hippocampus.[13,26]

Rakic has never published a labeling index in his postnatal studies, so that we can only speculate as to what values he considers negligible. Perhaps his use of intravenous [^{3}H]thymidine injections or his use of thick autoradiographic sections precludes any reasonable chance to accurately evaluate the rate of postnatal neurogenesis in the primate brain (see discussion above).

The concept of postnatal neurogenesis in fish, rodents, and cats (reviewed in Ref. 56) and its manifestation in birds[118] has gained generalized acceptance only within the last 10 years. With the advent of electron microscopic identification of [^{3}H]thymidine-labeled cells, we first demonstrated that mature neurons were formed in adult rodents.[57] Subsequent studies have shown that even though the labeling index in some species is very low after a single injection of [^{3}H]thymidine,[59] in other groups neurogenesis in adulthood can occur at a remarkably high rate.[118] In either case the number of new neurons added in adulthood can be significant.[59] More recently, the concept of postnatal neurogenesis has been further strengthened by the first identification of mitotic neuroblasts in young mice and adult rats.[56] Before we dismiss the possibility that neurogenesis occurs in adult *Rhesus*, we must be sure we have carefully investigated this issue. Indeed, light microscopy of thick sections cannot demonstrate unequivocally that neurons incorporate or do not incorporate [^{3}H]thymidine. Qualitative observations of labeling within tissue cannot replace rigorous quantitative morphometric analysis and accurate determination of labeling indices.

REFERENCES

1. ALTMAN, J. 1962. Are new neurons formed in the brains of adult mammals? Science **135:** 1127–1128.
2. ALTMAN, J. 1963. Autoradiographic investigation of cell proliferation in the brains of rats and cats. Anat. Rec. **145:** 573–591.
3. ALTMAN, J. 1966. Autoradiographic and histological studies of the postnatal neurogenesis. II. A longitudinal investigation of the kinetics, migration and transformation of cells incorporating tritiated thymidine in infant rats, with special reference to postnatal neurogenesis in some brain regions. J. Comp. Neurol. **128:** 431–474.
4. ALTMAN, J. 1967 Postnatal growth and differentiation of the mammalian brain, with implications for a morphological theory of memory. *In* The Neurosciences, a Study Program. G. C. Quarton, T. Melnechuck & F. O. Schmitt, Eds.: 723. Rockefeller University Press. New York, NY.
5. ALTMAN, J. 1969. Autoradiographic and histological studies of postnatal neurogenesis. III. Dating the time of production and onset of differentiation of cerebellar microneurons in rats. J. Comp. Neurol. **136:** 269–294.
6. ALTMAN, J. 1969. Autoradiographic and histological evidence of postnatal hippocampal neurogenesis. IV. Cell proliferation and migration in the anterior forebrain, with special reference to persisting neurogenesis in the olfactory bulb. J. Comp. Neurol. **137:** 433–458.
7. ALTMAN, J. & G. D. DAS. 1965. Postnatal origin of microneurons in the rat brain. Nature **207:** 953–956.
8. ALTMAN, J. & G. D. DAS. 1965. Autoradiographic and histological evidence of postnatal hippocampal neurogenesis in rats. J. Comp. Neurol. **124:** 319–335.

9. ALTMAN, J. & G. D. DAS. 1966. Autoradiographic and histological studies of postnatal neurogenesis. I. A longitudinal investigation of the kinetics, migration and transformation of cells incorporating tritiated thymidine in neonate rats, with special reference to postnatal neurogenesis in some brain regions. J. Comp. Neurol. **126:** 337–390.
10. ALTMAN, J. & G. D. DAS. 1967. Postnatal neurogenesis in the guinea pig. Nature **214:** 1098–1101.
11. ANDREWS, A. D., S. F. BARRETT & J. H. ROBBINS. 1976. Relation of DNA repair processes to pathological aging of the nervous system in xeroderma pigmentosum. Lancet **1** (7973): 1318–1320.
12. ANGEVINE, J. B., JR. 1965. Time of neuron origin in the hippocampal region, an autoradiographic study in the mouse. Exp. Neurol. **13** (Suppl. 2): 1–70.
13. BAYER, S. A., J. W. YACKEL & P. S. PURI. 1982. Neurons in the rat dentate gyrus granular layer substantially increase during juvenile and adult life. Science **216:** 890–892.
14. BAYER, S. A. 1983. ^{3}H-thymidine-radiographic studies of neurogenesis in the rat olfactory bulb. Exp. Brain Res. **50:** 329–340.
15. BOHN, R. C. & R. B. MITCHELL. 1976. Cytophotometric identification of tetraploid Purkinje cells in young and aged rats. J. Neurobiol. **7:** 255–258.
16. BOULDER COMMITTEE. 1970. Embryonic vertebrate central nervous system: Revised terminology. Anat. Rec. **166:** 257–262.
17. BRIGHTMAN, M. W. 1977. Morphology of blood-brain interfaces. *In* The Ocular and Cerebrospinal Fluids. L. Z. Bito, H. Davson & S. D. Fenstermacher, Eds.: 1–25. National Institutes of Health. Bethesda, MD.
18. BRIGHTMAN, M. W., I. KLATZO, Y. OLSSON & T. S. REESE. 1970. The blood-brain barrier to proteins under normal and pathological conditions. J. Neur. Sci. **10:** 215–239.
19. BRIZZEE, K. R. & J. M. ORDY. 1979. Age pigments, cell loss and hippocampal function. Mech. Age Devel. **9:** 143–162.
20. BRUCKNER, G. V., V. MARES & D. BIESOLD. 1976. Neurogenesis in the visual system of the rat. An autoradiographic investigation. J. Comp. Neurol. **166:** 245–256.
21. CALEY, D. W. & D. S. MAXWELL. 1968. An electron microscopic study of neurons during postnatal development of the rat cerebral cortex. J. Comp. Neurol. **133:** 17–44.
22. COWAN, W. M., B. B. STANFIELD & K. KISHI. 1980. The development of the dentate gyrus. Curr. Top. Dev. Biol. **15:** 103–159.
23. D'AGATA, P. M. 1950. Richerche sulla morfologia e classificazione dell' oligodendroglia. Riv. Neurol. **20:** 81–127.
24. DAS, G. D. & J. ALTMAN. 1971. Postnatal neurogenesis in the cerebellum of the cat and tritiated thymidine autoradiography. Brain Res. **30:** 323–330.
25. DECASTRO, F. 1946. Sobre el comportamiento y significacion de la oligodendroglia en la substancia gris central y de los gliocitos en los ganglios perifericos. Arch. Histol. Nor. Patol. **3:** 318–343.
26. DIAMOND, M. C., R. E. JOHNSON and C. A. INGHAM 1975 Morphological changes in the young, adult and aging rat cerebral cortex, hippocampus and diencephalon. Behav. Biol. **14:** 163–174.
27. DIAMOND, M. C., R. E. JOHNSON & M. W. GOLD. 1977. Changes in neuron number and size and glia number in the young, adult, and aging medial occipital cortex. Behav. Biol. **20:** 409–418.
28. FUJITA, S. 1974. DNA constancy in neurons of the human cerebellum and spinal cord as revealed by Feulgen cytophotometry and cytofluoromentry. J. Comp. Neurol. **155:** 195–202.
29. FUJITA, S., T. HATTORI, M. FUKUDA & T. KITAMURA. 1974. DNA contents in Purkinje cells and inner granule neurones in the developing rat cerebellum. Dev. Growth Differ. **16:** 205–211.
30. FUJITA, S., S. YOSHIDA & M. FUKUDA. 1971. Improvement of technique to minimize nonspecific absorption in microspectrophotometric measurement of nuclear DNA. Acta. Histochem. Cytochem. **4:** 126–136.
31. GOLDMAN, G. & P. D. COLEMAN. 1981. Neuron numbers in locus coerulus do not change with age in Fisher 344 rat. Neurobiol. Aging **2:** 33–36.

32. Graziadei, P. P. C. & G. A. Monti Graziadei. 1978. Continuous nerve cell renewal in the olfactory system. *In* Handbook of Sensory Physiology. Vol. 9: Development of Sensory Systems. M. Jacobson, Ed.: 55–83, Springer-Verlag. Berlin.
33. Graziadei, P. P. C. & G. A. Monti Graziadei. 1979. Neurogenesis and neuron regeneration in the olfactory system of mammals. I. Morphological aspects of differentiation and structural organization of the olfactory sensory neurons. J. Neurocytol. **8:** 1–18.
34. Gueneau, G., A. Privat, J. Drouet & L. Court. 1982. Subgranular zone of the dentate gyrus of young rabbits as a secondary matrix: A high-resolution autoradiographic study. Dev. Neurosci. **5:** 345–358.
35. Hain, R. F., W. O. Rieke & N. B. Everett. 1961. Evidence of mitosis in neuroglia as revealed by radioautography employing tritiated thymidine. J. Neuropathol. Exp. Neurol. **19:** 147–148.
36. Hamilton, A. 1901. The division of differentiated cells of the central nervous system of the white rat. J. Comp. Neurol. **11:** 297–324.
37. Hatai, S. 1901 Mitosis in the nerve cells of the cerebellar cortex of the foetal cat. J. Comp. Neurol. **11:** 277.
38. Hawkers, R., E. Niday & A. Matus. 1982. MIT-23: A mitochondrial marker for terminal neuronal differentiation defined by a monoclonal antibody. Cell **28:** 253–258.
39. Herman, C. J. & L. N. Lapham. 1968. DNA content of neurons in the cat hippocampus. Science **160:** 537.
40. Herman, C. J. & L. W. Lapham. 1969. Neuronal polyploidy and nuclear volume in cat central nervous system. Brain Res. **15:** 35–48.
41. Hinds, J. W. 1968. Autoradiographic study of histogenesis in the mouse olfactory bulb. I. Time of origin of neurons and neuroglia. J. Comp. Neurol. **134:** 287–304.
42. Hinds, J. W. 1972. Early neuron differentiation in the mouse olfactory bulb. I. Light microscopy. J. Comp. Neurol. **146:** 233–252.
43. Hinds, J. W. 1972. Early neuron differentiation in the mouse olfactory bulb. II. Electron microscopy. J. Comp. Neurol. **146:** 253–276.
44. Hinds, J. W. & N. A. McNelly. 1977. Aging of the rat olfactory bulb: Growth and atrophy of constituent layers and changes in size and number of mitral cells. J. Comp. Neurol. **171:** 345–368.
45. Hinds, J. W. & N. A. McNelly. 1981. Aging in the rat olfactory system: Correlation of changes in the olfactory epithelium and olfactory bulb. J. Comp. Neurol. **203:** 441–453.
46. Hinds, J. W., P. L. Hinds & N. A. McNelly. 1984. An autoradiographic study of the mouse olfactory epithelium: Evidence for long-lived receptors. Anat. Rec. **210:** 375–383.
47. Hommes, O. R. & C. P. Leblond. 1967. Mitotic division of neuroglia in the normal adult rat. J. Comp. Neurol. **129:** 269–278.
48. Howard, E. 1973. DNA content of rodent brains during maturation and aging, and autoradiography of postnatal DNA synthesis in monkey brain. Prog. Brain Res. **40:** 91–114.
49. Hughes, A. F. 1953. The growth of embryonic neurites. A study on cultures of chick neuronal tissue. J. Anat. **91:** 150–162.
50. Hughes, W. L., S. L. Commerford, D. Gitlin, R. C. Krueger, B. Schultze, V. Shah & P. Reilly. 1964. Deoxyribonucleic acid metabolism in vivo: I. Cell proliferation and death measured by incorporation and elimination of iododeoxyuridine. Fed. Prod. **23:** 640–648.
51. Jacobson, M. 1978. Differentiation, growth and maturation of neurons. *In* Developmental Neurobiology, Ed. 2.: 118. Plenum Press. New York, NY.
52. Kaplan, M. S. 1981. Neurogenesis in the 3-month-old rat visual cortex. J. Comp. Neurol. **195:** 323–338.
53. Kaplan, M. S. 1983. Proliferation of subependymal cells in the adult primate CNS: Differential uptake of DNA labeled precursors. J. Hirnforsch. **24:** 23–33.
54. Kaplan, M. S. & D. Bell. 1981. Neurogenesis in the dentate gyrus of the 9- and 11-month-old rat. Neurosci. Abstr. **7:** 62 (abstr. #8).

55. Kaplan, M. S. & D. H. Bell 1983. Neuronal proliferation in the 9-month-old rodent—radioautographic study of granule cells in hippocampus. Exp. Brain Res. **52:** 1–5.
56. Kaplan, M. S. & D. H. Bell. 1984. Mitotic neuroblasts in the 9-day-old and 11-month-old rodent hippocampus. J. Neurosci. **4:** 1429–1441.
57. Kaplan, M. S. & J. W. Hinds. 1977. Neurogenesis in the adult rat: Electron microscopic analysis of light radioautographs. Science **197:** 1092–1094.
58. Kaplan, M. S. & J. W. Hinds. 1980. Gliogenesis of astrocytes and oligodendrocytes in the neocortical grey and white matter of the adult rat: Electron microscopic analysis of light radioautographs. J. Comp. Neurol. **193:** 711–727.
59. Kaplan, M. S., N. A. McNelly & J. W. Hinds. 1985. Population dynamics of adult-formed granule neurons of the rat olfactory bulb. J. Comp. Neurol. **239:** 117–125.
60. King, J. S. 1968. A light and electron microscopic study of perineuronal glial cells and processes in the rabbit neocortex. Anat. Rec. **161:** 111–124.
61. Klatzo, I. 1952. A study of glia by the Golgi method. Lab. Invest. **1:** 345–350.
62. Klein, A. W. & M. Michel. 1977. A morphometric study of the neocortex of young adult and old maze-differentiated rats. Mech. Age. Devel. **6:** 441–452.
63. Konigsmark, B. W. & E. A. Murphy. 1970. Neuronal populations in the human brain. Nature **228:** 1335–1336.
64. Korr, H., B. Schultze & W. Maurer. 1973. Autoradiographic investigations of glial proliferation in the brain of adult mice. I. The DNA synthesis phase of neuroglia and endothelial cells. J. Comp. Neurol. **150:** 169–176.
65. Kusch, A. A. & V. N. Yarygin. 1965. Polyploid of mono- and binucleate neurons in upper cervical ganglion of rabbit. Tsitologia **7:** 228–233.
66. Lapham, L. W. 1965. The tetraploid DNA content of normal human Purkinje cells and its development during the perinatal period: A quantitative cytochemical study. Excerpta Med. **100:** 445–449.
67. Lapham, L. W. 1968. Tetraploid DNA content of Purkinje neurons of human cerebellar cortex. Science **159:** 310–312.
68. Lapham, L. W., R. D. Lentz, D. J. Woodward, B. J. Hoffer & C. J. Herman. 1971. Postnatal development of tetraploid DNA content in the Purkinje neuron of the rat: An aspect of cellular differentiation. *In* Cellular Aspect of Neural Growth and Differentiation. D. Pease, Ed.: 61–71. UCLA Forum in Medical Sciences No. 14. University of California Press. Berkeley, CA.
69. Leblond, C. P. & B. E. Walker. 1956. Renewal of cell populations. Physiol. Rev. **36:** 255–276.
70. Lee Ding-Jen, W. Prensky, G. Krause & W. L. Hughes. 1976. Blood thymidine level and iododeoxyuridine incorporation and reutilization in DNA in mice given long-acting thymidine pellets. Cancer Res. **36:** 4577–4583.
71. Lentz, R. D. & L. W. Lapham. 1969. A quantitative cytochemical study of the DNA content of neurons of rat cerebellar cortex. J. Neurochem. **16:** 379–384.
72. Lentz, R. D. & L. W. Lapham. 1970. Postnatal development of tetraploid DNA content in rat Purkinje cells: A quantitative cytochemical study. J. Neuropathol. Exp. Neurol. **29:** 43–56.
73. Levitt, P. & P. Rakic. 1980. Immunoperoxidase localization of glial fibrillary acidic protein in radial glial cells and astrocytes of the developing rhesus monkey brain. J. Comp. Neurol. **193:** 815–840.
74. Levitt, P., M. L. Cooper & P. Rakic. 1981. Coexistence of neuronal and glial precursor cells in the cerebral ventricular zone of the fetal monkey: An ultrastructural immunoperoxidase analysis. J. Neurosci. **1:** 27–39.
75. Lewis, P. D. 1968 Mitotic activity in the primate subependymal layer and the genesis of gliomas. Nature **217:** 974–975.
76. Ling, E. A., J. A. Paterson, A. Privat, S. Mori & C. P. Leblond. 1973. Investigation of glial cells in semithin sections. I. Identification of glial cells in the brain of young rats. J. Comp. Neurol. **149:** 43–72.
77. Mann, D. M. A. & P. O. Yates. 1973. Polyploidy in the human nervous system. I. The DNA content of neurons and glia of the cerebellum. J. Neurol. Sci. **18:** 183–196.

78. MANN, D. M.A., P. O. YATES & C. M. BARTON. 1978. The DNA content of Purkinje cells in mammals. J. Comp. Neurol. **180:** 345–348.
79. MANUELIDIS, L. & E. E. MANUELIDIS. 1974. On the DNA content of cerebellar Purkinje cells in vivo and in vitro. Exp. Neurol. **43:** 192–206.
80. MARANGOS, P. J., D. E. SCHMECHEL, A. M. PARMA & F. K. GOODWIN. 1980. Developmental profile of neuron-specific (NSE) and non-neuronal (NNE) enolase. Brain Res. **190:** 185–193.
81. MAREŚ, V., Z. LODIN & S. SACHA. 1973. A cytochemical and autoradiographic study of nuclear DNA in mouse Purkinje cells. Brain Res. **53:** 273–289.
82. MAREŚ, V. & Z. LODIN. 1974. An autoradiographic study of DNA synthesis in adolescent and adult mouse forebrain. Brain Res. **76:** 557–561.
83. MAREŚ, V., Z. LODIN & M. JILEK. 1975. An estimate of the number of cells arising by division in mouse cerebral hemispheres from age one to 12 months: An autoradiographic study of DNA synthesis. J. Comp. Neurol. **161:** 471–482.
84. MAREŚ, V., B. SCHULTZE & W. MAURER. 1974. Stability of DNA in Purkinje cell nuclei of the mouse. J. Cell Biol. **63:** 665–674.
85. MATSUYAMA, S. S. 1980. Cell proliferation and the aging brain. Age **3:** 43–47.
86. MESSIER, B. & C. P. LEBLOND. 1960. Cell proliferation and migration as revealed by radioautography after injection of H^3-thymidine into male rats and mice. Am. J. Anat. **106:** 247–285.
87. MESSIER, B., C. P. LEBLOND & I. SMART. 1958. Presence of DNA synthesis and mitosis in the brain of young adult mice. Exp. Cell Res. **14:** 224–226.
88. MORSELT, A. F. W., D. J. BRAAKMAN & J. JAMES. 1972. Feulgen DNA and fast green histone estimations in individual cell nuclei of the cerebellum of young and old rats. Acta Histochem. **43:** 281–286.
89. NOETZEL, J. & J. ROX. 1964. Autoradiographische Untersuchungen über Zellteilung und Zellentwicklung im Gehirn der erwachsenen Maus und der erwachsenen Rhesus-Affen nach Injektion von radioakitivem Thymidin. Acta Neuropathol. **3:** 326–342.
90. NOVÁKOVÁ, V., W. SANDRITTER & G. SCHLUETER. 1970. DNA content of neurons in rat central nervous system. Exp. Cell Res. **60:** 454–456.
91. NOWAKOWSKI, R. S. & P. RAKIC. 1979. The mode or migration of neurons to the hippocampus: A Golgi and electron microscopic analysis in fetal rhesus monkey. J. Neurocytol. **8:** 697–718.
92. NOWAKOWSKI, R. S. & P. RAKIC. 1981. The site of origin and route and rate of migration of neurons to the hippocampal region of the Rhesus monkey. J. Comp. Neurol. **196:** 129–154.
93. ORDY, J. M., K. R. BRIZZEE, B. KAACK & J. HANSCHE. 1978. Age differences in short term memory and cell loss in the cortex of the rat. Gerontology **24:** 276–285.
94. PENFIELD, W. 1932. Neuroglia: Normal and pathological. *In* Cytology and Cellular Pathology of the Nervous System, Vol. II, W. Penfield, Ed.: 423–479. Hoeber. New York, NY.
95. PETERS, A., S. L. PALAY & H. DEF. WEBSTER. 1976. *In*: The Fine Structure of the Nervous System: The Neurons and Supporting Cells. W. B. Saunders. Philadelphia, PA.
96. RAKIC, P. & R. S. NOWAKOWSKI. 1981. The time of origin of neurons in the hippocampal region of the rhesus monkey. J. Comp. Neurol. **196:** 99–128
97. REZNIKOV K. YU, L. B. VERBITSKAYA, V. S. KESAREV & I. V. VIKTOROV. 1978. Postnatal histogenesis and proliferation of cells and the parietal neocortex in normal mice and after brain trauma. Bull. Exp. Biol. Med. **85:** 242–244.
98. RÍO-HORTEGA, P. DEL. 1928. Tercera aportación al conocimiento morfológico e interpretactión functional de la oligodendroglia. Arch. Histol. Nor. Patol. **6:** 132–183 and 239–306 (reprinted in 1956).
99. ROSSELLI-AUSTIN, L. & J. ALTMAN. 1979. The postnatal development of the main olfactory bulb of the rat. J. Dev. Physiol. **1:** 295–313.
100. SANDRITTER, W., V. NOVÁKOVÁ, J. PILNY & G. KIEFER. 1967. Cytophotometrische Messungen des Nukleinsäure und Proteingehaltes von Ganglienzellen der Ratte während der postnatalen Entwicklung und im Alter. Z. Zellforsch. **80:** 145–152.

101. Schaper, A. 1894. Die morphologische und histologische Entwicklung des Kleinhirns der Teleostiere. Anat. Anz. **9:** 489.
102. Schaper, A. 1897. Die frühesten differenzierungsvorgänge im Zentral Nervensystems. Arch. Entwicklungsmech. Org. **5:** 81.
103. Schlessinger, A. R., W. M. Cowan & D. I. Gottlieb. 1975. An autoradiographic study of the time of origin and the pattern of granule cell migration in the dentate gyrus of the rat. J. Comp. Neurol. **159:** 149–176.
104. Schmechel, D. E., M. W. Brightman & P. J. Marangos. 1980. Neurons switch from non-neuronal enolase to neuron-specific enolase during differentiation. Brain Res. **190:** 195–214.
105. Schultz, R. L. 1964. Macroglial identification in electron micrographs. J. Comp. Neurol. **122:** 281–295.
106. Schultze, B., B. Nowak & W. Maurer. 1974. Cycle times of the neural epithelial cells of various types of neurons in the rat. An autoradiographic study. J. Comp. Neurol. **158:** 207–218.
107. Shoukimas, G. M. & J. W. Hinds. 1978. The development of the cerebral cortex of the embryonic mouse: An electron microscopic serial section analysis. J. Comp. Neurol. **179:** 795–830.
108. Sidman, R. L. 1970. Autoradiographic methods and principles for study of the nervous system with H^3-thymidine. *In* Contemporary Research Methods in Neuroanatomy. W. J. H. Nauta & S. O. E. Ebbeson, Eds.: 252–274. Springer. Berlin.
109. Sidman, R. L. 1970. Cell proliferation, migration and interaction in the developing mammalian central nervous system. *In* The Neurosciences: Second Study Program. F. O. Schmitt, Ed.: 100–107. Rockefeller University Press. New York, NY.
110. Slater, E. & M. Roth. 1969. Clinical Psychiatry, 3rd ed.: 543. Williams and Wilkins. Baltimore, MD.
111. Smart, I. 1961. The subependymal layer of the mouse brain and its cell production as shown by radioautography after H^3-thymidine injection. J. Comp. Neurol. **116:** 325–347.
112. Smart, I. & C. P. Leblond. 1961. Evidence for division and transformation of neuroglia cells in the mouse brain as dervied from radioautography after injection of H^3-thymidine. J. Comp. Neurol. **116:** 349–367.
113. Spiedel, C. C. 1933. Studies of living nerves. II. Activities of ameboid growth cones, sheath cells, and myelin segments, as revealed by prolonged observations of individual nerve fibers in frog tadpoles. Am. J. Anat. **52:** 1–79.
114. Stanfield, B. & W. M. Cowan. 1979. The development of the hippocampus and dentate gyrus in normal and reeler mice. J. Comp. Neurol. **185:** 423–460.
115. Terry, R. D. & H. M. Wisniewski. 1975. Structural and chemical changes of the aged human brain. *In* Aging, vol. 2. S. Gershon & A. Raskin, Eds.: 127–141. Raven Press. New York, NY.
116. Warwick, R. & P. Williams. 1973. Gray's Anatomy. 35th ed. W. B. Saunders. Philadelphia, PA.
117. Yamada, K. M., B. S. Spooner & N. K. Wessells. 1971. Ultrastructure and function of growth cones and axons of cultured nerve cells. J. Cell Biol. **49:** 614–635.
118. Nottebohm, F. 1985. Neuronal replacement in adulthood. Ann. N.Y. Acad. Sci. **457:** 143–161 (this volume).

DNA Synthesis and Cell Division in the Adult Primate Brain[a]

PASKO RAKIC

Section of Neuroanatomy
Yale University School of Medicine
New Haven, Connecticut 06510

HISTORICAL PERSPECTIVE

It is generally accepted that the adult human brain is incapable of producing new neurons. Even cursory examination of neurologic, neuropathologic, or neurobiological textbooks published during the past 50 years will testify that this belief is deeply entrenched,[1,24,27,31] In his classification of cell populations on the basis of their proliferative behavior, Leblond[36] regarded neurons of the central nervous system as belonging to a category of static, nonrenewing epithelial tissue incapable of expanding or replenishing itself. This belief, however, needs to be reexamined for two major reasons: First, as reviewed below, a number of reports have provided evidence of neurogenesis in adult brain of several vertebrate species. Second, the capacity for neurogenesis in the adult primate central nervous system has never been examined by modern methods. In this article I will describe our recent results from an extensive autoradiographic analysis performed on twelve rhesus monkeys injected with the specific DNA precursor [^{3}H]thymidine at ages ranging from 6 postnatal months to 17 years.[56]

Impetus for the present study came from numerous reports which indicate that in the rodent brain new neurons may be continuously produced throughout the animals' lifespan.[2,23,28–30,41,50,52,63] Postdevelopmental neurogenesis has also been regarded in the Russian literature[42] as an important repair mechanism of the injured mammalian brain. These results, obtained mostly from [^{3}H]thymidine autoradiographic studies, appear to be supported by several recent reports claiming that the number of neurons in the hippocampal formation, olfactory bulb, and cerebellum increases substantially in normal adult rodents.[5,6,11,25] Both undifferentiated stem cells[24] as well as fully mature, synaptically connected neurons[29] were considered to be possible sources of neurons generated *de novo* in the mature organism. Furthermore, in the course of an extensive electron microscopic analysis of the cytologic and synaptic organization of various brain structures in normal adult rhesus monkeys conducted in my laboratory over the last decade, we occasionally have encountered cells in various phases of their mitotic cycle.

[a] This work was supported by Grants NS 14841 and EY 02593. Rhesus monkeys were obtained from the colonies at Yale Medical School, which is in part supported by the U.S. Public Health Service Grant NS 22807, and from the New England Regional Primate Research Center, Southborough, Massachusetts.

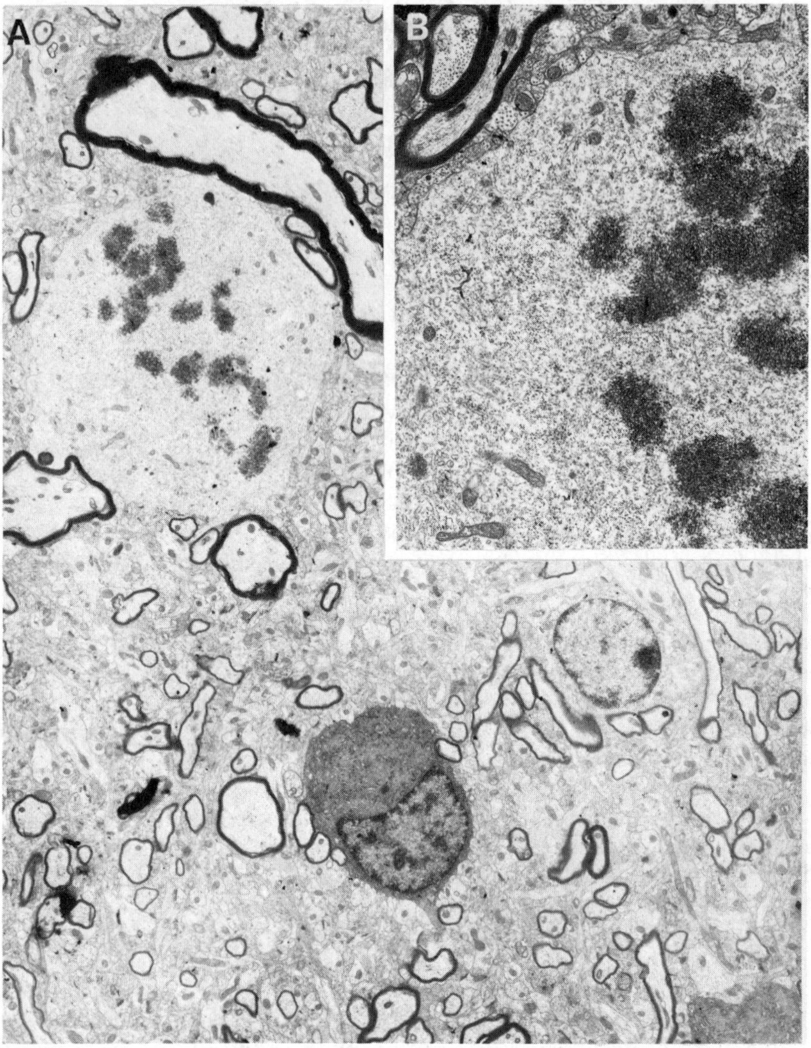

FIGURE 1. (**A**) Example of dividing cell encountered in the primary motor cortex (Brodmann's area 4) in a normal 7-month-old rhesus monkey. This is the only mitotic figure encountered during a survey of more than 10,000 electron micrographs taken from the four major cytoarchitectonic cortical fields for quantitative analysis in twelve juvenile and adult rhesus monkeys.[69] (**B**) Higher magnification electron micrograph ($\times$ 12,000; reduced by 40%) showing a part of the cell illustrated in **A** demonstrates that a dividing cell cannot be classified as to its prospective phenotype by the ultrastructural characteristics during mitosis. The dividing cell has to be labeled by [^{3}H]thymidine and examined by the autoradiographic method after an interval that allows expression of its phenotype by specific characteristics such as presence of dendrites, axons and synapses, or by synthesis of neuron- or glia-specific antigens detectable by the immunoreactivity method.

The mitotic figures are found extremely rarely and, although we regard them as a curiosity, their presence raises questions about the nature of their progeny. For example, a cell in the metaphase illustrated in FIGURE 1A was observed in the primary motor cortex of a 7-month-old rhesus monkey, but transmission electron microscopy, even at higher magnification, does not provide any clue as to whether the progenies of this cell will eventually become neurons or glial cells (FIG. 1B).

Since even a small capacity for postdevelopmental neurogenesis may play a significant role in neural repair after mechanical, chemical, radiologic, or viral injury to the adult human brain, it is essential to examine critically whether any neurons are being added or replaced in the mature central nervous system in primates. The most reliable method for detecting new neurons in the brain of a given animal is systemic injections of the specific DNA precursor, [^{3}H]thymidine. This radioactive nucleotide becomes incorporated into the nucleus of all dividing cells during the S-phase of DNA synthesis (FIG. 2). The duration of this phase of the cell's cycle is relatively stable[1] and it varies little from one to another brain structure or between

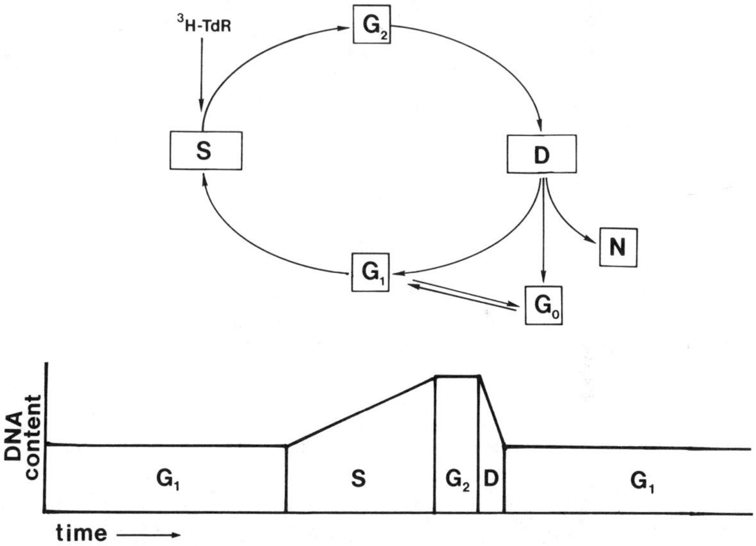

FIGURE 2. Graphic illustration of compartments of a cell proliferation cycle. Phases of the cycle are designated according to Howard and Pelc.[26] G_1, presynthetic (gap) phase; S, phase of DNA synthesis; G_2, gap between phases of DNA synthesis and cell division; D, phase of cell division. Neuronal precursors in the proliferative zones pass repeatedly through this cycle (*top*) until a given cell enters its last division and becomes a permanently postmitotic neuron (N) or dies. One of the questions addressed in this symposium is whether some precursor cells may withdraw transiently into the quiescent compartment (G_0) and later be induced to reenter the cycle again. The bottom drawing provides schematic representation of the relative duration of each phase and content of nuclear DNA. The duration of G_1 is the most variable, while the length of S phase is remarkably constant and in the mammalian central nervous system lasts about 8 to 10 hours.[17,33]

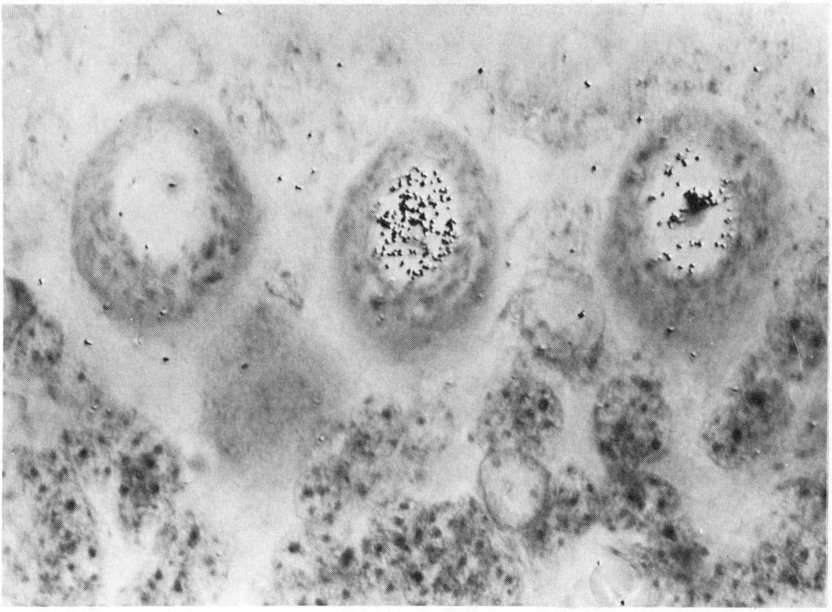

FIGURE 3. Autoradiogram of the cerebellar cortex from a postnatal monkey that was exposed to [^{3}H]thymidine on the 40th embryonic day illustrates principles of autoradiographic detection of DNA replication. Differential interference contrast (Nomarski) photomicrograph is focused on the silver grains situated in the photosensitive emulsion coating the section; therefore the outline of cell bodies and organelles are only vaguely indicated by the relief of their membranes. The Purkinje cell situated in the middle, which contains more than 60 grains over its nucleus, was in the S-phase of its last division at the time of [^{3}H]thymidine injection. The cell situated on the right, which contains about 30 grains, has presumably divided one more time and therefore is at least 12 hours younger. The unlabeled Purkinje cell on the left must have completed its last division either before or considerably later than the 40th embryonic day. Systematic timetable of injections at various embryonic days enables precise delineation of the span of neurogenesis for each neuronal class.[53–55,64]

neuronal and glial cell lineages.[17,33] All cells in the proliferative pool which leave the dividing cycle to become a neuron will retain this radioactivity and can be detected in histologic sections coated with photosensitive emulsion (FIG. 3). Counterstaining of sections with cresyl violet allows easy recognition of labeled neurons and glial cells. The half-life of tritium (^{3}H), which ranges between 12–14 years, is adequate even for long-term experiments in primates.

EXPERIMENTAL DESIGN AND METHOD OF ANALYSIS

Since the principal conclusion of this study depends on our ability to detect the presence or absence of only a few radiolabeled neurons among millions of unlabeled cells in the large primate brain, it is essential to examine large populations of cells in an adequate number of animals prepared by the proper method. A total of twelve rhesus monkeys of both sexes ranging in age from 6 months to 5 years of age were injected, one to seven times, with [^{3}H]thymidine (10 mCi/kg) and sacrificed after intervals between 3 days and 6 years (TABLE 1). Variable and lengthy intervals between injections and sacrifice allow dividing cells to express their postmitotic phenotype and to differentiate into specific classes, while the shorter intervals eliminate the possibility of missing neurons that may have divided several times after the injection. Furthermore, as evident from the dates of injection (columns 1–7 in TABLE 1), animals were exposed to [^{3}H]thymidine at different times of the year, i.e., at least one animal was injected during each month (with the exception of December). Thus, every season was covered by several injections of [^{3}H]thymidine.

After fixation, brain specimens were blocked, embedded in paraffin, cut serially at 8 μm, and every second to tenth section (depending on size of the region) was processed for fine-resolution light microscopic autoradiography.[53,55] Tissue samples from other organs of the body (skin, intestine, spleen, kidney, liver) were also processed for light microscopic autoradiography and served as controls for the autoradiographic method.

In selected brain structures, small blocks of tissue were osmicated, embedded in Epon-Araldite, and processed for combined autoradiographic and electron microscopic analysis.[9] Vibratome sections of the hippocampal region from selected monkeys were reacted with antibodies against glial fibrillary acidic protein (GFAP) and processed for EM analysis to determine the glial or neuronal nature of labeled cells that were difficult to distinguish in sections stained with cresyl violet or toluidine blue.[14,16]

Exposure of emulsion-coated sections ranged from 12 to 18 weeks for light microscopic autoradiography, and more than 24 weeks for electron microscopic autoradiography. This lengthy exposure time was necessary because [^{3}H]thymidine is quickly destroyed in the blood stream of rhesus monkeys and is available for incorporation only during a fraction of the time that DNA synthesis in any given cell occurs.[45] Nine animals (cases 3–11 in TABLE 1) were pregnant at the time of injection and the presence of heavily labeled neurons in the brains of their offspring served as a test of the availability and specificity of the isotope, and adequacy of the autoradiographic technique. In addition this material provided useful data on the amount of radioactivity that is indicative of DNA replication in mothers of these offspring.

The lowest level of radiolabeling accepted as evidence that a given cell was in the S-phase preceding its last mitotic division at the time of the [^{3}H]thymidine injection was determined for each animal separately (see, for example, FIGURE 3). This level (usually more than 15–20 silver grains per nucleus) was considered to be one-half of the maximum count of reduced silver grains present in the emulsion situated over postmitotic neurons, glial and endothelial cells in the brain, or in the cells of renewable non-brain tissue (e.g., epithelial cells, fibroblasts, corneal endothelium, intestinal cells, hepocytes) obtained from the same specimen. Nuclei containing fewer than half the maximum count, but more than five grains, were considered to be

TABLE 1. Schedule of [^{3}H]Thymidine Injections and Sacrifice[a]

Case	Sex	Date of Death	Age at Death	Date of [^{3}H]Thymidine Injection(s) 1	2	3	4	5	6	7	Interval between Injection and Death
1	F	3/07/83	7 mo	1/31/83							35 days
2	M	3/16/83	19 mo	2/09/83							35 days
3	F	2/25/76	6 yr	5/16/74							1.8 yr
4	F	9/09/78	6 yr	10/14/75							2.9 yr
5	F	10/07/79	6 yr	11/12/73							5.8 yr
6	F	3/12/80	8 yr	11/05/73							6.3 yr
7	F	5/02/69	4 yr	4/30/69							3 days
8	F	02/15/83	17 yr	10/11/76							6 yr
9	F	10/07/77	6 yr	3/16/73	6/23/74						3.2 yr
10	F	1/29/80	10 yr	6/27/75	3/06/76	4/08/77					2.8 yr
11	F	1/23/76	10 yr	1/05/73	10/23/73	7/21/74	5/27/74	1/19/76			14 days
12	M	11/28/83	5 yr	8/26/83	8/27/83	8/28/83	8/29/83	8/30/83	8/31/83	9/01/83	3 mo

[a] From Rakic.[56]

lightly labeled (FIG. 3, middle cell). Light labeling may occur because of dilution of radioactivity produced by additional divisions of precursor cells after the [^{3}H]thymidine injection. However, light label could also be caused by several other biological factors that are unrelated to cell division, as well as by various technical artifacts.[60,64] The same criteria for the classification of [^{3}H]thymidine radioactive cells into categories of heavily and lightly labeled cells have been routinely used in the analysis of developing brain in our own as well as in other laboratories.[4,53,55,57,59,65,68] As a rule, nuclei containing less than 5 grains were not considered as indicative of cell division, even though theoretically some of these cells may be far-removed offspring of initially heavily labeled cells. However, as discussed in the next section, the scheduling of injection and sacrifice in our experiments allows us to exclude this possibility. Furthermore, even in autoradiograms with the lowest background, an occasional cluster of silver grains can occur in the photosensitive emulsion over an area roughly equal to the surface of a nucleus. Since a large surface area in each specimen was surveyed to examine approximately 10^8 cells, one cannot rule out the possibility that clusters of 5 grains can occur by chance over a given nucleus. For these reasons, the presence of grains slightly above background level over an occasional cell nucleus can be considered either an artifact, the expression of "polyploidyzation," or DNA repair. As to the latter cause, a growing body of evidence indicates that a small quantity of nucleotides may be constantly replaced in the nuclear and mitochondrial DNA of nondividing cells including neurons.[34,51,67] Repair of DNA by normal metabolic processes or by various mutagenic agents (including ionizing radiation, heat, carcinogens, and viruses) probably occurs in neurons as in any other class of cells. The level of repair as well as the possibility for incorporation of radioactive nucleotide might be enhanced in cases that received multiple injections of [^{3}H]thymidine.

INCIDENCE AND NATURE OF RADIOLABELED CELLS

All major areas of the brain including visual, motor, and association neocortex, hippocampus, olfactory bulb, basal ganglia, thalamus, retina, cerebellum, brain stem, and spinal cord were processed for autoradiography and thoroughly analyzed. Between 500 and 1000 sections in each case were first scanned with a low-power objective in darkfield illumination and all cells suspected of being radiolabeled by the above-delineated criteria were examined in detail in lightfield illumination using a 63X oil immersion objective with normal and Nomarski interference illumination. This procedure makes it possible to scan over more than 10^8 cells in each specimen. Given the number of almost 10,000 sections surveyed in 10 mature monkeys that received a total of 23 individual [^{3}H]thymidine injections, the probability of missing heavily radiolabeled neurons is infinitesimal.

In most structures of the primate central nervous system, neurons can be rather easily recognized in autoradiograms prepared from well-fixed tissue counterstained with the cresyl violet or toluidine blue method because of

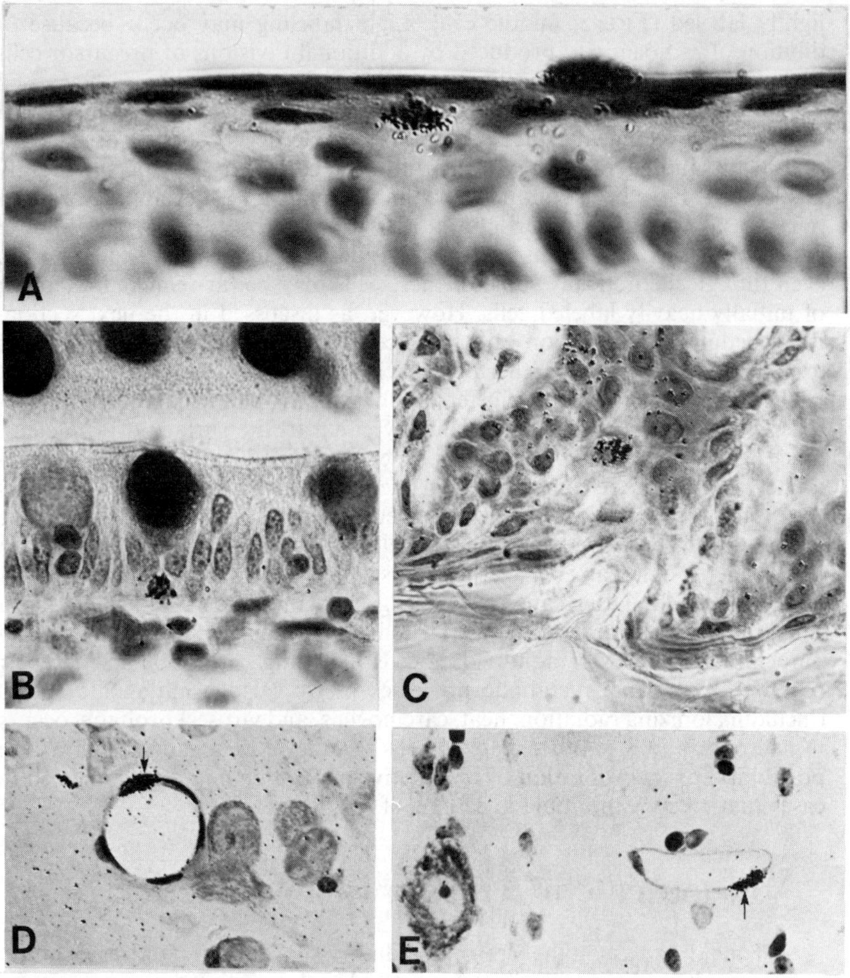

FIGURE 4. Photographs using Nomarski optics show intensity of labeling in various renewing non-neuronal cells after [^{3}H]thymidine injection. (**A**) Two heavily labeled corneal endothelial cells in a 5-year-old monkey exposed to seven injections of [^{3}H]thymidine three months before sacrifice. (**B**) The lining of the small intestine in $1\frac{1}{2}$-year-old monkey showing [^{3}H]thymidine-labeled cells in the epithelium of the villi. (**C**) Facial epidermis with a heavily labeled basal cell. (**D**) Heavily labeled endothelial cells in blood vessels of the caudate nucleus in the 7-month-old monkey injected 1 month earlier with [^{3}H]thymidine. (**E**) Heavily labeled vascular endothelial cell in the neocortex of the occipital lobe of the same specimen.

their location, size, shape, and the abundance of Nissl substance in their karyoplasm. It is significant that not a single heavily labeled cell with the distinct morphologic characteristics of a neuron was observed in any specimen of this series. [^{3}H]Thymidine, however, easily passed the blood–brain barrier since it was available for dividing glial cells in the same series of specimens.

Low levels of radioactivity (5 grains and less) observed over some neurons could not be the result of the dilution of radioactivity caused by the subsequent divisions of initially heavily labeled cells because specimens sacrificed at various short intervals after [^{3}H]thymidine injections also contained a few such neurons (with less than 5 grains), but not a single heavily labeled one.

In the juvenile monkeys injected at 6 and 18 months of age, comprehensive examination of autoradiograms revealed an occasional small cell in the caudate nucleus and the dentate gyrus of the hippocampus that are clearly labeled but were difficult to classify as belonging to a neuronal or glial cell lineage (FIG. 4). The number of such labeled cells, however, was extremely small to begin with and decreased further by age: only 6 cells were observed in more than 100 sections cut across the caudate nucleus in 6-month-old monkeys; and only 2 cells were seen in 18-month-old monkeys. It is important to underscore that no such cells have been encountered in postpubertal monkeys.

In the dentate gyrus, the incidence of radiolabeled cells of undetermined category was somewhat higher in juvenile monkeys: more than 50 cells were observed at 6 months and about 20 in specimens from 18-month-old monkeys in 100 randomly selected coronal sections across hippocampal regions in each specimen. Most of these labeled cells were located at the bottom of the dentate plate, in the so-called subgranular zone. This proliferative zone can be considered as a displaced subventricular zone of the hippocampal region.[12,15,46] It is formed during embryonic life and remains relatively prominent during the first 3 postnatal months, diminishing considerably during adolescence. However, the subgranular zone persists in the adult monkey as a single, broken-down row of small, dark cells.[14,16] In fully sexually mature monkeys (more than 4 years of known age or with a history of pregnancy), only an occasional radiolabeled cell was present in the subgranular zone of the dentate gyrus. These cells are as a rule smaller, have densely stained nuclei, a characteristic distribution of nuclear chromatin, and scanty cytoplasm, which makes them distinct from the larger and paler granule cells (FIG. 5C). During embryonic life and the first 2 to 3 months of postnatal age this zone produces both astroglial elements and dentate granule neurons.[14,15,53] However, after 6 months of age, the use of routine autoradiograms counterstained with the cresyl violet method does not allow determination of the nature of the labeled cells in this zone.

In order to distinguish between the somas of the dentate granule neurons and of the astrocytes or radial glial cells in the subgranular zone, we performed an immunocytochemical analysis using polyclonal antibody prepared against glial acidic fibrillary protein (GFAP), a specific astroglial marker, alone and in combination with [^{3}H]thymidine autoradiography. The localization of immunoreactivity at both the light and electron microscopic levels clearly demonstrates that the subgranular zone diminishes drastically with time, and that in postpubescent monkeys, a larger proportion of cells in this zone become GFAP-positive (FIG. 6). This study was followed by a combined [^{3}H]thymidine–immunocytochemical analysis, again at both light and

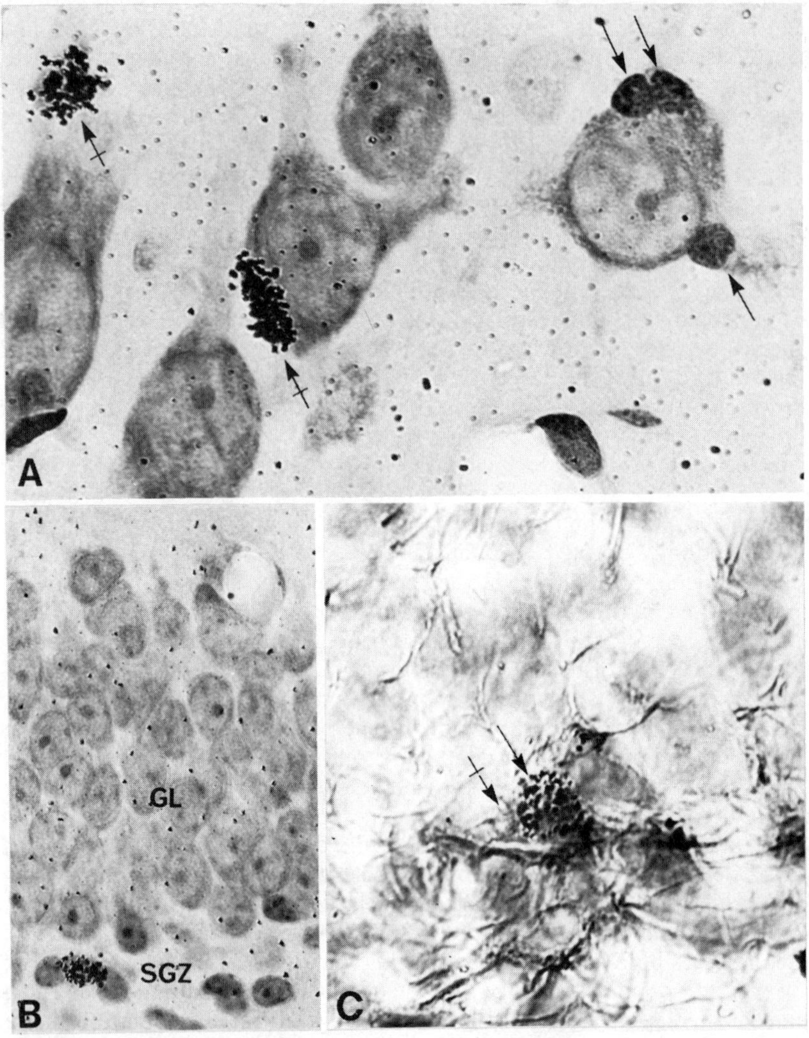

FIGURE 5. (**A**) Autoradiogram of the heavily labeled glial satellite cells in the neocortex of the frontal lobe in the 7-month-old monkey that was exposed to [^{3}H]thymidine at 6 months of age. The two radiolabeled cells (*crossed arrows*) are classified as glial in cresyl-violet-counter-stained autoradiograms on the basis of their size, shape, staining properties, and position in relation to the neuronal soma. Unlabeled satellite glial cells (*arrows*) attached to other neurons in the vicinity serve as a useful control. (**B**) Labeled cell in the subgranular zone of the dentate gyrus of the same monkey. (**C**) An example of double-labeled cell radiolabeled with [^{3}H]thymidine (*arrow*) and immunolabeled with anti-GFAP serum (*crossed arrow*) in the subgranular zone of the 5-year-old monkey.

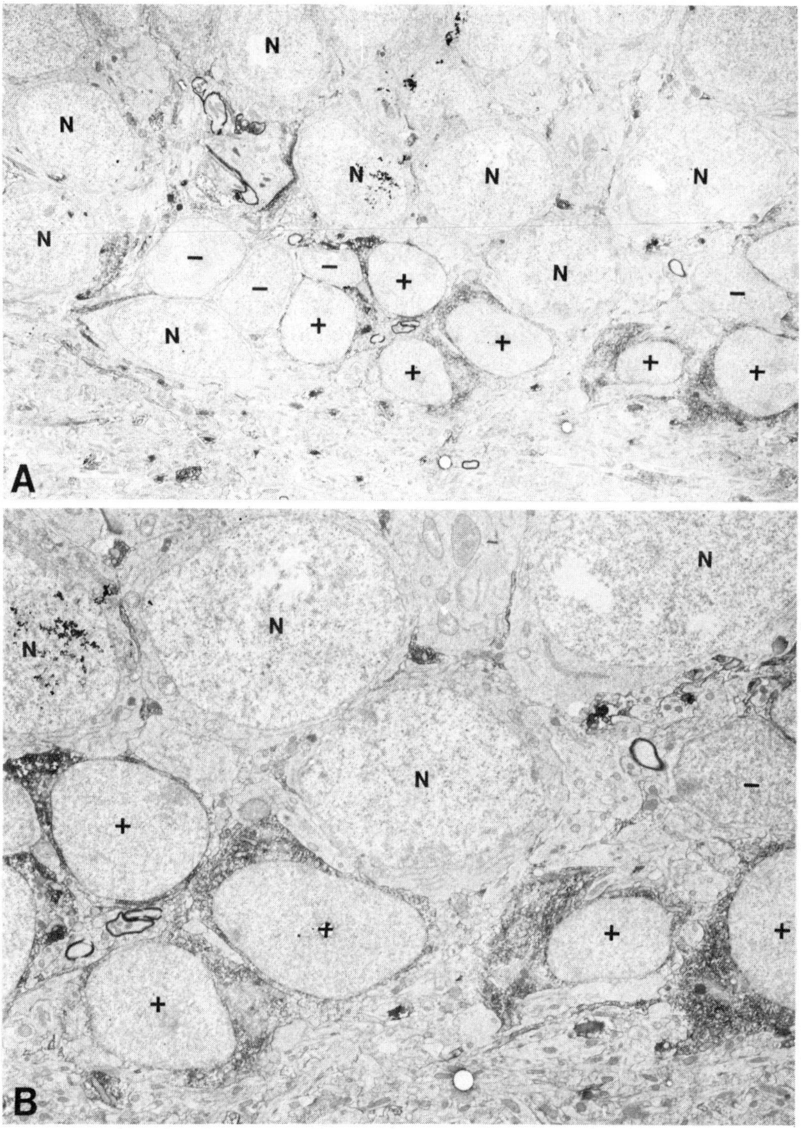

FIGURE 6. (**A**) An electron micrograph of the granular layer and subgranular zone of the hippocampal dentate gyrus in a 7-month-old monkey. GFAP-positive astroglial cells (+) and GFAP-negative stem cells (−) are situated in the subgranular zone while neurons (N) lie mostly above. (From Eckenhoff and Rakic.[16] Reproduced by permission.) (**B**) Enlargement of the area illustrated in **A** to show that, once identified immunocytochemically, stem cells, glial cells, and neurons can be distinguished on the basis of the ultrastructural characteristics, including electron density and distribution of nuclear chromatin.

electron microscopic levels, designed to determine the exact relationship between radiolabeled and immunolabeled cells.[16] Furthermore, in order to increase the incidence of radiolabeled cells, one monkey was injected seven times with [^{3}H]thymidine (TABLE 1). In the material from adult monkeys processed so far, all radiolabeled cells were either GFAP-positive (FIG. 5D) or had the morphologic characteristics of proliferative stem cells (FIG. 6). It is significant that not a single labeled cell in material processed thus far showed neuronal properties.[16] Although negative, these results are highly significant since multiple injections of [^{3}H]thymidine provided a reasonable sample of radiolabeled cells.

In contrast to neurons, cells of glial lineage in the primate brain display different proliferative behavior. The size, tinctorial properties, distribution, and density of nucleochromatin and karyoplasm in most instances provide sufficient cues for identification of glial cells in cresyl-violet-counterstained autoradiograms. Radiolabeled astrocytes were frequently observed in the two youngest monkeys of our series, but, although rare, they nevertheless can also be regularly found in older animals (FIG. 5A). The incidence of radiolabeled astrocytes was, of course, the largest in the 5-year-old monkey injected seven times. They were most often present in a satellite position to neurons. The close apposition of some satellite cells to neurons occasionally posed a problem for distinguishing whether the radioactivity emanated from the nucleus of an astrocyte or from an underlying neuronal nucleus. However, the use of high-power oil immersion objectives or Normarski interference contrast illumination enabled a clear distinction in each case. Thus, unlike neurons, astrocytes in primates should be classified as a renewing cell population.

A number of oligodendrocytes were heavily labeled in the specimens from the 6- and 18-month-old animals. The labeled oligodendrocytes were particularly numerous in the white matter of the forebrain, corpus callosum, and throughout the length of the pyramidal tract, which are still being myelinated at these ages (FIG. 7). However, an occasional small radiolabeled cell that has the characteristics of an oligodendrocyte could be found also in the autoradiograms prepared from multiply injected postpubertal animals, indicating that under the living conditions in a primate colony a small number of oligodendrocytes may also be replenished. Since oligodendroglial cells represent almost half of the total number of cells in the primate central nervous system, three or four labeled cells suspected to be oligodendrocytes is infinitesimally small. It was recently reported that mature oligodendrocytes may be induced to enter the proliferative cycle after the occurrence of mechanical lesions.[40] It was not possible to determine whether the few labeled oligodendrocytes in our material represented a response to some viral or toxic injury that could occur under normal laboratory conditions. The experimental design of the present study does not allow any conclusion about the origin of the newly formed astrocytes or oligodendrocytes.

Another issue which is equally important to the main subject of this symposium, but which has been less thoroughly analyzed, is whether a lesion of the brain could induce formation of new neurons from dormant stem cells

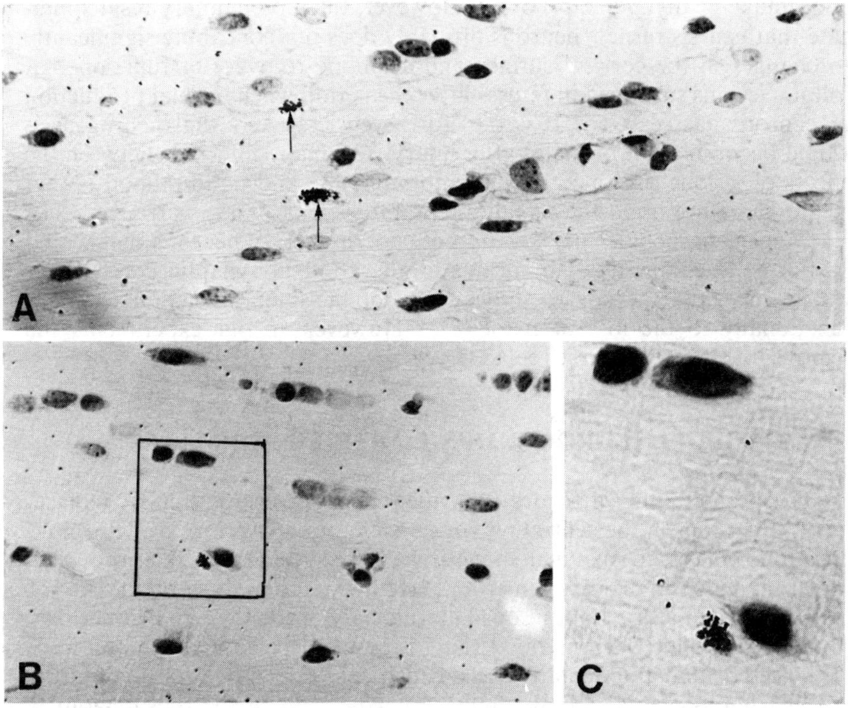

FIGURE 7. Heavily labeled oligodendroglial cell situated within the corpus callosum (**A**) and pyramidal tract (**B**) of the 7-month-old monkey exposed to [^{3}H]thymidine 35 days before death. (**C**) Higher magnification photograph of labeled oligodendrocytes enclosed in the rectangle in **B** to show its cytologic characteristics.

(e.g., G_0 in FIGURE 2). From all that is known about recovery of function in primates, the chances for this phenomenon to occur are higher if the lesion is made in younger animals.[19] Data relevant to this issue came from the analysis of monkeys that sustained resection of cerebral cortex before birth, but after the completion of neurogenesis for the ablated region.[18] In recent years we have used a surgical procedure that allows removal of substantial areas of the cerebral cortex in a monkey fetus, which is then returned to the uterus, subsequently delivered at term, and allowed to mature.[19,20] This type of prenatal neurosurgery is usually performed during the second half of pregnancy after the full complement of neocortical neurons has been achieved.[54] When a part of the cortex is removed from one hemisphere, new sulci and gyri as well as new patterns of connectivity are observed in the adult cerebrum on both sides in areas distant from the lesion.[18,19] Although two of these monkeys were injected with [^{3}H]thymidine 1 to 3 days after surgery, they nevertheless failed to show any radiolabeled neurons.[18] Obviously, additional experiments with different combinations of timing of surgery, injection of isotopes, and sacrifice should be performed and uptake of thymidine followed. However, these preliminary results indicate that genesis of new neurons probably does not contribute significantly to changes in the cortical surface and dramatic recovery of function that follows lesions sustained in fetuses after the period when normal production of neurons has ceased.[18] It is therefore even less likely that neurogenesis would occur in adult primates after injury. The main difference between the effects of lesions sustained during embryonic life and in adulthood is that in the immature brain the remaining brain tissue becomes rearranged. The rearrangement includes preservation of supernumerary neurons that would be normally eliminated[58] or dramatic alteration in synaptic connectivity which may hold the key to the capacity of the immature brain to adapt functionally to the loss of tissue.[18–20] However, in our experiments the removed neurons were not replaced.

WHY IS NEUROGENESIS LIMITED IN PRIMATES?

The present study provides no evidence for either addition or replacement of neurons in the central nervous system of adult primates. The onset, duration, and cessation of neurogenesis vary in a systematic and reproducible way from region to region. Numerous [^{3}H]thymidine analyses on the time of neuronal origin carried out in our laboratory on more than 25 distinct neuronal classes have demonstrated that, with the exception of granule cells of the cerebellum and dentate gyrus, which continue to be produced during the first few postnatal months, most other neurons in the rhesus monkey are generated within the first half of gestation.[8–10,22,35,37,38,46,48,53–55,57] In each case, prospective neurons irreversibly enter the G_1 phase of their generation cycle prior to the onset of migration, differentiation, and elaboration of axons and dendrites and establishment of their synaptic connectivity.[46,53,65] Experiments using supravital DNA synthesis in human fetal brain slices[60] indicate that the human brain develops according to remarkably similar principles.[65] When a given cell becomes committed to a specific neuronal class and begins the synthesis of specific neurotransmitters, it loses its capacity for DNA replication. If we take into account the experimental design and the scope of our experiments, there seems little doubt that the full complement of neurons in the primate brain is generated during a restricted developmental period.

Increase and/or turnover of neurons appear to occur during postembryonic stages in most nonprimate species analyzed so far. From the available literature on invertebrates it appears that at least certain populations of neuronal cells can be added during postembryonic life in a variety of species.[3,39,47,49,66] The evidence on this issue, however, is rather sporadic, incomplete, and difficult to evaluate. For example, the mode and length of the life cycle is variable and in some species includes metamorphosis, while in the others there is continuous growth. As a result, the definition of the postdevelopmental stage is rather arbitrary. Furthermore, with the exception of the work by Technau in *Drosophila*,[66] the [^{3}H]thymidine autoradiography technique has not been used in the analysis of neurogenesis in adult invertebrates. It needs to be emphasized that adult neurogenesis occurs only among some cell classes in selected structures, while other cell classes within the same organism remain fixed in number. Furthermore, in each case new neurons appear to be generated from dormant stem cells. The factors that induce cell division of progenitor cells are unknown, but there seems to be a correlation with increased functional needs[66] or continuous growth.[47]

In submammalian vertebrates, postdevelopmental neurogenesis is best documented in several species of fishes[7,43,61] and amphibia.[32] Although it was generally believed that the adult avian brain does not acquire new neurons, postembryonic neurogenesis has been recorded in some singing birds, such as canaries.[21,44] As reviewed in the first section of this article, postdevelopmental neurogenesis has been also reported for certain classes of neuron in several nonprimate mammals[3,28–30,41,50,52,63] In some of these studies all the criteria necessary to prove neurogenesis, which were discussed above, have not been satisfied; nevertheless many investigators believe that certain classes of neuron, including neocortical cells,[28] can be produced in adult rodents.

Although the majority of species have not been examined by [^{3}H]thymidine autoradiography, the examples of postdevelopmental neurogenesis that have come to light have been obtained across a rather wide range of animals representing different levels of the evolutionary scale. If the findings of postdevelopmental neurogenesis in rodents and other mammals prove to be correct, and I am not as yet fully convinced that they are, then the possibility has to be considered that the primate brain is significantly different from the brain of nonprimates in that it does not normally produce new neurons once it reaches the adult form. This, perhaps, should not be surprising since there are many reasons to expect major differences between the development and organization of the brain in primate and nonprimate species.

What is the biological significance of the early completion of genesis of neurons and strict limits of neurogenesis in adult primates? One possibility is that the large, synaptically interconnected brain would not allow migration of newly formed neurons across long distances and would be resistant to subsequent growth of axons to distant synaptic targets. For example, neurons constituting the neocortex of the rhesus monkey that are thought to be of principal importance in higher brain functions are all generated and have completed their migration during the first half of pregnancy.[54] Once afferent, efferent, and intrinsic synaptic contacts between these neurons become established, it is likely that new neurons cannot be incorporated into the appropriate cortical layers or succeed in sending their axons to some distant targets. Indeed, postdevelopmental neurogenesis is most prominent in those nonmammalian vertebrate species that have a capacity for regeneration of axons, such as fish and amphibians,[32,43,61,62] or in the avian brain with particular seasonal changes of brain structures.[21,44] This is an important point since the addition of new neurons that occurs in adult fish is followed by growth of new axons, resulting in a constant rearrangement of synapses in terminal structures.[13] However, a stable population of neurons may be an essential prerequisite for social and cognitive behavior in primates. For example, one can entertain the possibility that an extensive interaction with the environment requires a stable set of neurons that would retain acquired experiences in the pattern of synaptic connectivity. The very survival of primates depends on accurate maintenance of records stored in the integrity of their neuronal connectivity. Structural, biochemical, and functional properties of synapses can change, but the basic set of connections cannot. The addition of new, "naive" neurons into existing circuits would interfere with retention of acquired experience and learned behavior that is evolutionarily the most significant advantage of all primate species including humans. One might suppose the very same advantages are shared by all mammals, but studies of neurogenesis apparently suggest otherwise.

SUMMARY

Autoradiographic analysis of juvenile and adult monkeys that received single or multiple injection of the specific DNA precursor, [^{3}H]thymidine, demonstrates slight turnover of glial cells, but failed to provide any evidence of either neuronal addition or replacement. Therefore, while the brains of nonmammalian vertebrates and possibly some nonprimate mammals may display variable degrees of postembryonic neurogenesis, all neurons of the primate central nervous system are generated during restricted developmental periods, mostly before birth and not after infancy. It is not surprising that a stable population of neurons in mature primates, including man, may be essential for the retention of memory and learned behavior.

REFERENCES

1. Alberts, B., D. Bray, J. Lewis, M. Raff, K. Roberts & J. Wietson. 1983. The Molecular Biology of the Cell. Garland. London and New York.
2. Altman, J. 1962. Are neurons formed in the brains of adult mammals? Science **135:** 1127–1128.
3. Anderson, H. 1978. Postembryonic development of the visual system of locust, *Schistocerca gregaria*. J. Embryol. Exp. Morphol. **45:** 55–83.
4. Angevine, J., Jr. 1965. Time of neuron origin in the hippocampal region. An autoradiographic study in the mouse. Exp. Brain Res. (Suppl.) **2:** 1–70.
5. Bayer, S. A. 1982. Changes in the total number of dentate granule cells in juvenile and adult rats: A correlated volumetric and ^{3}H-thymidine autoradiographic study. Exp. Brain Res. **46:** 315–323.
6. Bayer, S. A., J. Yakel & P. Puri. 1982. Neurons in the rat dentate gyrus granular layer substantially increase during juvenile and adult life. Science **216:** 890–892.
7. Birse, C. S., R. L. Leonard & R. E. Coggeshall. 1980. Neuronal increase in various areas of the nervous system of the guppy, *Lebistes*. J. Comp. Neurol. **194:** 291–301.
8. Brand, S. & P. Rakic. 1979. Genesis of the primate neostriatum: [^{3}H]-thymidine autoradiographic analysis of the time of neuron origin in the rhesus monkey. Neuroscience **4:** 767–778.

9. BRAND, S. & P. RAKIC. 1980. Neurogenesis of the nucleus accumbens septi and neighboring septal nuclei in the rhesus monkey: A combined [^{3}H]-thymidine and electron microscopic study. Neuroscience **5:** 2125–2138.
10. COPPER, M. L. & P. RAKIC. 1981. Neurogenetic gradients in the superior and inferior colliculi of the rhesus monkey. J. Comp. Neurol. **202:** 309–334.
11. DIGLIO, T. & K. HERRUP. 1982. A significant fraction of the adult number of mature cerebellar Purkinje cells appears between postnatal day 16 and 30 in the mouse. Soc. Neurosci. Abstr. **8:** 636.
12. DUFFY, J. C. & P. RAKIC. 1983. Differentiation of granule cell dendrites in the dentate gyrus of the rhesus monkey: A quantitative Golgi study. J. Comp. Neurol. **214:** 224–237.
13. EASTER, S. S. 1983. Postnatal neurogenesis and changing connections. Trends Neurosci. **6:** 53–56.
14. ECKENHOFF, M. & P. RAKIC. 1983. Composition of the proliferative subgranular zone of the developing and mature dentate gyrus in the rhesus monkey: EM-immunocytochemical (anti-GFAP) and autoradiographic (^{3}H-TdR) analysis. Soc. Neurosci. Abstr. **9:** 900.
15. ECKENHOFF, M. & P. RAKIC. 1984. Radial organization of the hippocampal dentate gyrus: A Golgi, ultrastuctural and immunocytochemical analysis in the developing rhesus monkey. J. Comp. Neurol. **223:** 1–21.
16. ECKENHOFF, M. & P. RAKIC. 1985. The nature of the proliferative cells in the dentate gyrus in the prenatal and adult rhesus monkeys: A combined immunocytochemical, ^{3}H-thymidine autoradiographic and electromicroscopic study. J. Neurosci. Submitted for publication.
17. FJUITA, S. 1962. Kinetics of cellular proliferation. Exp. Cell Res. **28:** 52–60.
18. GOLDMAN-RAKIC, P. S. 1980. Morphological consequences of prenatal injury to the primate brain. Prog. Brain Res. **53:** 3–19.
19. GOLDMAN-RAKIC, P. S. 1982. Neuronal development and plasticity of association cortex in primates. Neurosci. Res. Program Bull. **20:** 520–532.
20. GOLDMAN-RAKIC, P. S. & P. RAKIC. 1984. Experimental modification of gyral patterns. *In* Cerebral Dominance: Biological Foundation. N. Geschwind & A. M. Galaburda, Eds.: 193–211. Harvard University Press. Cambridge, MA.
21. GOLDMAN, S. A. & F. NOTTEBOHM. 1983. Neuronal production, migration and differentiation in a vocal control nucleus of the adult female canary brain. Proc. Natl. Acad. Sci. USA **80:** 2390–2394.
22. GOULD, B. B. & P. RAKIC. 1981. The total number, time of origin and kinetics of proliferation of neurons comprising the deep cerebellar nuclei in the rhesus monkey. Exp. Brain Res. **44:** 195–206.
23. GRAZIADEI, P. P. C. & G. A. MONTI-GRAZIADEI. 1979. Neurogenesis and neuron regeneration in the olfactory system of mammals. I. Morphological aspects of differentiation and structural organization of the olfactory sensory neurons. J. Neurocytol. **8:** 1–18.
24. HAYMAKER, W. & R. D. ADAMS. 1982. Histology and Histopathology of the Nervous System. Charles C Thomas, Springfield, IL.
25. HINDS, J. W. & N. A. MCNELLY. 1977. Aging of the rat olfactory bulb. Growth and atrophy of constituent layers and changes in size and number of mitrotic cells. J. Comp. Neurol. **171:** 345–368.
26. HOWARD, A. & C. R. PELC. 1953. Synthesis of deoxyribonucleic acid in normal and irradiated cells and its relation to chromosome breakage. Heredity (Suppl.) **6:** 261–273.
27. JACOBSON, M. 1978. Developmental Neurobiology. Plenum. New York, NY.
28. KAPLAN, M. S. 1981. Neurogenesis in the 3-month-old rat visual cortex. J. Comp. Neurol. **195:** 323–338.
29. KAPLAN, M. S. & D. BELL. 1981. Neurogenesis in the dentate gyrus of the 8 and 11 month old rat. Soc. Neurosci. Abstr. **7:** 184.
30. KAPLAN, M. S. & J. W. HINDS. 1977. Neurogenesis in the adult rat: Electron microscopic analysis of light radiographs. Science **197:** 1092–1094.
31. KANDEL, E. R. & J. H. SCHWARTZ. 1981. Principles of Neural Science. Elsevier. New York and Amsterdam.

32. KIRSCHE, W. 1967. Über postembryonale matrixzonen in Gehirn verschiedener Vertebrate und deren Beziehung zur Hirnbauplanlehre. Z. Mikroskop. Anat. Forsch. **77:** 313–406.
33. KORR, H., B. SCHULTZE & W. MAURER. 1975. Autoradiographic investigations of glial proliferation in the brain of adult mice. J. Comp. Neurol. **160:** 477–490.
34. KRONBERG, A. 1980. DNA Replication. Freeman. San Francisco, CA.
35. LAVAIL, M., D. YASUMURA & P. RAKIC. 1983. Cell genesis in the rhesus monkey retina. Invest. Ophthal. **24:** 7.
36. LEBLOND, C. P. 1964. Classification of cell populations on the basis of their proliferative behavior. Natl. Cancer Inst. Monogr. **14:** 119–150.
37. LENN, W. J., N. HALFON & P. RAKIC. 1978. Development of the interpeduncular nucleus in the midbrain of rhesus monkey and human. Anat. Embryol. **152:** 273–289.
38. LEVITT, P. & P. RAKIC. 1982. The time of genesis, embryonic origin and differentiation of the brainstem monoamine neurons in the rhesus monkey. Dev. Brain Res. **4:** 35–57.
39. LUSCHER, M. 1967. Insects as a medium for study of differentiation. *In* Insects and Physiology. J. W. L. Beamont & J. E. Treherme, Eds.: 39–51. Oliver and Boyd. Edinburgh.
40. LUDWIN, S. K. 1984. Proliferation of mature oligodendrocytes after trauma to the central nervous system. Nature **308:** 274–275.
41. MESSIER, B., C. P. LEBLOND & J. SMART. 1958. Presence of DNA synthesis and mitosis in the brain of young adult mice. Exp. Cell Res. **14:** 224–226.
42. MEPISASHVILLI, I. S. 1971. Reactive and Regenerative Processes in the Nervous System. [Collection of papers dealing with this subject (in Russian)]. Sabchota Sakartvelo. Tbilisi.
43. MEYER, R. L. 1978. Evidence from thymidine labeling for continuing growth of retina and tectum in juvenile goldfish. Exp. Neurol. **59:** 99–111.
44. NOTTEBOHM, F. & S. KASPARIAN. 1983. Widespread labeling of avian forebrain neurons after systemic injections of ^{3}H-thymidine in adulthood. Soc. Neurosci. Abstr. **9:** 380.
45. NOWAKOWSKI, R. S. & P. RAKIC. 1974. Clearance rate of exogenous ^{3}H-thymidine from the plasma of pregnant rhesus monkeys. Cell Tissue Kinet. **7:** 189–194.
46. NOWAKOWSKI, R. S. & P. RAKIC. 1981. The site of origin and route and rate of migration of neurons to the hippocampal region of the rhesus monkey J. Comp. Neurol. **196:** 129–154.
47. OGAWA, F. 1939. The nervous system of the earthworm (*Pheretina communissima*) in different ages. Sci. Rep. Res. Inst. Tohoku Univ. **13:** 395–488.
48. OGREN, M. & P. RAKIC. 1981. The prenatal development of the pulvinar in the monkey. ^{3}H-thymidine autoradiographic and morphometric analyses. Anat. Embryol. **162:** 1–20.
49. PANOV, A. A. 1963. The origin and fate of neuroblasts, neurons, and neuroglial cells in the central nervous system of the china oak silkworm *Antheraea perhyi guer* (Lepidoptera, attacidae). Entomol. Rev. **42:** 337–350.
50. PELC, S. R. 1972. Metabolic DNA in ciliated protozoa, salivary gland chromosomes and mammalian cells. Int. Rev. Cytol. **32:** 327–355.
51. PERONE-CAPANO, C., G. D'ONOFRIO & A. GIUDITTA. 1982. DNA turnover in rat cerebral cortex. J. Neurochem. **38:** 52–56.
52. RAHMANN, H. 1968. Autoradiographische Untersuchungen zum DNS-soffwechsel (mitosehanfigkeit) im ZNS von *Brachydamo rerio*. J. Hirnforsch. **10:** 279–284.
53. RAKIC, P. 1973. Kinetics of proliferation and latency between final division and onset of differentiation of the cerebellar stellate and basket neurons. J. Comp. Neurol. **147:** 523–546.
54. RAKIC, P. 1974. Neurons in rhesus monkey visual cortex: Systematic relation between time of origin and eventual disposition. Science **183:** 425–427.
55. RAKIC, P. 1977. Genesis of the dorsal lateral geniculate nucleus in the rhesus monkey: Site and time of origin, kinetics of proliferation, routes of migration and pattern of distribution of neurons. J. Comp. Neurol. **176:** 23–52.
56. RAKIC, P. 1985. Limits of neurogenesis in primates. Science **227:** 154–156.
57. RAKIC, P. & R. S. NOWAKOWSKI. 1981. Time of origin of neurons and route and rate of migration of neurons to the hippocampal region of the rhesus monkey. J. Comp. Neurol. **196:** 99–128.

58. RAKIC, P. & K. P. RILEY. 1983. Regulation of axon number in primate optic nerve by binocular competition. Nature (London) **305:** 135–137.
59. RAKIC, P. & R. L. SIDMAN. 1968. Subcommissural organ and adjacent ependyma: Autoradiographic study of their origin in the mouse brain. Am. J. Anat. **122:** 317–335.
60. RAKIC, P. & R. L. SIDMAN. 1968. Supravital DNA synthesis in the developing human and mouse brain. J. Neuropath. Exp. Neurol. **27:** 246–276.
61. RAYMOND, P. A. & S. S. EASTER, JR. 1983. Postembryonic growth of optic tectum in goldfish. I. Location of germinal cell and numbers of neurons produced. J. Neurosci. **3:** 1077–1091.
62. RAYMOND, P. A., S. S. EASTER, JR., J. A. BURNAM & M. K. POWERS. 1983. Postembryonic growth of the optic tectum in goldfish. II. Modulation of cell proliferation by retinal fiber input. J. Neurosci. **3:** 1092–1099.
63. REINS, S. 1972. Autoradiographic study of ^{3}H-thymidine incorporation into brain DNA during learning. Physiol. Chem. Phys. **4:** 391–397.
64. SIDMAN, R. L. 1970. Autoradiographic methods and principles for study of the nervous system with thymidine-H^3. *In* Contemporary Research Methods in Neuroanatomy. W. J. H. Nauta & J. O. E. Ebbesson, Eds.: 25–274. Springer. Berlin.
65. SIDMAN, R. L. & P. RAKIC. 1982. Development of the human central nervous system. *In* Cytology and Cellular Neuropathology, 2nd ed. W. Haymaker & R. D. Adams, Eds.: 3–145. Charles C Thomas, Springfield, IL.
66. TECHNAU, G. M. 1984. Fiber number in the mushroom bodies of adult *Drosophila melanogaster* depends on age, sex and experience. J. Neurogenetics **1:** 113–126.
67. WINTZERISH, M., E. WITTERNDORP, R. V. RECHENMANN & P. MANDEL. 1977. Nuclear, nucleolar repair, or turnover of DNA in adult rat brain. J. Neurosci. Res. **3:** 217–230.
68. WYSS, J. M., B. SPIRANDIKULACHAI & T. L. HICKEY. 1983. An analysis of the time of origin of neurons in the enthorinal and subicular cortices in the cat. J. Comp. Neurol. **221:** 341–357.
69. ZECEVIC, N., J.-P. BOURGEOIS & P. RAKIC. Unpublished observations.

Neurogenesis in Adult Vertebrate Spinal Cord *in Situ* and *in Vitro*: A New Model System[a]

MARILYN J. ANDERSON AND STEPHEN G. WAXMAN[b]

Department of Neurology
Stanford University School of Medicine, and
Veterans Administration Medical Center
Palo Alto, California 94304

INTRODUCTION

Current clinical management of neurologic disorders, including cerebrovascular disease, degenerative disorders such as amyotrophic lateral sclerosis, and central nervous system trauma, is limited as a result of the fact that, under usual conditions, the number of neurons in the mammalian nervous system is fixed at, or shortly after, birth. Nevertheless, since production of new neurons could, in a manner similar to that of neural transplantation, lead to some degree of functional recovery after damage to the CNS, a number of research groups have recently begun to examine the mechanisms that underlie neurogenesis (production of new neurons) in those sites where it does occur, either as a normal process or in response to CNS injury. To date, the number of demonstrations of postnatal neurogenesis in mammalian CNS has been small; and these have been restricted, moreover, to a limited number of sites, such as rodent olfactory epithelium[1,2] and hippocampus.[3,4] Careful studies of postnatal neurogenesis have also been carried out in other vertebrate systems, such as the telencephalic vocal control nucleus of adult female canaries.[5,6] Nevertheless, the cellular mechanisms controlling postnatal neurogenesis remain poorly understood. In this regard, the development of accessible models of neurogenesis would be of great value.

Phylogenetically lower species in some cases exhibit *compensatory neurogenesis* after injury to the CNS; these species include urodele amphibians and teleosts.[7–10] Furthermore, even though postnatal neurogenesis is absent from most regions of the mammalian CNS, new neurons are produced in adulthood in fish and amphibians.[11] Thus, for example, there is clear evidence that new neurons are added in the retina[12–14] and its projection zone, the

[a] This work was supported in part by the Medical Research Service, Veterans Administration, by Grant NS-15320 from the National Institute of Neurological and Communicative Disorders and Stroke, and by the Folger Foundation.

[b] Address for correspondence: Dr. Stephen G. Waxman, Stanford University Neurological Unit, Veterans Administration Medical Center (127), 3801 Miranda Avenue, Palo Alto, California 94304

optic tectum,[15–17] in adult fish and amphibia. An increase in the number of neurons in several other areas of postnatal CNS, including spinal cord, has been reported in the guppy,[18] stingray,[19] and gymnotiform teleosts.[29] Since teleosts exhibit compensatory neurogenesis after injury and postnatal neurogenesis during normal growth in the adult, they may provide useful model systems for the study of this process. In the present report, we describe neurogenesis from adult tissue, both *in situ* and *in vitro*, in the spinal cord of *Sternarchus albifrons*.

THE *STERNARCHUS* ELECTROMOTOR SYSTEM

In the weakly electric gymnotiform teleost *Sternarchus albifrons*, the spinal electromotor system exhibits striking regeneration (FIG. 1) after injury or extirpation in the adult.[9,10,21] In contrast to other vertebrate species in which neurites may regenerate but where neuronal perikarya are not replaced after injury, spinal cord regeneration in *Sternarchus* includes an initial phase of neurogenesis, which is followed by neuronal differentiation and selective neuronal cell death.[22] Synaptic connections, presumably from the appropriate brainstem nuclei, are established with many of these regenerated neurons.[9,22] Moreover, neurogenesis in *Sternarchus* is not limited to the response to injury. In adult *Sternarchus*, ongoing growth of the spinal cord and electric organ, including the production and differentiation of new neurons, occurs concomitant with continued increase in length of the mature adult animal.[20,23] These newly added neurons are contacted by descending axons,[9] and apparently are recruited into functional neural circuits.

The spinal electromotor system in *Sternarchus albifrons*[24–27] contains electromotor neurons (which are specialized spinal motor neurons) clustered in paired medial columns, located on either side of the central canal and

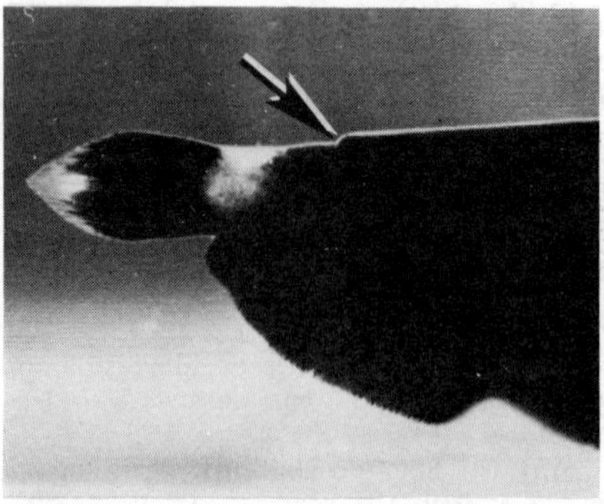

FIGURE 1. Regenerated tail of *Sternarchus albifrons*. Nine months after amputation of the tail, 2.8 cm of tail has regenerated from the amputation site, demarcated by the notch (*arrow*) at the dorsal surface.

dorsal to the ventral gray matter (FIG. 2A). Within the normal spinal cord (except the terminal spinal segment, where neurons are produced; see description below), each transverse section contains profiles of 4–12 electromotor neurons. The cell bodies of electromotor neurons exhibit a characteristic morphologic pattern which permits their identification in normal[28] and regenerated[9,22] spinal cord. In particular, the cells are relatively large and spherical in shape and lack dendrites, and the initial myelin segment extends up to or partially over the cell body so that there is no unmyelinated initial segment. This mode of cell architecture closely reflects the functional role of these cells in terms of firing in response to incoming synaptic information.[28] Cell bodies are contacted by descending bulbospinal axons and are electrically coupled via a presynaptic pathway. While some presumably chemical synapses are present, most axosomatic synapses are characterized by gap junctions.[28,29] Single axons can form gap junctions with several neighboring electromotor neurons.[28] The presynaptic fibers arise as blunt projections from large myelinated fibers, in some cases forming *en passant* synapses (arising from nodes of Ranvier) with the electromotor neurons. Gap junctions at these synapses are relatively large, often occupying all of the area of apposition between the presynaptic ending and the neuronal cell body. This characteristic morphologic structure facilitates electron microscopic identification of these descending electromotor junctions.

After amputation of the tail in *Sternarchus*, there is a striking degree of spinal cord regeneration.[9,22,30] While individual fish vary significantly with respect to the rate of regeneration, in most fish maintained at 26°C, 1.0–4.0 cm of tail regenerates in the first year post amputation (FIG. 1). Regeneration of the spinal cord initially occurs at a rate of 0.6–1.5 mm per week; after a period of 3–5 months, the rate slows somewhat. Regenerated cord usually exhibits one or two segmental-type swellings; spinal nerves emerge from the regenerated cord at irregular intervals along the rostral portion. Notably, while ongoing growth of the normal (not operated on) spinal cord occurs in the caudalmost spinal segment (see below), spinal cord regeneration occurs after amputation at levels more than 5 cm rostral to the caudal tip,[30] i.e., from regions of the cord that are no longer actively growing and that are histologically stable. This observation indicates that some cells, even in the mature (rostral) spinal cord, retain the ability to generate new neurons and glia under appropriate conditions.

COMPENSATORY NEUROGENESIS *IN SITU*

After amputation of the tail, new spinal cord is produced from the regenerated ependymal tube, which is continuous with ependymal tube surrounding the central canal in the spinal cord at the site of injury.[30] Neurogenesis occurs in the caudal region (limited to the caudalmost several millimeters) of the regenerating cord, while rostral to this, cells differentiate into neurons and glia. Thus, there is a rostrocaudal gradient of development along the regenerated cord. As judged along this gradient, rostral regions

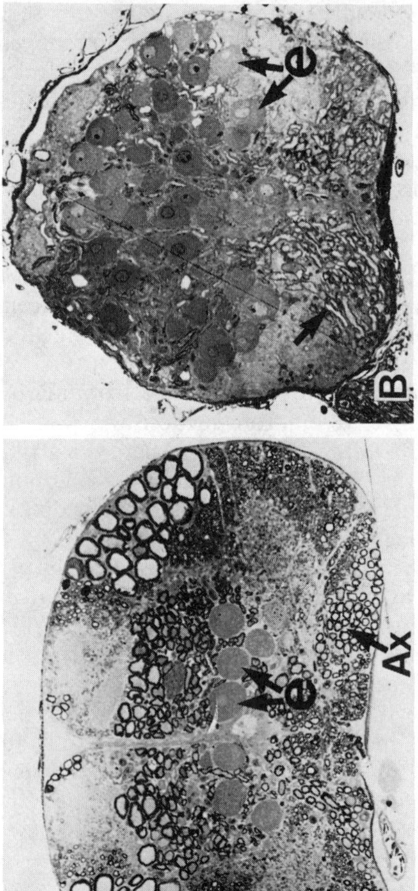

FIGURE 2A and B. A series of transverse sections through regenerated spinal cords. (**A**) Normal, unregenerated spinal cord. Cell bodies of the electromotor neurons (e) are clustered in a medial column. Axons of the electromotor neurons (Ax) are grouped at the ventral border, prior to exit in the ventral root. Large-diameter myelinated axons are grouped in a dorsolateral column; small-diameter myelinated fibers line the ventrolateral border of the cord. Magnification ×130. (**B**) Two-month regenerated cord. Note the large number of electromotor neurons (e) which virtually fill the dorsal half of the cord. Organized groupings of axons are lacking except for the electrocyte axons (*arrow*), which run towards the ventral roots (one visible at lower left). Magnification ×160.

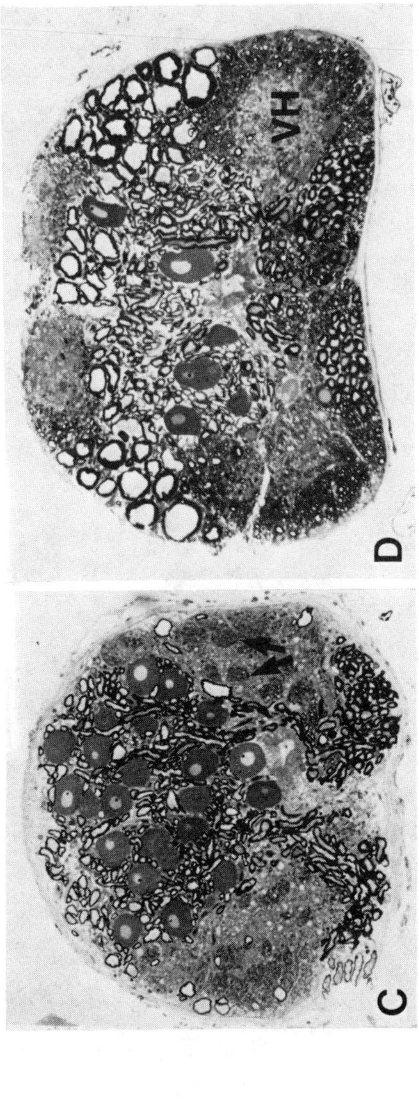

FIGURE 2C and D. Transverse sections through regenerated spinal cords. (**C**) Section from the mid-regenerated region of a 12-month regenerated cord. The number of electromotor neurons is decreased (compared to the early-regenerated stage in FIGURE 2B) and small groups of myelinated axons (*arrow*) are present. Magnification ×120. (**D**) Rostral region of 29-month regenerated cord. Overall morphology is indistinguishable from that of normal cord shown in FIGURE 2A. This section contains the normal number of electromotor neurons, dorsolateral tracts of large-diameter myelinated axons, small myelinated axons lining the ventrolateral border, and a distinct ventral horn (VH) region. Magnification ×120.

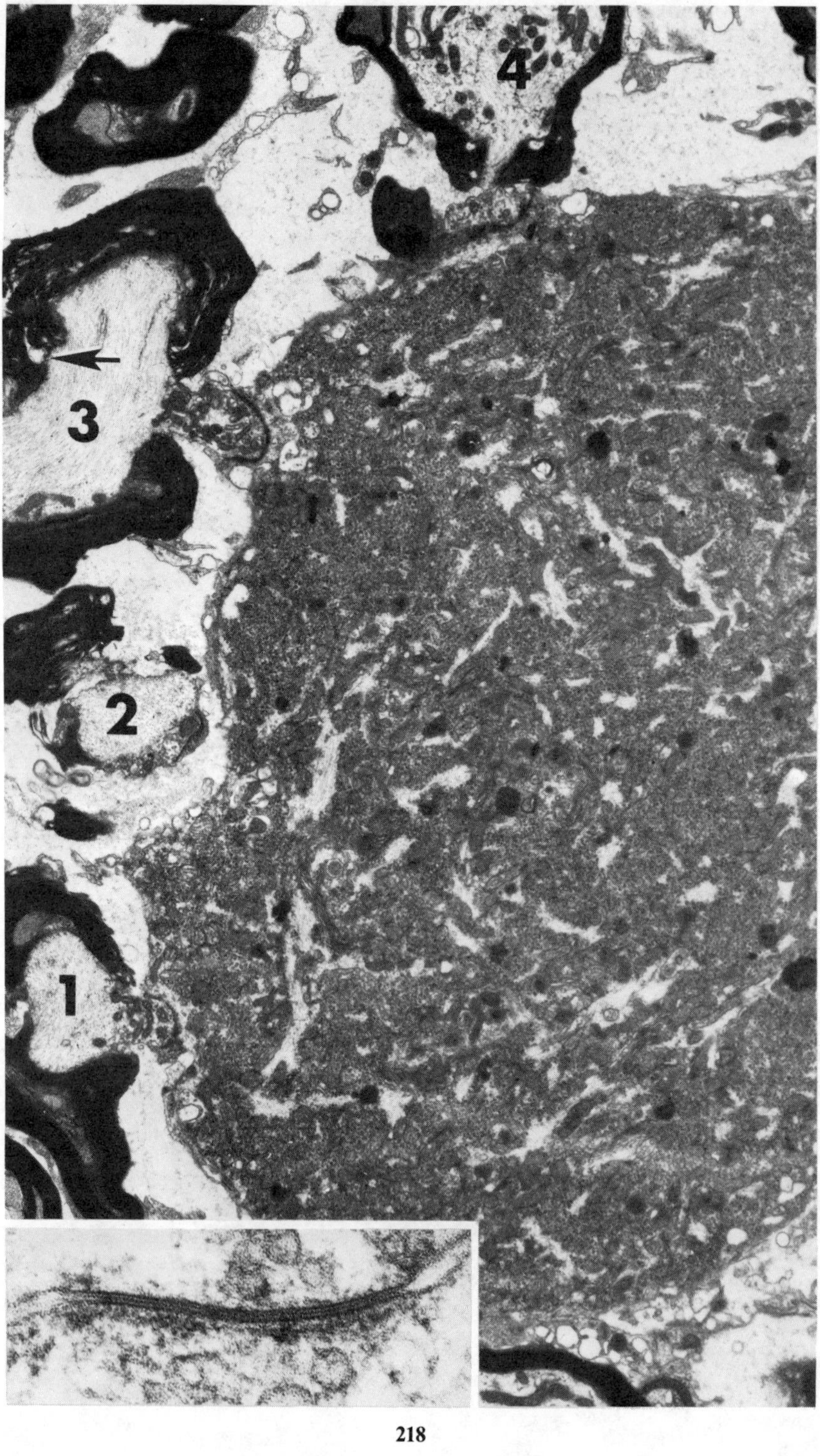
4
3
2
1

are more highly differentiated and organized, since they have regenerated for longer periods of time than caudal regions. This report will first briefly describe the morphologic structure of rostral regenerated spinal cord, where the morphologic pattern approaches that of the normal spinal cord. We will then turn attention to caudal zones, where neurogenesis begins.

After long-term regeneration of *Sternarchus* spinal cord, the most mature regenerated tissue (just behind the transition zone between regenerated and nonregenerated cord) exhibits a normal morphology.[22] The rostral, long-term regenerated cord (FIG. 2D) contains the normal number of electromotor neurons, located lateral and dorsal to the central canal (as in normal cord). Axon tracts in rostral long-term regenerated cord are indistinguishable from normal ones (FIG. 2A) in numbers and placement. Moreover, synapses (both chemical and electrical) with a normal morphologic structure are established within the regenerated cord.

In contrast to the rostral long-term regenerated spinal cord, more caudal cord, which has regenerated for shorter periods of time, exhibits a very different morphologic pattern. Cross sections of *Sternarchus* cords which have regenerated for up to 6 months (or sections in the middle of long-term regenerated cords) show an excess number of the electromotor neurons, with neuronal perikarya often filling the dorsal half of the regenerating cord (FIG. 2B and C). Thus, many more electromotor neurons are produced within the regenerating cord than are present in normal cord.[9,22] This overproduction of neurons during spinal cord regeneration *in situ* can result in a five-fold excess of electromotor neurons. However, continuing morphogenesis of the regenerating cord over time leads to a modulation of the number of electromotor neurons and the establishment of a normal spinal cord organization. Excess electromotor neurons are eliminated by a process of cell death, which results in the normal number of electromotor neurons in long-term regenerated cord. Cell elimination is selective, in that neurons in abnormal locations are eliminated, while neurons in appropriate locations are retained. This process of selective neuronal death in the regenerating spinal cord is described in detail by Anderson *et al.*[22] Similar processes of cell death play a role in regulating neuronal numbers in a number of developing systems.[31–34]

The recapitulation of normal morphologic structure in the regenerated spinal cord extends to the structure of the electromotor neurons and their afferent synapses.[9,22] Regenerated electromotor neurons, like normal ones,[28] are spherical in shape, between 25–50 μm in diameter, and lack dendrites. As in the normal cord, myelin extends over the initial segment to contact, or partially cover, the electromotor neuron. Perikarya of the regenerated electromotor neurons receive electrotonic synapses (FIG. 3), as do normal

FIGURE 3. Regenerated electromotor neuron receiving four axosomatic synapses. The synapses all arise from large myelinated axons and contain extensive areas of gap junction (*inset*). One of the synapses (number 3) arises *en passant*, from a node of Ranvier (*arrow* denotes other side of node). Ultrastructure of the regenerated electromotor neuron is identical to that of normal cells. Magnification $\times 6100$; that of *inset* $\times 92{,}400$.

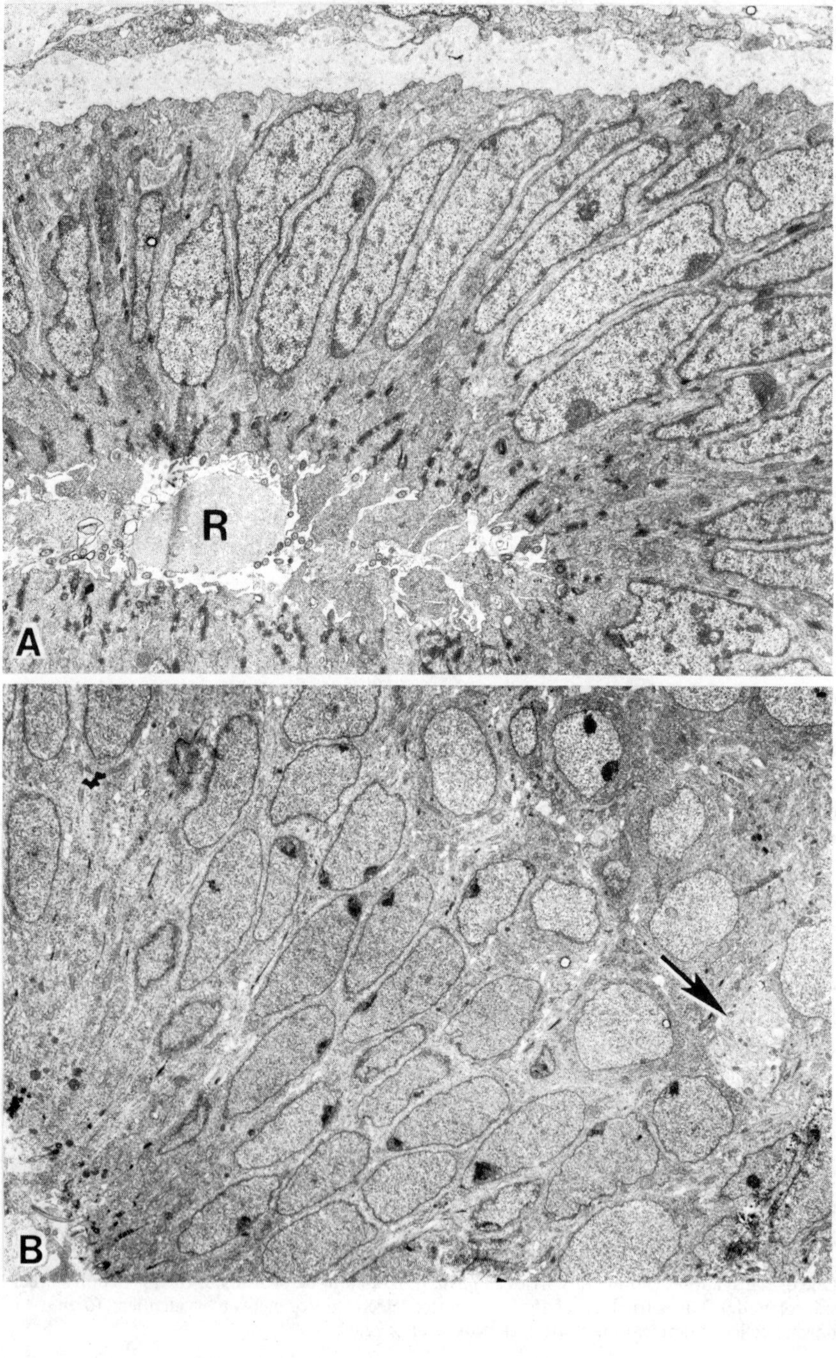
R
A
B

Sternarchus electrocytes. These synapses, as in the normal *Sternarchus* spinal cord, arise as blunt endings derived from large myelinated fibers or as *en passant* synapses which originate at nodes of Ranvier. Extensive gap junctions (FIG. 3, inset) are present at these synapses on the electromotor cell bodies, as in normal spinal cord. In addition, after regeneration *in situ*, the peripheral axons of the electromotor neurons develop a normal ultrastructure; this recapitulation of morphologic structure includes the establishment of several classes of nodes of Ranvier and normal axoglial relationships.[21]

EPENDYMAL CELLS AS NEURONAL PROGENITORS

Morphologic studies have indicated that cells in the ependymal layer constitute the source of the new neurons (and glia) in the regenerating cord in *Sternarchus*.[9,30] The ependymal layer similarly serves as a source of neurons during embryogenesis in a variety of species, a fact that has led some authors to refer to it as the "generative neuroepithelium."[35] Since development proceeds in a rostrocaudal sequence, the caudalmost cord contains the "youngest" (most recently generated) elements. The caudalmost region of regenerated spinal cord, in fact, consists of a single tubular layer of ependymal cells (FIG. 4A). The caudal ependymal cells in regenerating cord are enlarged and are more numerous (80–90 per transverse section) than are those in the unregenerated spinal cord (30–40 per transverse section).[30] The cells in this generative neuroepithelial layer do, however, continue to exhibit the morphologic characteristics of ependymal cells: they give rise to microvillae and cilia which extend into the central canal, they exhibit the cytoplasmic characteristics of ependymal cells, and they are joined via junctional complexes.[30,36]

Rostral to the single-cell ependymal layer, undifferentiated cells radiate away from the ependyma (FIG. 4B) and subsequently differentiate into the neurons and glia of the regenerating spinal cord. Neurites and axons from the rostral part of the regenerated cord and from undamaged cord rostral to the extirpation site grow caudally into and through the regenerating cord, where they establish synapses which exhibit a normal ultrastructure.[9,30] The progression of cell generation from the ependymal layer in *Sternarchus*

FIGURE 4. Ependymal layer in caudal regenerated cord. (**A**) Caudalmost regenerated cord, which is constituted solely of a tube of ependymal cells. Ependymal cells are large and nuclei contain patchy or dispersed chromatin. Processes of the ependymal cell cytoplasm extend into the central canal, which also contains numerous ependymal cell cilia and the Reissner's fiber (R). Magnification ×5330. (**B**) A section of caudal regenerated cord from a specimen with a 3-week regeneration period. Undifferentiated cells radiate away from the cells surrounding the central canal (*lower left*), creating a multilayered cord. Groups of longitudinally oriented axons (*arrow*) are present amidst the cells. At this stage there is no clear distinction between the ependymal cells and other cells that have moved away from the ependymal layer. Magnification ×2640.

is very similar to that observed in regenerating spinal cord of urodele amphibians.[7,37]

These results in both urodele amphibians and teleosts indicate that some of the ependymal cells in adult spinal cord of these species retain the ability to undergo mitosis and produce new neurons as well as glial cells, given the proper stimulus. In this regard, the presence of ependyma has been shown to be a necessary prerequisite for regeneration of spinal axons and non-neuronal structures in the tail of the lizard *Lygosoma*.[38] In addition, the course of generation of cells from the ependymal layer in regenerating spinal cords of amphibians and teleosts is very similar to the sequence of maturation during normal embryonic development of the spinal cord in some species.[39,40] A comparison with embryonic development in *Sternarchus* is not presently possible since the fish have not been bred in captivity. However, as described below, ependyma constitutes the stem-cell population from which neurons arise during postnatal growth of the spinal cord in this species.

POSTNATAL NEUROGENESIS DURING NORMAL GROWTH *IN VIVO*

Teleosts exhibit growth in size, which continues into adult life; as part of this postnatal growth, neurons are added to many parts of the teleost CNS throughout adult life.[11,18,19] This aspect of teleost growth provides the opportunity to study neurogenesis from adult tissues. In *Sternarchus*, addition of spinal cord tissue and generation of new neurons during ongoing growth of the adult occurs in the caudalmost segment of spinal cord.[20,23] The source of the new neurons and glia in the caudalmost segment of cord is the ependymal layer,[23] which shows striking morphologic similarity to the ependyma of regenerating cord.[30]

The caudalmost spinal segment in normal adult *Sternarchus*[23] consists of a single layer of ependymal cells. These cells, as in regenerating cord, are radially enlarged and more numerous than in the more rostral (mature) cord (50–55 cells versus 30–40 cells in rostral cord). Within 1–2 mm rostral from the caudalmost tip, numerous undifferentiated cells are generated from the innermost ependymal layer. Somewhat more rostral, neurons and glia begin to differentiate, while longitudinally oriented axons have grown in from the more rostral cord. Morphologic structure of the cord thus undergoes a gradual transition in the caudalmost two spinal segments from the single-cell layer of ependymal tube to the "mature" morphologic pattern of more rostral, histologically unchanging cord.

Although in most respects the caudalmost (generative) segment of spinal cord in normal adult *Sternarchus* resembles the caudal portion of regenerating spinal cord, it is interesting that the massive overproduction and subsequent cell death of electromotor neurons that are seen in regenerated cord do not occur in the processes of ongoing growth at the tip of normal cord.[20] Apparently, the mechanisms by which neuronal number is modulated are different in normally growing spinal cord compared with regenerating cord. This interesting difference between regeneration and normal growth is currently under study.

The background of demonstrated neurogenesis, which occurs both *in situ* in normal adult *Sternarchus* cord and during regeneration after injury, suggested that *Sternarchus* spinal cord might also carry on neurogenesis *in vitro*. Accordingly, an explant culture system was developed in our laboratory and [^{3}H]thymidine incorporation was examined in cultured explants from *Sternarchus* spinal cord.

NEUROGENESIS FROM ADULT TISSUE *IN VITRO*

Previous *in vitro* studies on CNS neurons have been carried out almost entirely with embryonic tissue, since adult avian or mammalian neuronal tissue has been extremely difficult to grow in culture. Besides, with a few exceptions,[41,42] studies of neuronal tissue *in vitro* have led to the general conclusion that the growth observed in cultures of even embryonic neuronal tissue represents an outgrowth of neurites from postmitotic neurons, rather than production of neurons *in vitro*. Thus, *in vitro* studies have provided an extremely useful model for the study of neuronal differentiation, growth, and interaction with other cells; however, it has not been possible to study neurogenesis *in vitro*. Recently, however, Kriegstein and Dichter[43] provided autoradiographic evidence for the generation of new neurons in cultures of embryonic brain tissue. This study is important since it demonstrated the possibility of studying *in vitro* the factors controlling neurogenesis from embryonic CNS tissue.

Whereas *in vitro* systems for studying CNS tissue (in contrast to embryonic tissue) from adult mammals or birds have not been readily available, CNS tissue from adult teleosts has proved amenable to tissue culture.[44,45] Recently, a culture system has been developed for spinal cord explants from adult *Sternarchus albifrons*.[46] The explants are grown in Leibovitz's L-15 medium on plastic tissue-culture dishes coated with polylysine or polyornithine.[47] These spinal cord cultures have been examined to determine whether neurogenesis occurs *in vitro* in this system. Examination of the spinal cord explants with [^{3}H]thymidine and antineuronal monoclonal antibodies has demonstrated that thymidine incorporation occurs in cells which, after a further growth period, can unequivocally be identified as neurons.[48] Notably, the neurogenesis occurs in cultures derived from both normal adult spinal cord (i.e., from tissue derived from mature spinal cord regions located rostral to the growing tip) and from regenerated spinal cord.

Neurons in the cultures were identified by a combination of morphologic and behaviorial characteristics and by staining with neuron-specific monoclonal antibodies.[49,50] Neurites could be observed in the cultures after 3–6 days, and typical networks of neurites were formed in the cultures after 6–9

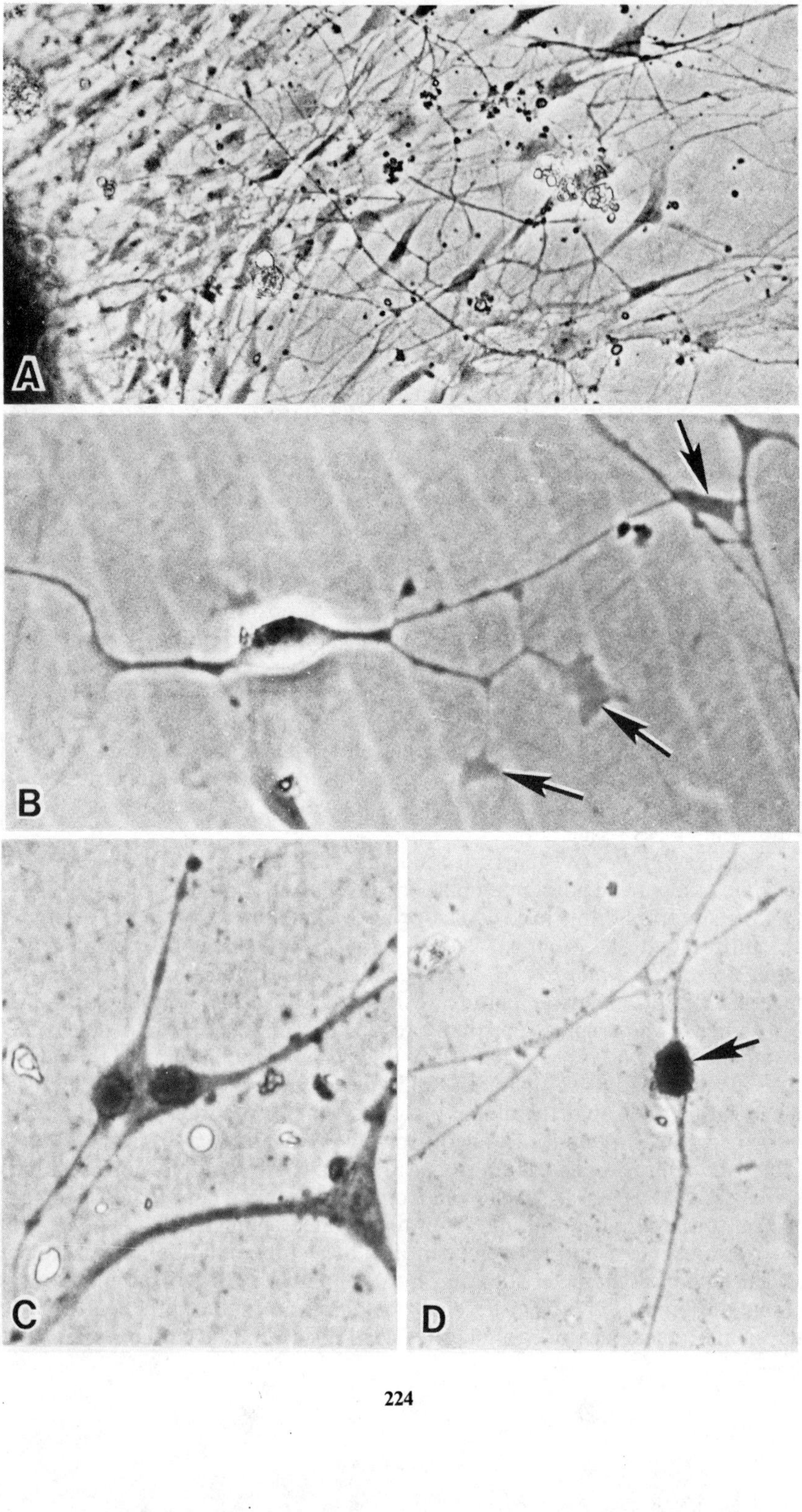
A
B
C
D

days (FIG. 5A). Despite the formation of neurite networks, individual neurons could clearly be observed at the edges of the outgrowth area or in areas of less dense outgrowth. Cells were identified as neurons (FIG. 5B) on the basis of the following characteristics: rounded cell bodies, the presence of neurites and growth cones, branching and fasciculation of the neurites, and contacts of the cell body or neurites with non-neuronal cells. The morphologic identification of neurons was confirmed, in some cultures, by positive staining with monoclonal antibodies against neurofilaments (FIG. 6A).

Explants derived from regenerating spinal cord start neurite outgrowth sooner (2–4 days versus 5–9 days for normal cord) and show a denser outgrowth than do explants from unregenerated normal adult cord.[46] However, both types of cultures clearly show dense neurite outgrowth after 2–3 weeks. At 3–10 days in culture, groups of closely apposed rounded cells, which are presumably undergoing mitosis, are observed. Cells with short neurites, probably in early stages of outgrowth, are present at the edges of these groups of presumptively postmitotic cells. Mitosis is, in fact, demonstrated by tritiated thymidine autoradiography.[48]

For demonstration of neurogenesis, tritiated thymidine (0.5–5 μCi/ml) was added to the culture medium between days 7–14 in culture. After a labeling period of 24–72 hr, the [^{3}H]thymidine was washed out and fresh medium containing 100 × cold unlabeled thymidine was added. The explants were cultured for a period of 2–8 more days, to allow neuronal differentiation, before fixation and autoradiography. Some cultures were fixed in methanol and stained with neuron-specific antineurofilament antibody (RT-97 [Ref. 49] or 02–40 [Ref. 50]) prior to application of the autoradiographic emulsion.

In cultures that were incubated with [^{3}H]thymidine, dense nuclear labeling is observed in cells that can unequivocally be identified as neurons by both morphologic criteria (FIG. 5C and D) and by staining with antineuronal monoclonal antibody (FIG. 6B and C). ^{3}H-labeled neurons are present in cultures from both unregenerated adult spinal cords and regenerating cords. Many ^{3}H-labeled neurons can be clearly identified by morphologic criteria alone; however, colabeling with antineurofilament antibody (FIG. 6) makes the case unequivocal. A total of 110 cultures were examined in this study: 98 cultures were ^{3}H-labeled cultures and 12 cultures were colabeled with tritum plus antibody.[48] Double-labeled neurons were present in each of the

FIGURE 5. *Sternarchus* spinal cord in tissue culture. (**A**) Outgrowth of neurites and non-neuronal cells from explant of normal adult spinal cord after 1½ weeks in culture. Explant proper is at left (*dark area*). Magnification ×265. (**B**) Bipolar neuron from a 4-week culture of regenerated cord. Several prominent growth cone areas (*arrows*) are present on this neuron. Magnification ×530. (**C**) and (**D**) Autoradiograms of neurons from cultures labeled with [^{3}H]thymidine. (**C**) Two neurons showing dense nuclear labeling with tritium grains. This 18-day culture was from regenerated cord. Magnification ×540. (**D**) Neuron from a 30-day culture from normal adult cord. A dense cap of tritium grains (*arrow*) is visible over the nuclear area. One neurite from this cell fasciculates with several neurites from other cells near top of figure. Magnification ×450.

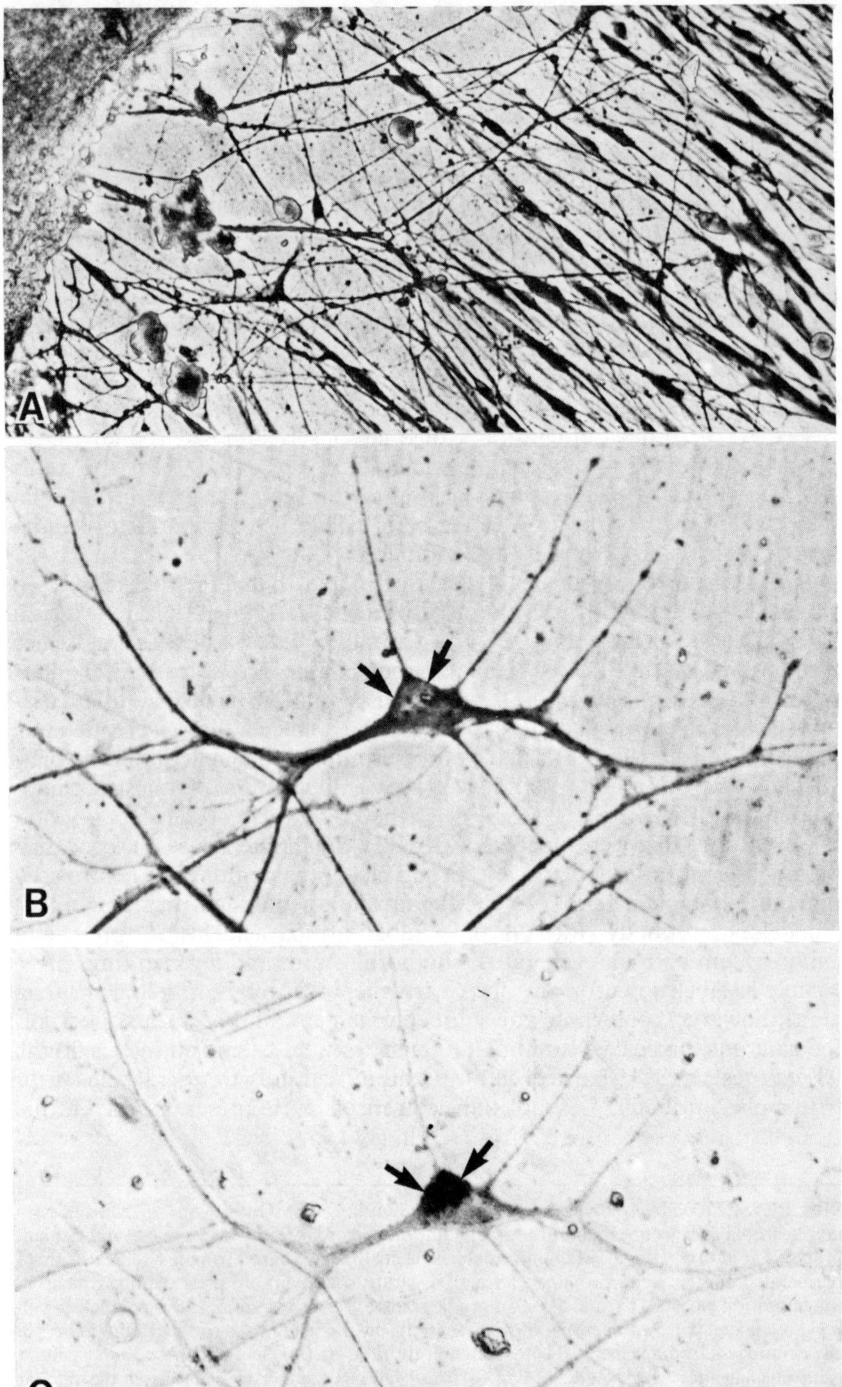
A
B
C

12 antibody-stained cultures that were examined. In counts of 826 normal neurons and 952 regenerated neurons, a mean value of 15% of the neurons are labeled with [^{3}H]thymidine in the cultures derived from normal adult spinal cord. A mean value of 45% of the neurons are ^{3}H-labeled in cultures derived from regenerating cords.

In order to rule out the possibility that [^{3}H]thymidine could be taken up by already differentiated neurons, autoradiography was carried out on a culture that was exposed to [^{3}H]thymidine for a shorter time period (17 hr) and was fixed immediately; another culture was exposed to [^{3}H]thymidine for 20 hours and then allowed to grow for 4 more days (to allow neuronal differentiation) prior to fixation and autoradiography. In the culture that was fixed immediately after the labeling period, no differentiated neurons exhibited ^{3}H-labeled nuclei; only rounded cells and non-neuronal cells were labeled with tritium. This finding demonstrates that tritium labeling is not due to uptake of [^{3}H]thymidine into already differentiated neurons. The sister culture, which was allowed to grow for 4 days subsequent to the labeling period, did contain ^{3}H-labeled neurons. These results indicate that tritiated thymidine incorporation takes place prior to neuronal differentiation.

The results of this study provide strong evidence that neurogenesis occurs in the cultures from both normal adult and regenerating *Sternarchus* spinal cord. The possibility of thymidine incorporation into already differentiated neurons is very unlikely for several reasons. First, as noted above, the cultures fixed immediately after the thymidine-labeling period show no tritium-labeled neurons. Instead, the tritium appears only in rounded non-neuronal cells and glia. However, when time is allowed after thymidine uptake, neuronal differentiation occurs in some of the labeled cells. Second, a mitotic origin for the thymidine-labeled neurons is suggested by the appearance of groups of rounded, apparently dividing cells in the cultures at the times when thymidine labeling is obtained. Many of these rounded cells are labeled in cultures fixed immediately after incubation with [^{3}H]thymidine.Third, the *in situ* evidence for neurogenesis in normal adult and regenerating *Sternarchus* cord strongly implies that some of the ependymal cells within histologically mature cord remain capable of mitosis and the generation of new neurons. The demonstration of thymidine incorporation into cultured *Sternarchus* neurons now suggests that this process can also proceed *in vitro*.

A prior study by de Boni and coworkers[44] failed to demonstrate thymidine incorporation in cultures of adult goldfish brain. However, species

FIGURE 6. Tritiated thymidine labeling in culture stained with RT-97 antineuronal monoclonal antibody. (**A**) Overview of an explant from regenerated cord fixed and stained with RT-97 after 18 days in culture. The neurite network and neuronal cell bodies stain darkly with the antineurofilament antibody. Non-neuronal cells, not clearly visible in this figure, do not stain with the antibody. Magnification ×235. (**B**) and (**C**) Double-labeled neurons from the culture in (**A**). (**B**) Neuron stained with antineurofilament antibody, but before autoradiography. The cell body and neurites are positively stained by the antibody. The nuclear area (*arrows*) is clear, except for two dark inclusions (nucleoli). Magnification ×470. (**C**) The same cell after autoradiography to visualize [^{3}H]thymidine labeling. Dark tritium grains now cover the nuclear area (*arrows*). Magnification ×470.

differences or differences in the methods used could account for the disparity between their report and the present results in *Sternarchus* spinal cord cultures. *Sternarchus* spinal cord may have greater capability for regeneration than does goldfish brain. The study on goldfish brain employed a different medium and different timing of ^{3}H-labeling and autoradiography. And, interestingly, despite their failure to demonstrate [^{3}H]thymidine incorporation, de Boni *et al.* observed that fragments of goldfish brain that did not contain a portion of the ventricular and subventricular zones resulted in cultures that contained mesenchymal and glial cells, but not neurons.[44]

As in previously reported studies on amphibian[51] and fish[45] retina in culture, neuritic outgrowth was more rapid and more dense from explants of regenerated *Sternarchus* spinal cord as compared to nonregenerated cord. In effect, the explantation procedure to tissue culture may initiate the process of regeneration, which we know occurs *in vivo* in response to cellular injury. In this sense, the explantation procedure for tissue culture may "prime" the neuronal precursor cells in the explants derived from normal cord to initiate regeneration. Explants from regenerated cord would be expected to grow faster in tissue culture because they are already "primed" and regenerating. The nature of the priming stimulus is not known, although it may be related to tissue injury. With respect to neurogenesis, however, it should be noted that ependymal cells do not give rise to axons, and thus the priming mechanism involved in neurogenesis may not be the same as the mechanism involved in the "priming lesions" which have been shown to stimulate regeneration of axons.[45,51,52]

FUNCTIONAL CORRELATES AND IMPLICATIONS FOR REPAIR OF THE NERVOUS SYSTEM

As shown above, postnatal neurogenesis continues as an ongoing process in the caudal spinal cord of *Sternarchus*. One obvious question concerns the functional implications of this ongoing production of neurons. Electromotor neurons in *Sternarchus* constitute the effector cells of the electromotor system[26,27] These cells generate an electric field which is sensed by electroreceptors distributed along the sides of the fish. Given the source-sink arrangement of current flow in the electric organ,[26,27] it is functionally advantageous for the electric organ to increase in size by addition of electromotor neurons concomitant with growth of the fish. Thus, neurogenesis in *Sternarchus* serves to optimize function of the electromotor system.

Compensatory neurogenesis and regeneration after injury have obvious evolutionary advantages. The tail in *Sternarchus* is marked by several white bands (FIG. 1) and these distinguish the tail from the rest of the fish, which is covered with dark skin, and make it a more attractive target for predators. Since the caudal region of the spinal cord is a site of ongoing neurogenesis, it might be speculated that regeneration after injury should occur more rapidly at caudal than at rostral levels of the spinal cord. According to this hypothesis, *Sternarchus* would offer, as a target for predators, caudalmost regions, where the capability for regeneration is greatest. Importantly, however, regeneration after injury is not confined to this caudal region; on the contrary, regenerative capacity is retained even at rostral levels of the spinal cord.

During growth and regeneration of the *Sternarchus* electromotor system, it appears that a basic structural plan is conserved, so that growth yields more neurons of the same type, rather than neurons with an intrinsically different structure or type of connectivity. These new neurons are incorporated into the electromotor circuit in a manner similar to that of preexisting cells, and thus do not appear to qualitatively alter the input-output function of the system in question (in contrast to the example of postnatal neurogenesis in the avian vocal control nuclei[6]). Nevertheless, the important point is that the electromotor system in *Sternarchus* demonstrates the *modifiability of the adult CNS in terms of production of new neurons*. This modifiability may provide an important degree of freedom in terms of functional characteristics, and may have important implications with respect to mechanisms by which the CNS can adapt to injury.

Since the electromotor neurons exhibit a relatively simple and stereotyped morphology, it might be assumed that their production, or regeneration, would require one basic set of genetic instructions, which are expressed iteratively in the production of multiple neurons. Even in this respect, however, neurogenesis must involve a significant degree of regulation in terms of neuronal differentiation. The generation of new electromotor neurons, showing normal relationships with presynaptic fibers (at the cell body) and with myelin-forming oligodendrocytes (at the initial segment) or Schwann cells (in the regenerated electric organ[21]), suggests that the neuronal plasma membrane of newly generated electromotor neurons differentiates in a normal manner with respect to the distribution of "recognition molecules."[53–55] It should also be recalled that the electromotor neurons exhibit a complex and highly specific pattern of synaptic innervation by descending fibers (see below); this implies the need for a more complex set of instructions that can regulate the development of a spectrum of axonal characteristics.

Since electromotor neurons are innervated by medullary control neurons,[26] the occurrence of postnatal neurogenesis in the caudal region of spinal cord leads to a requirement for plasticity at more rostral levels in the medulla. The necessity for reorganization at higher levels is even more acute in the case of regenerating spinal cord, where up to five times the normal number of electromotor neurons can be produced[9] and where synapses are established with at least some of these regenerated neurons. While the functional properties of the regenerated *Sternarchus* spinal cord and electric organ have not yet been examined, both of these regenerated neural systems do achieve an apparently normal morphologic structure over time. Descending synaptic inputs onto regenerated electromotor neurons are indistinguishable from normal ones in terms of the ultrastructure of the synapses.[22] The relatively sudden introduction of large numbers of new neurons during spinal cord regeneration would, moreover, be expected to place an immediate and increased (relative to normal) demand on higher centers for production and integration of new descending connections.

In normal adult *Sternarchus*, there is morphologic[28] and physiological[26,56] evidence for synaptic projection of the medullary command nucleus to caudal (more recently generated) electromotor neurons as well as to rostral neurons. Thus, during growth and concomitant addition of neurons to the caudal spinal cord, there is continuing formation of new axonal projections to, and synaptic connection with, the newly formed neurons in the spinal cord. It is not at present clear whether the new projections reflect production of additional relay neurons in the medulla[56] or collateral formation or branching from preexisting bulbospinal axons that arise from these medullary cells. Irrespective of which of these mechanisms is shown to be correct, reorganization of neural structures in adult *Sternarchus* must occur at a variety of levels to accommodate newly generated neurons. In this regard, the situation in *Sternarchus* may be similar to that in telencephalic vocal control nucleus in canaries, where newly generated neurons in the adult brain have been shown to be recruited into functional synaptic circuits.[6] It should be recalled, moreover, that the morphologic pattern (and conduction velocity) of bulbospinal fibers in the *Sternarchus* electromotor system are matched to functional requirements so that the axons can function as time-delay lines to mediate synchronous firing of electromotor neurons.[57,58] Thus, the ongoing reorganization of the caudal spinal cord and descending projections involves a high degree of specificity at the cellular level.

In summary, spinal cord from the adult teleost *Sternarchus albifrons* shows a high capacity for neurogenesis, which occurs *in situ* as an ongoing process and in response to injury, as well as *in vitro* in explant cultures of spinal cord. Moreover, both regeneration *in situ* and neurogenesis *in vitro* can occur from mature spinal cord tissue which is not normally a site of neuron production. This raises the possibility of study of the signals by which neurogenesis is initiated and controlled. In this respect, the *Sternarchus* culture system should provide a very useful model in which the determinants of neurogenesis and neuronal differentiation can be examined. The occurrence of neurogenesis and regeneration in the *Sternarchus* electromotor system provides an ideal system in which to address basic questions of neuronal recovery after injury and plasticity in the adult vertebrate central nervous system.

SUMMARY

Phylogenetically "lower" species in some cases use different biological strategies for recovery after injury to the CNS than do "higher" species. One approach that we have taken in our laboratory has been to study the mechanisms of functional recovery of the CNS after injury in those vertebrate species where recovery does occur. The present report reviews recent studies on a model system, the spinal electromotor system of the gymnotiform teleost *Sternarchus albifrons*, which exhibits regeneration and neurogenesis after injury. Regeneration in this system leads to a recapitulation of relatively normal morphologic structure by the damaged or extirpated spinal cord. In

Sternarchus, new spinal cord is generated from ependymal cells; some ependymal cells in the adult remain pluripotent and retain the capability to generate new neurons. The *Sternarchus* spinal cord thus represents an especially useful model for the study of neurogenesis after injury to the CNS.

Recent studies in our laboratory indicate that neurogenesis in adult *Sternarchus* spinal cord tissue occurs both *in vivo* and *in vitro*. Neurogenesis has been demonstrated by incorporation of tritiated thymidine into explant cultures from the spinal cord of adult *Sternarchus*. Autoradiography reveals the presence of thymidine-labeled neurons. Neuronal identity of ^{3}H-labeled cells has been confirmed by positive staining with neuron-specific monoclonal antibodies. Thymidine labeling occurs in cultured neurons derived from both normal (histologically and functionally mature) and regenerating spinal cord of adult *Sternarchus albifrons*. These results provide evidence that some cells in spinal cord of adult *Sternarchus* retain the ability to incorporate thymidine and undergo neuronal differentiation *in vitro*. This system provides a new model in which neurogenesis from adult tissue can be studied *in vivo* and *in vitro*.

ACKNOWLEDGMENTS

C. Choy and H. L. Fong provided excellent technical assistance for this research. The RT-97 antibody was the generous gift of Dr. John Wood; 02-40 was the generous gift of Drs. Nancy and Ludwig Sternberger.

REFERENCES

1. Graziadei, P. P. C. & G. A. Graziadei. 1979. Neurogenesis and neuron regeneration in the olfactory system of mammals. I. Morphological aspects of differentiation and structural organization of the olfactory sensory neurons. J. Neurocytol. **8:** 1–18.
2. Wilson, K. C. P. & G. Raisman. 1980. Age-related changes in the neurosensory epithelium of the mouse vomeronasal organ: Extended period of postnatal growth in size and evidence for rapid cell turnover in the adult. Brain Res. **185:** 103–113.
3. Altman, J. & G. D. Das 1965. Postnatal origin of microneurones. Nature **207:** 953–956.
4. Kaplan, M. S. & J. W. Hinds. 1977. Neurogenesis in the adult rat: Electron microscopic analysis of light autoradiographs. Science **197:** 1092–1094.
5. Goldman, S. A. & F. Nottebohm. 1983. Neuronal production, migration and differentiation in a vocal control nucleus of the adult female canary brain. Proc. Natl. Acad. Sci. USA **80:** 2390–2394.
6. Paton, J. A. & F. N. Nottebohm. 1984. Neurons generated in the adult brain are recruited into functional circuits. Science **225:** 1046–1048.
7. Nordlander, R. H. & M. Singer. 1978. The role of ependyma in regeneration of the spinal cord in the urodele amphibian tail. J. Comp. Neurol. **180:** 349–374.
8. Kirsche, W. 1965. Regenerative Vorgange im Gehirn und Rukkenmark. Ergeb. Anat. Entwicklungsgesch. **38:** 143–194.
9. Anderson, M. J. & S. G. Waxman. 1981. Morphology of regenerated spinal cord in *Sternarchus albifrons*. Cell Tissue Res. **219:** 1–8.
10. Anderson, M. J. & S. G. Waxman. 1983. Regeneration of spinal neurons in inframammalian vertebrates: morphological and developmental aspects. J. Hirnforsch. **24:** 371–398.
11. Easter, S. S., Jr. 1983. Postnatal neurogenesis and changing connections. Trends Neurosci. **6:** 53–56.

12. Johns, P. R. 1982. Formation of photoreceptors in larval and adult goldfish. J. Neurosci. **2:** 178–198.
13. Johns, P. R. & S. S. Easter. 1977. Growth of the adult goldfish eye. II. Increase in retinal cell number. J. Comp. Neurol. **176:** 331–342.
14. Straznicky, K. & R. M. Gaze. 1971. The growth of the retina in *Xenopus laevis*: An autoradiographic study. J. Embryol. Exp. Morphol. **26:** 67–79.
15. Raymond, P. A. & S. S. Easter, Jr. 1983. Postembryonic growth of the optic tectum in goldfish. I. Location of germinal cells and numbers of neurons produced. J. Neurosci. **3:** 1077–1091.
16. Stevenson, J. & M. G. Yoon. 1980. Kinetics of cell proliferation in the halved tectum of adult goldfish. Brain Res. **184:** 11–22.
17. Straznicky, K. & R. M. Gaze. 1972. Development of the optic tectum in *Xenopus laevis*. An autoradiographic study. J. Embryol. Exp. Morphol. **28:** 87–115.
18. Birse, S. C., R. B. Leonard & R. E. Coggeshall. 1980. Neuronal increase in various areas of the nervous system of the guppy, *Lebistes*. J. Comp. Neurol. **194:** 291–301.
19. Leonard, R. B., R. E. Coggeshall & W. D. Willis. 1978. A documentation of an age related increase in neuronal and axonal numbers in the stingray. J. Comp. Neurol. **179:** 13–22.
20. Waxman, S. G. & M. J. Anderson. 1985. Generation of electromotor neurons in *Sternarchus albifrons*: Differences between normally growing and regenerating spinal cord. Dev. Biol. **112:** in press.
21. Waxman, S. G. & M. J. Anderson. 1980. Regeneration of spinal electrocyte fibers in *Sternarchus albifrons*: Development of axon-Schwann cell relationships and nodes of Ranvier. Cell Tissue Res. **208:** 343–352.
22. Anderson, M. J., S. G. Waxman & C. H. Tadlock. 1984. Cell death of asynaptic neurons in regenerating spinal cord. Dev. Biol. **103:** 443–455.
23. Anderson, M. J. & S. G. Waxman. 1983. Caudal spinal cord of the teleost *Sternarchus albifrons* resembles regenerating cord. Anat. Rec. **205:** 85–92.
24. Oliviera Castro, G. de 1955. Differentiated nervous fibers that constitute the electric organ of *Sternarchus albifrons*. Linn. Anais Acad. Brasil Cien. **4:** 557–562.
25. Bennett, M. V. L. 1970. Comparative physiology: Electric organs. Ann. Rev. Physiol. **32:** 471–528.
26. Bennett, M. V. L. 1971. Electric organs. *In* Fish Physiology. W. S. Hoar & D. J. Randall, Eds. Vol. **5:** 347–491. Academic Press. New York, NY.
27. Waxman, S. G., G. D. Pappas & M. V. L. Bennett. 1972. Morphological correlates of functional differentiation of nodes of Ranvier along single fibers in the neurogenic electric organ of the knife fish *Sternarchus*. J. Cell Biol. **53:** 210–224.
28. Pappas, G. D., S. G. Waxman & M. V. L. Bennett. 1975. Morphology of spinal electromotor neurons and presynaptic coupling in the gymnotid *Sternarchus albifrons*. J. Neurocytol. **4:** 469–478.
29. Bennett, M. V. L., C. Sandri & K. Akert. 1978. Neuronal gap junctions and morphologically mixed synapses in the spinal cord of a teleost, *Sternarchus albifrons* (Gymnotoidei). Brain Res. **143:** 43–60.
30. Anderson, M. J., S. G. Waxman & M. Laufer. 1983. Fine structure of regenerated ependyma and spinal cord in *Sternarchus albifrons*. Anat. Rec. **205:** 73–83.
31. Hamburger, V. 1975. Cell death in the development of the lateral motor column of the chick embryo. J. Comp. Neurol. **160:** 535–546.
32. Cowan, W. M. 1973. Neuronal death as a regulative mechanism in the control of cell number in the nervous system. *In* Development and Aging in the Nervous System. M. Rockstein, Ed.: 19–41. Academic Press. New York, NY.
33. Oppenheim, R. W. 1981. Neuronal cell death and some related regressive phenomena during neurogenesis: A selective historical review and progress report. *In* Studies in Developmental Neurobiology: Essays in Honor of Viktor Hamburger. W. M. Cowan, Ed.: 74–133. Oxford University Press. London.
34. Cunningham, T. J. 1982. Naturally occurring neuron death and its regulation by developing neural pathways. Int. Rev. Cytol. **74:** 163–186.

35. JACOBSON, M. 1978. Developmental Neurobiology, 2nd ed.: 1–42. Plenum Press. New York, NY.
36. SANDRI, C., K. AKERT & M. V. L. BENNETT. 1978. Junctional complexes and variations in gap junctions between spinal cord ependymal cells of a teleost, *Sternarchus albifrons* (Gymnotoidei). Brain Res. **143:** 27–41.
37. EGAR, M. & M. SINGER. 1972. The role of ependyma in spinal cord regeneration in the urodele, *Triturus*. Exp. Neurol. **37:** 422–430.
38. SIMPSON, S. B. 1964. Analysis of tail regeneration in the lizard *Lygosoma laterale*. I. Initiation of regeneration and cartilage differentiation: The role of ependyma. J. Morphol. **114:** 425–436.
39. SINGER, M., R. H. NORDLANDER & M. EGAR. 1979. Axonal guidance during embryogenesis and regeneration in the spinal cord of the newt: The blueprint hypothesis of neuronal patterning. J. Comp. Neurol. **185:** 1–22.
40. NORDLANDER, R. H. & M. SINGER. 1982. Spaces precede axons in *Xenopus* embryonic spinal cord. Exp. Neurol. **75:** 221–228.
41. JUURLINK, B. & S. FEDERHOFF. 1982. The development of mouse spinal cord in tissue culture. II. Development of neuronal precursor cells. In Vitro **18:** 179–182.
42. SENSENBRENNER, M., E. WITTENDORP, I. BARAKAT & R. Rechenmann. 1980. Autoradiographic study of proliferating brain cells in culture. Dev. Biol. **75:** 268–277.
43. KRIEGSTEIN, A. & M. A. DICHTER. 1984. Neuron generation in dissociated cell cultures from fetal rat cerebral cortex. Brain Res. **295:** 184–189.
44. DE BONI, U., M. SEGER, J. W. SCOTT & D. R. CRAPPER. 1976. Neuron cultures from adult goldfish. J. Neurobiol. **7:** 495–512.
45. LANDRETH, G. E. & B. W. AGRANOFF. 1976. Explant culture of adult goldfish retina: Effect of prior optic nerve crush. Brain Res. **118:** 299–303.
46. ANDERSON, M. J. 1985. Neuronal growth in cultures from adult teleost spinal cord. Submitted for publication.
47. LETOURNEAU, P. C. 1975. Possible roles for cell-to-substrate adhesion in neuronal morphogenesis. Dev. Biol. **44:** 77–91.
48. ANDERSON, M. J. & S. G. WAXMAN. 1985. Neurogenesis in tissue cultures of adult teleost spinal cord. Dev. Brain Res. **20:** 203–212.
49. WOOD, J. N. & B. H. ANDERTON. 1981. Monoclonal antibodies to mammalian neurofilaments. Biosci. Rep. **1:** 263–268.
50. STERNBERGER, L. A., L. W. HARWELL & N. H. STERNBERGER. 1982. Neurotypy: Regional individuality in rat brain detected by immunochemistry with monoclonal antibodies. Proc. Natl. Acad. Sci. USA **79:** 1326–1330.
51. AGRANOFF, B. W., P. FIELD & R. M. GAZE. 1976. Neurite outgrowth from explanted *Xenopus* retina: an effect of prior optic nerve crush. Brain Res. **113:** 225–234.
52. MCQUARRIE, I. G. & B. GRAFSTEIN. 1981. Effect of a conditioning lesion on optic nerve regeneration in goldfish. Brain Res. **216:** 253–264.
53. GOODMAN, C. S., M. J. BASTIANI, C. Q. DOE, S. DU LAC, S. L. HELFORD, J. KUWADA, & J. B. THOMAS. 1984. Cell recognition during neuronal development. Science **225:** 1271–1279.
54. WAXMAN, S. G. & R. E. FOSTER. 1980. Development of the axon membrane during differentiation of myelinated fibres in spinal nerve roots. Proc. Roy. Soc. London, Ser. B **209:** 441–446.
55. SMITH, M. E., J. D. KOCSIS, & S. G. WAXMAN. 1983. Myelin protein metabolism in demyelination and remyelination in the sciatic nerve. Brain Res. **270:** 37–44.
56. TOKUNAGA, A., K. AKERT, C. SANDRI & M. V. L. BENNETT. 1980. Cell types and synaptic organization of the medullary electromotor nucleus in a constant frequency weakly electric fish, *Sternarchus albifrons*. J. Comp. Neurol. **192:** 407–426.
57. BENNETT, M. V. L. 1968. Neural control of electric organs. *In* The Central Nervous System and Fish Behavior. D. Ingle, Ed.: 147–169. The University of Chicago Press. Chicago, IL.
58. WAXMAN, S. G. 1975. Integrative properties and design principles of axons. Int. Rev. Neurobiol. **18:** 1–40.

Index of Contributors

Subject Index